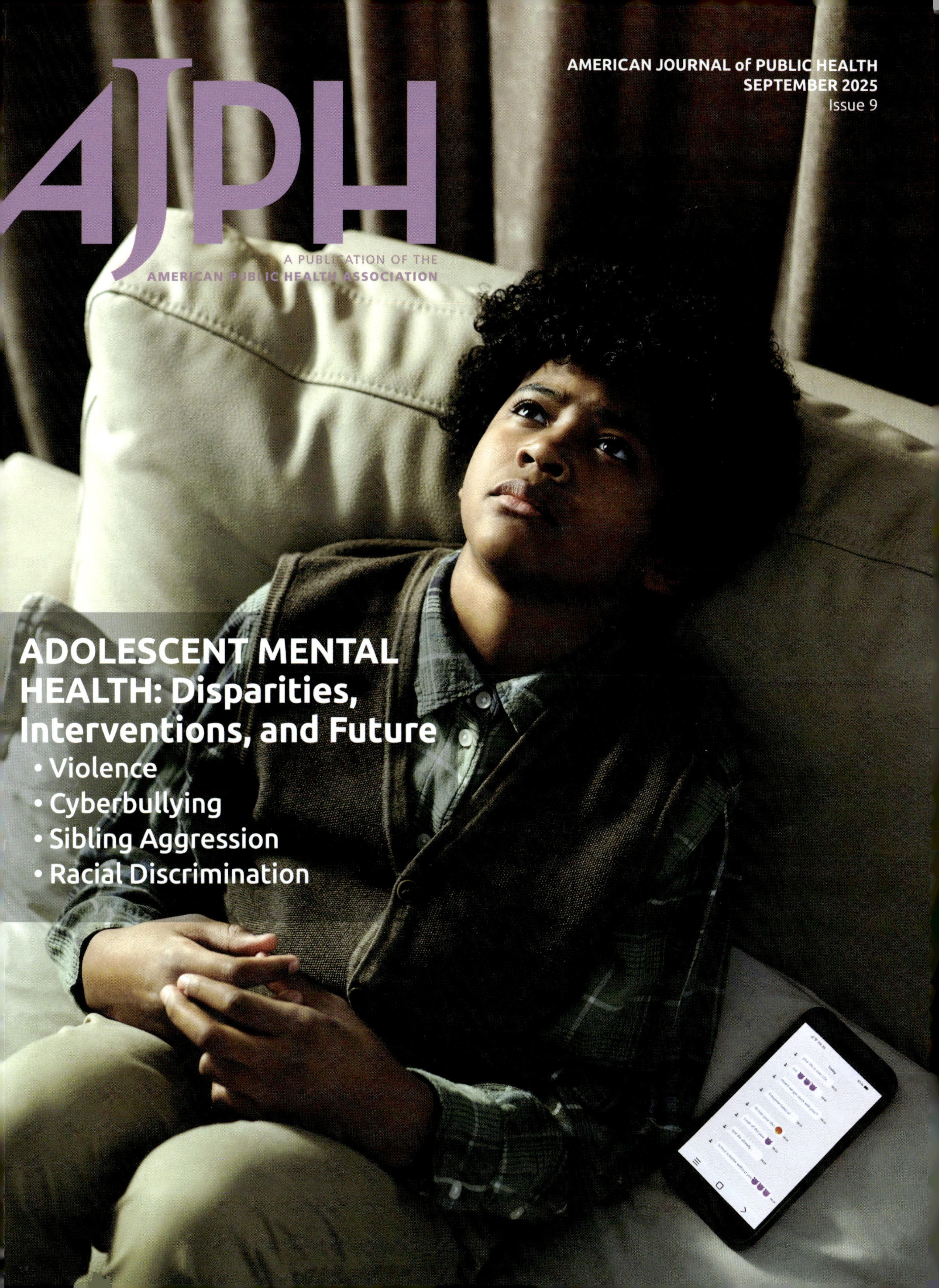

AJPH
A PUBLICATION OF THE
AMERICAN PUBLIC HEALTH ASSOCIATION

AMERICAN JOURNAL of PUBLIC HEALTH
SEPTEMBER 2025
Issue 9

ADOLESCENT MENTAL HEALTH: Disparities, Interventions, and Future

- Violence
- Cyberbullying
- Sibling Aggression
- Racial Discrimination

APHA
AMERICAN PUBLIC HEALTH ASSOCIATION
For science. For action. For health.

AJPH®, published monthly, is the official Journal of the American Public Health Association®, 800 I St NW, Washington, DC 20001-3710; (202) 777- APHA; TDD (202) 777-2500. APHA is a nongovernmental professional society founded in 1872, representing all disciplines and specialties in public health.

The *American Journal of Public Health*® (*AJPH*) (print ISSN: 0090-0036; electronic ISSN: 1541- 0048), first published in 1911, is the official journal of the American Public Health Association® (APHA). The oldest and largest organization of public health professionals in the world, APHA represents approximately 30 000 members from more than 50 occupations of public health.

Submissions: Visit www.editorialmanager.com/ajph or ajph.edmgr.com for online manuscript preparation and submission guidelines. Contributions of original unpublished research, social science analyses, scholarly essays, critical commentaries, departments, and letters to the editor are welcome. Questions? Write ajph.submissions@apha.org or call APHA at (202) 777-2469.

Print plus online subscriptions: Institutional price (print copy with online access for a single institution and all authorized users, regardless of geographic location) varies by size of organization and ranges from $993–$1445 for US organizations, and $1073–$1526 for international organizations (air delivery); multiple campuses not permitted without special arrangement. Details of the tiered pricing system at https://subscriptionoffice.com/pages/apha-landing-page. To order, write apha.subscriptions@apha.org.

Online-only subscriptions: Institutional price for one institution and its authorized users (regardless of geographic location) is $878–$1307. To order, write apha.subscriptions@apha.org. For academic consortia or multisite corporate subscriptions, contact apha.subscriptions@apha.org.

Print-only subscriptions: Institutional price is US $701, $782 international.

Back print issues: A limited number of print issues are for sale. Single copies are US $65, $75 international (air delivery). Shipping included; prepay only. To order, write apha.subscriptions@apha.org.

Reprints: For prices and ordering information on 50 or more reprints, check the Reprints section at www.ajph.org. To order smaller quantities of reprints (rush delivery), use the "Purchase Article" link on the article site itself.

Electronic access: Online articles more than 10 years old are available free for personal use at www.ajph.org. Recent articles are available through pay-per-view: single PDF article for $24, single issue access for 24 hours for $33, or entire site access for 24 hours for $38.

Postal information: Periodicals postage paid at Washington, DC, and additional mailing offices. Postmaster: Send address changes to American Journal of Public Health, 800 I St NW, Washington, DC 20001-3710.

Address changes: Send to AJPH, Membership Department (members) or AJPH Subscriptions (subscribers), APHA, 800 I St NW, Washington, DC 20001-3710. Or write to membership.mail@apha.org (members) or apha.subscriptions@apha.org (subscribers).

Advertising: For pricing and other information, see www.ajph.org. Please write to brian.selzer@apha.org or call (202) 777-2470 for other advertising opportunities. Ask about special exhibit packages and sponsorships. Acceptance of advertising by the *Journal* does not imply endorsement of products.

Indexes: Publications that index or abstract articles from *AJPH* include the following: Ageline, Assia (Applied Social Science Index and Abstracts), Biological Abstracts, Chemical Abstracts, CINAHL, Criminal Justice Abstracts, EMBASE, EMCare, Environmental Abstracts, e-psyche, ERIC, ETOH (Alcohol and Alcohol Problems Science Database), Excerpta Medica, Food Science and Technology, General Science Index, Grateful Med, Hospital Literature Index, Human Resources Abstracts, International Pharmaceutical Abstracts (IPA), Medline, Physical Education Index, Pollution Abstracts, Psychological Abstracts, PsychINFO, Safety Science Abstracts, Sage Family Studies Abstracts, Sage Human Resources Abstracts, Science Citation Index, SCOPUS, SIIC Data Bases, Social Work Research and Abstracts, and Statistical Reference Index (SRI)/LexisNexis.

AJPH

A PUBLICATION OF THE
AMERICAN PUBLIC HEALTH ASSOCIATION

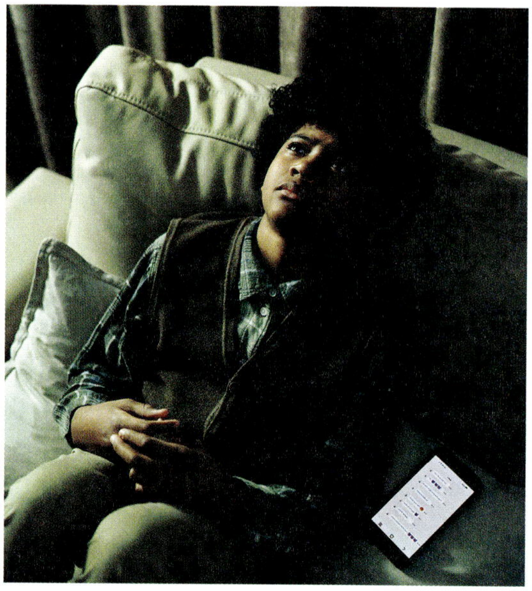

COVER: In the United States, both depression and suicide rates are on the rise among young Black men. However, feelings of authenticity can offer an envelope of protection from the rising tide of suicidal ideation and depression. Understanding this, public health practitioners can create evidence-based support systems that address systemic inequities, bolster resilience, and improve mental health outcomes.

Cover concept and selection by Aleisha Kropf. Photo by press master/ Adobe Stock. Printed with permission.

APHA
AMERICAN PUBLIC HEALTH ASSOCIATION
For science. For action. For health.

Promoting public health research, policy, practice, and education is the *AJPH* mission. As we widen our scope to embrace global issues, we also sharpen our focus to support the needs of public health practitioners. We invite contributions of original unpublished research, opinion and commentary, and letters to the editor.

The *Journal* is printed on acid-free recycled paper.

OPEN ACCESS | ONLINE ONLY | PODCAST | DATA SUPPLEMENT AVAILABLE

EDITOR'S CHOICE

1342 My Vision for *AJPH*
D. T. Lau

BOOKS & MEDIA

1344 Urban Health in Africa: Implications for Global Public Health
N. Freudenberg

OPINIONS, IDEAS, & PRACTICE

EDITORIALS

1346 Medicaid Expansion Prevents Human Papillomavirus Cancers for Everyone
H. M. Brandt

1349 A Measure Aligned With Reproductive Justice, Human Rights, and Sexual Well-Being ... ? Yes Please, and Here's Why
J. A. Higgins, D. N. Carvajal, and L. Senderowicz

1352 Gun-Free Zones in Sensitive Places
L. Klarevas

1354 Did COVID-19 Slow Our Progress Toward Ending the HIV Epidemic?
A. E. Nijhawan

1357 Hidden in Plain Sight: The Case for Disaggregated HIV Data and Tailored Interventions for African Immigrants
O. Okoro

PERSPECTIVES

1360 Food Is Medicine: Prioritizing Equitable Implementation
M. J. Landry and K. Hollis-Hansen

1364 School Nurses: An Upstream Investment for Achieving Menstrual Equity
S. Bergen, E. D. Maughan, M. Secor, K. E. Johnson, R. Cogan, and M. Sommer

1368 The FDA Acts to Eliminate Asbestos in Talc: A Half-Century–Long Struggle
G. Markowitz and D. Rosner

IMAGES OF HEALTH

1371 Is Your Home Making You Sick? Health Risks Associated With Black Mold in Air Vents
O. B. Novoa

HISTORY

1373 James P. Keogh, MD: Advocate for Bringing Environmental Medicine to Worker Protection
E. Persaud

ADOLESCENT MENTAL HEALTH

1377 Adolescents' Mental Health: Disparities, Prevention Strategies, and Future Directions
T. T. LeBlanc, J. Liu, H. He, and M. Livings

1379 Wellness Coaching in a Summer Internship Program to Address the Mental Health Pandemic Among College Students, 2022–2023
S. Mulkey, C. Knaub, M. Rodriguez, D. Thomas, H. Williams, M. Bahrenburg, and P. J. Fleming

1383 Sibling Aggression and Abuse: Invisible and Widespread Public Health Problems
C. J. Tucker, T. R. Whitworth, and N. H. Perkins

RESEARCH & ANALYSIS

ADOLESCENT MENTAL HEALTH

1388 Adolescent Dating Violence and Suicide Planning Among Girls in US High Schools: An Intracategorical Intersectional Analysis by Race and Ethnicity
L. Sharpless, K. Alvarez, T. Kershaw, and T. C. Willie

1397 Persistent Sadness, Violence, and Bullying and Associations With Screen Time Among New York City Public High School Students, 2021
J. Jackson, M. Hamwey, N. Stratton, and A. Vasan

1408 Cost-Effectiveness of an Economic Empowerment and Family Intervention on Mental Health Among School-Going Adolescent Girls in Uganda, 2017–2022
F. M. Ssewamala, Y. Tozan, R. Brathwaite, J. Kiyingi, P. Namatovu, O. S. Bahar, P. Nabunya, P. B. Nartey, and T. B. Neilands

1417 Authenticity, Racial Discrimination, Depression, and Suicidal Ideation Among Young Black Men, United States, 2024
D. T. Boyd, M. I. Durkee, D. W. Brown, and A. S. Constant

1426 Mental Health of Emerging Adults in New York City in 2023
R. Suss, J-A. Caton, M. Close, D. Sihaloho, E. Tuazon, and C. Norman

1436 Social Vulnerability and Racial Disparities in Depression Screening of US Adolescents, 2016 to 2021
K. Galper, J. M. Rung, A. Shergill, T. S. Barrett, D. Marousis, and E. Brignone

1445 Violence and Depression Among Adolescent Boys in Soweto, South Africa, 2020–2023
E. M. Inman, G. Leshabane, A. Kalegina, A. Violari, and R. Kidman

POLICY

1454 Effects of Medicaid Expansion on HPV Vaccination Uptake Among Adolescents in the United States: Difference-in-Differences Analyses From 2011 to 2022
A. W. Chen, T. L. Amberson, H. F. Adhiambo, and B. H. Wagenaar

OPEN-THEMED RESEARCH

1463 Advancing a Measure of Sexual and Reproductive Well-Being Aligned With Core Values of Reproductive Justice and Human Rights
C. Dehlendorf, S. Desai, J. Danaux, C. Green, S. Sarnaik, J. Crear-Perry, and J. Hart

1472 Public Firearms Carriage and Public Opinion, National Gun Policy Survey, 2023
C. K. Crifasi, K. E. W. Roskam, and A. D. McCourt

1480 HIV Care Linkage and Initial Viral Suppression Among Persons Newly Diagnosed With HIV in North Carolina Before and After the Start of the COVID-19 Pandemic
C. N. Maierhofer, B. W. Pence, E. Samoff, A. N. Turner, V. Mobley, J. Maxwell, W. C. Miller, and K. A. Powers

1490 African Immigrants and the End of the HIV Epidemic in the United States: Actionable Recommendations to Enhance Equity
G. Aidoo-Frimpong, E. Koku, N. Malika, C. Nnaji, and R. Kerani

1500 Critical Reflections From the Black Women First Initiative
L. S. Sprague Martinez, J. C. Scott, M. Rocco, M. Miranda, C. Tucker, and A. W. Walter

1508 Primary Prevention of Drug Overdoses in Rural Low-Resource and Tribal Communities: A Cluster Randomized Trial
K. A. Komro, M. D. Livingston, J. R. Skinner, B. J. Livingston, T. K. Kominsky, A. Jagtiani, C. M. Barry, A. C. Wagenaar, H. L. F. Cooper, M. Harmon, E. Ivanich, H. LaBounty, A. N. Gassaway, and S. L. Talavera-Brown

1518 Excess Mortality and Containment Performance During the COVID-19 Pandemic: Evidence From 34 Countries
C. Cheng, H-Y. Wu, S-C. Kuo, B. Fan, Y-T. Hsu, Y-K. Chen, B. Fan, Y-A. Jang, C-F. Hung, W-M. Jiang, H-Y. Chiou, W. J. Chen, and H-H. Tsou

CLIMATE CHANGE

1529 The Citizens Air Complaint Program: Laypeople Reporting Air Pollution Violations in New York City
C. Hartmann

HISTORY

1536 Promulgating Joy and Expiating Guilt: Camp and LGBTQ+ Health Education in the History of The Sisters of Perpetual Indulgence
T. J. Fuller

My Vision for *AJPH*

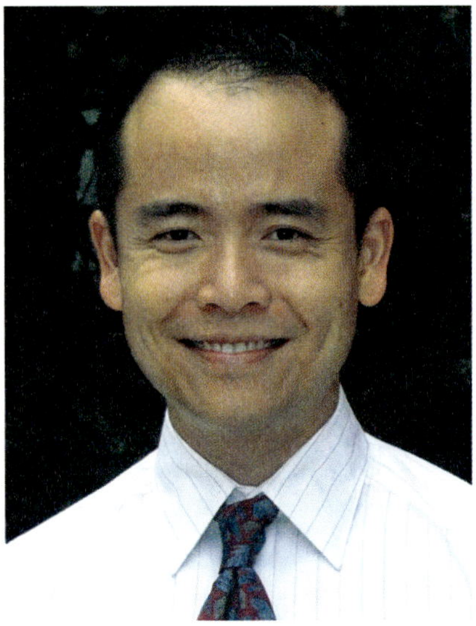

Denys T. Lau, PhD
AJPH Incoming Editor-in-Chief

Furthering the success that Alfredo Morabia has built for the *Journal* during his 10-year leadership, I am excited to take the helm as the new Editor-in-Chief of the *American Journal of Public Health* (*AJPH*). During this extraordinary time, I am committed to position and maintain the *Journal* as one of the most trusted sources of up-to-date scientific information in public health. All *AJPH* content will satisfy this essential question for our readers: "Why should I trust this resource as authoritative?" The following highlights my overall approach.

First is my commitment to high-quality scientific content. All original research, research methods, and program evaluations will meet rigorous quality standards of scientific inquiry and reporting. *AJPH* will continue to refuse publishing pilot studies or quantitative studies of small convenience samples as research articles. Analytical essays will bring new evidence-based insights to significantly move the field forward. *Journal* policy statements on the use of artificial intelligence in submissions will be developed and enforced to safeguard published research integrity.

Research papers will be critically evaluated to determine if their methods and results are transparent and replicable, their interpretation is strictly derived from the study data and analyses, and their study implications and recommendations do not extend beyond the study's scope, while acknowledging the limitations. Research that does not include at least one year of data collected within the last three years will be rejected without review, except under rare, exceptional circumstances.

Opinion pieces will be scientifically accurate, thorough, well-balanced, evidence-based views that include all perspectives. *AJPH* will not publish one-sided or baseless viewpoints. In addition, the *Journal* will seek actionable and impactful scientific papers that effectively drive nonpartisan policies and programs aimed at improving population health.

Second is my commitment to diversity in topics and reach. Although the scope of all *AJPH* studies addresses individual, community, or population health, the *Journal* will seek seminal research from disciplines across the broad field of public health—including epidemiology, health services and policy research, survey data and monitoring methods, law and ethics, population health, social and behavioral sciences, global health, and environmental health. In essence, *AJPH* will aim to be

Continued on page 1343...

HISTORY CORNER

34 YEARS AGO

Risk Factors for Suicide Attempts Among Navajo Adolescents

Among a cohort of American Indian high school students attending a boarding school in the southeast US, 23 percent had attempted suicide during their lifetime. This high rate of self-destructive behavior among Native American adolescents warrants further investigation and culturally appropriate intervention. The 1988 Navajo Adolescent Health Survey offered an opportunity to examine a set of traditional risk factors that are thought to be important in the general population. . . .Of all respondents, 6,637 (92 percent) answered the question about suicide attempts; 971 (15 percent) admitted to a past attempt to kill themselves. . . .An important finding of this study is the link between the suicide attempts of the respondents and those of their friends and family. Because prevalence of exposure was the highest for these risk factors and because of their strong association with suicide attempts, these risk factors have the greatest public health importance.

From *AJPH*, July 1991, pp. 870–872

the top choice for public health investigators seeking a home to publish their innovative, high-quality scientific work.

AJPH will intentionally publish papers about public health topics that are relevant to different subpopulations, including persons who historically have been understudied, underrepresented, or discriminated against, as well as persons who traditionally have not been considered underrepresented but feel that they have been left out of diversity or health equity discussions. Publishing diverse topics that are relevant to different audiences will broaden public trust in the *Journal*.

AJPH will expand its reach to scientific and nonscientific audiences through various platforms, including podcasts, online videos, and social media. Authors of accepted papers will be encouraged to leverage *AJPH* online platforms to amplify their published work and make their research more understandable and accessible to the general public.

Third is my commitment to stakeholder engagement. *AJPH* will actively seek submissions from public health thought-leaders, practitioners, educators, and policymakers at local, state, and federal levels to increase stakeholders' confidence in the *Journal*. The *Journal* will invest in long-term strategies to connect with future generations of researchers and leaders. *AJPH* will continue its successful Student Think Tank and Student Editorship, while exploring additional opportunities to promote student input, involvement, and submissions to the *Journal*. *AJPH* will aim to be the model educational tool for use in public health curricula.

This is my vision for the *Journal*. I look forward to working with my team of editors and production staff to ensure that the *AJPH* mission is met—that is, to uphold the *Journal* as the most current, authoritative, and in-depth source of scientific information in the public health field. In doing so, we will work toward an even greater goal of strengthening public trust in the public health science enterprise. AJPH

DOI: https://doi.org/10.2105/AJPH.2025.308238

HISTORY CORNER

60 YEARS AGO

Adolescent Patients Served in Outpatient Psychiatric Clinics

Outpatient psychiatric clinics in the United States serve more persons in the 10 through 19-year-age group than in any other decade of life. . . A major finding, that the 14 to 15- year-olds have the highest clinic utilization rates, may represent a higher true incidence of emotional disorders or may reflect increased anxiety on the part of significant adults at their inability to cope with the adolescent when he reaches this age, particularly in the case of boys. . . . The consistently higher rates for boys than girls in mid-adolescent years correspond with their relatively high rate of "appearance" at other "trouble handling" agencies-the police, juvenile court, the principal's office. The clinic may be used by school, police, and court personnel as an extension of their attempts to control or modify behavior, particularly of mid-adolescent boys. Though the clinic may relieve the child's disturbance, despondency, and anger, his behavior often is in response to the lack of meaningful educational or job training opportunities and of a satisfying role in the community, thus requiring society-wide action.

From *AJPH*, October 1965, pp. 1563–1569

Urban Health in Africa: Implications for Global Public Health

Nicholas Freudenberg, DrPH, MPH

ABOUT THE AUTHOR

Nicholas Freudenberg is with the Graduate School of Public Health and Health Policy, City University of New York, New York.

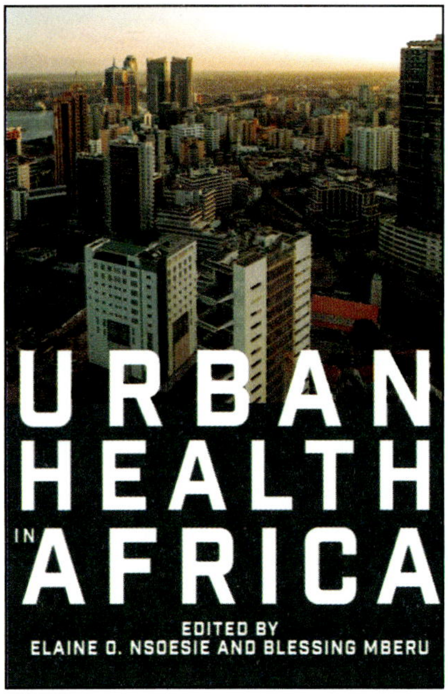

Urban Health in Africa
Edited by Elaine O. Nsoesie and Blessing U. Mberu
Baltimore, MD: Johns Hopkins University Press; 2025
360 pp; $74.95
ISBNs: 10: 1421451158; 13: 9781421451152

Several recent developments make the topic of improving the health of people living in cities in Africa timely and urgent. Although Africa is the continent with the lowest proportion of its population living in cities, its urban population is the world's fastest growing. Increasingly, cities are where emerging global public health crises grow and spread and where they are effectively tackled or not. Almost one quarter of the world's populations living in informal settlements (also known as slums) are in sub-Saharan Africa. And recent decisions by the United States to slash its funding and other support for improving global health will have dire consequences on the urban populations of Africa and therefore the world.

OVERVIEW

For these reasons, *Urban Health in Africa*, edited by Elaine O. Nsoesie and Blessing U. Mberu, scholars at the Boston University School of Public Health and the African Population and Health Research Center in Nairobi, Kenya, respectively, is a timely contribution to the literature on the health of people living in African cities. The book's 20 chapters, authored by 38 public health researchers, practitioners, and activists, 26 with appointments in African institutions, provide a comprehensive overview of key issues.

To set the stage, the book begins with a brief history of African cities and a discussion of the varying definitions of cities across Africa. Several chapters then review the impact on African urban populations of major social determinants of health such as housing, food security and diet, access to health care, military and civil conflicts, water and sanitation, transportation, and environmental pollution. Other chapters examine the impact of demographic changes on the sexual and reproductive health of young people and on the prevalence and prevention of chronic diseases. Case studies of efforts to improve health in specific cities examine air quality in Kampala, Uganda; mental health in Yaoundé, Cameroon; the role of education in health in Arusha, Tanzania; planning for health in informal settlements in Nairobi, Kenya; and the prospects for digital health in Nairobi, Kenya. A final section examines educating the next generation of urban health scholars for Africa and thinking about urban health in Africa in the coming decades.

This brief summary shows that *Urban Health in Africa* provides a useful introduction to urban health in Africa for students in Africa and beyond and a concise synopsis of what is known and what needs further investigation for urban health scholars in Africa and around the world. In totality, the book offers a more complex and comprehensive narrative than either the crisis and doom picture of the health of African cities often shown in mainstream media or the overly cheery stories of resilience and innovation sometimes offered as an antidote to the gloomier scenarios. By examining the differences in health across African cities, periods, and levels of economic development, the authors paint a more nuanced portrait of the variations and consistencies across the continent.

FUTURE RESEARCH ON URBAN HEALTH IN AFRICA

Although no single book can fully cover a topic as complex as urban health in Africa, this book raises several questions that warrant additional consideration. These include the following:

- What are the value and limits of studying urban health at various levels, such as the continent, the nation, the region, the city, and the community? This book illustrates both the insights and the drawbacks of looking at the entire African continent, a region as diverse as Latin America and Asia and therefore as subject to glib stereotyping.[1]
- How do changes in global economies, politics, and demographics influence African cities and their health? As many scholars predict the demise of neoliberalism,[2] we need to ask what will be the impact of the next global regime on the health of people living in African cities?
- How does the growing attention to the role of commercial determinants of health, how market economies and the profit motive influence health, affect the health of African cities?[3,4] What strategies will be most effective in protecting urban populations in Africa against harmful commercial determinants?[5]
- What role do the many military and civil conflicts now being waged in Africa have on the health of cities and the physical and mental health of the continent's people? What practical strategies can reduce these clashes and the harm they impose?[6]
- More urgently, as the United States and other Western countries eliminate or reduce their support for public health services and research in the Global South, how can health professionals and scholars concerned about urban health monitor the impact of these reductions and provide evidence to support activism to reverse this trend?

The editors and authors of *Urban Health in Africa* acknowledge these questions but do not address them in depth. However, by summarizing the evidence that can shape the next round of research, practice, and activism that seeks to improve the health of people living in cities in Africa, the book makes a vital contribution to charting urban health in Africa and global health and health equity more broadly. AJPH

CORRESPONDENCE

Correspondence should be sent to Nicholas Freudenberg, CUNY School of Public Health, 55 West 125th St, New York, NY 10027 (e-mail: nick.freudenberg@sph.cuny.edu). Reprints can be ordered at https://www.ajph.org by clicking the "Reprints" link.

PUBLICATION INFORMATION

Full Citation: Freudenberg N. Urban health in Africa: implications for global public health. *Am J Public Health*. 2025;115(9):1344–1345.

Acceptance Date: June 16, 2025.

DOI: https://doi.org/10.2105/AJPH.2025.308223

CONFLICTS OF INTEREST

The author has no conflicts of interest to disclose.

REFERENCES

1. Doh EF. *Stereotyping Africa. Surprising Answers to Surprising Questions*. East Lansing, MI: Michigan State University Press; 2009.
2. Davies W, Gane N. Post-neoliberalism? An introduction. *Theory, Cult. Soc.* 2021;38(6):3–28. https://doi.org/10.1177/02632764211036722
3. Friel S, Collin J, Daube M, et al. Commercial determinants of health: future directions. *Lancet*. 2023; 401(10383):1229–1240. https://doi.org/10.1016/S0140-6736(23)00011-9
4. Loewenson R, Godt S, Chanda-Kapata P. Asserting public health interest in acting on commercial determinants of health in sub-Saharan Africa: insights from a discourse analysis. *BMJ Glob Health*. 2022;7(7):e009271. https://doi.org/10.1136/bmjgh-2022-009271
5. African Commission on Human and Peoples' Rights. Resolution on States' Obligation to Regulate Private Actors Involved in the Provision of Health and Education Services. ACHPR/Res. 420 (64), 2019. Available at: https://achpr.au.int/en/adopted-resolutions/420-resolution-states-obligation-regulate-private-actors-involved-prov. Accessed March 29, 2022.
6. Carpiniello B. The mental health costs of armed conflicts—a review of systematic reviews conducted on refugees, asylum-seekers and people living in war zones. *Int J Environ Res Public Health*. 2023;20(4):2840. https://doi.org/10.3390/ijerph20042840

Medicaid Expansion Prevents Human Papillomavirus Cancers for Everyone

Heather M. Brandt, PhD

ABOUT THE AUTHOR

Heather M. Brandt is with the HPV Cancer Prevention Program, St. Jude Comprehensive Cancer Center, St. Jude Children's Research Hospital, Memphis, TN.

See also Chen et al., p. 1454.

Human papillomavirus (HPV) vaccination coverage in the United States remains below the *Healthy People 2030* national goal of having 80% of adolescents aged 13 to 15 years old fully vaccinated. Considerable and growing scientific evidence shows tremendous reductions in HPV prevalence, HPV infections, and actual cases of HPV cancer in populations with high vaccination coverage, and even in the United States, which has suboptimal coverage.[1] Medicaid expansion under the provisions of the Affordable Care Act (ACA) has been associated with increased HPV vaccination initiation and completion rates among children and adults in the United States based on previously published research.[2–10] This increase is attributed most often to mitigation of financial barriers, such as reductions in the number of uninsured people and greater access to health care services, including preventive care like HPV vaccination. Importantly, as a result of expansion, increased HPV vaccination coverage was observed among minoritized and marginalized groups experiencing strains on access to preventive health care.[11] To date, 41 states (including the District of Columbia), comprising a combination of so-called red and blue states, have adopted Medicaid expansion. Ten states have not adopted Medicaid expansion; seven of those states are in the South, which is a region with the lowest rates of HPV vaccination and highest rates of HPV cancers in the United States.

However, previously published studies lacked comprehensive analysis of subgroups. Chen et al. (p. 1454) examined changes in rates of HPV vaccination between Medicaid expansion states and nonexpansion states using difference-in-difference analyses of National Immunization Survey-Teen (NIS-Teen) data for the period 2011 to 2022. Difference-in-difference analyses are designed to estimate causal (or temporal) effects when a randomized controlled trial is not feasible. Results showed increases in HPV vaccination initiation among adolescents in the United States, with some of the largest increases among Black adolescents, consistent with previously published research.[2–11] This new article by Chen et al. adds to the literature because of its focus on subgroup analysis by sex, race, and ethnicity. In particular, the finding that male adolescents had the highest increases in HPV vaccination initiation highlights the role of Medicaid expansion in decreasing differences between females and males. Females have traditionally had variably higher rates of HPV vaccination compared with males as a result of the initial routine recommendation for HPV vaccination among females only. Furthermore, increases in HPV vaccination initiation among males were observed for all racial subgroups, with the largest increases among Black, Latino, and Other/Multiple races, reinforcing the added benefits of Medicaid expansion for those from minoritized groups. The focus of Chen et al. on initiation only offers the opportunity to extend this research methodology to examining the influence of Medicaid expansion on HPV vaccination series completion, which has previously been shown to lag among adolescents from minoritized groups.[11]

In addition to the role of dichotomous determination of Medicaid expansion on explaining HPV vaccination coverage, researchers previously examined the influence of the federal poverty level (FPL).[12] The provisions of the ACA offered states the option to extend access to health insurance coverage through Medicaid expansion to low-income adults earning up to 138% of the FPL. Medicaid income eligibility varies, with some states having much lower eligibility limits than others. A cost savings analysis estimated that increasing Medicaid eligibility to 200% of the FPL in 32 states with lower eligibility levels could generate approximately $9 million in cost savings by avoiding medical expenses that are typically incurred during the first two years after an HPV cancer diagnosis. Such savings would be realized as a result of increased HPV vaccination series

AJPH September 2025, Vol. 115, No. 9

completion and the subsequent reduced incidence of HPV cancers. Cost savings are likely underestimated because precancers of the cervix were not included in the study. These findings demonstrated that increased access through Medicaid expansion, coupled with eligibility levels at 200% of the FPL, increased HPV vaccination coverage and offered cost savings benefit. Chen et al. did not examine FPL among Medicaid expansion and nonexpansion states. Future research should examine the role of Medicaid expansion and FPL to further determine how setting the FPL at 200% might provide access to HPV vaccination for additional children and adults.

Chen et al. also did not attend to the influence of school-entry requirements. For other routinely recommended childhood and adolescent vaccinations, school-entry requirements have been a primary strategy for driving coverage. Coverage for two other routinely recommended vaccinations for adolescents—tetanus, diphtheria, and acellular pertussis vaccine (Tdap) and quadrivalent meningococcal conjugate vaccine (MenACWY)—are 89.0% and 88.4%, respectively, according to 2023 NIS-Teen data.[13] Every state requires Tdap for school entry, and all but 15 states have school-entry requirements for MenACWY.[14] For HPV vaccination, only three states (Hawaii, Rhode Island, and Virginia) and two jurisdictions (the District of Columbia and Puerto Rico) have school-entry requirements in place. HPV vaccination coverage among this same age group of adolescents is 76.8% for initiation and 61.4% for completion, which are significantly lower than for Tdap and MenACWY. Previous research has identified school-entry requirements for MenACWY as a policy strategy to increase HPV vaccination coverage.[12] Given the current climate regarding vaccination requirements, it is unlikely that additional states will adopt school-entry requirements for any vaccinations, including HPV vaccination, in the near future. Therefore, the role of policies such as Medicaid expansion are even more important.

Although Medicaid expansion has shown positive results, ongoing efforts are needed to further improve HPV vaccination coverage and ensure that all individuals have access to this crucial cancer prevention tool. Medicaid expansion has the potential to reduce cancer disparities, particularly among states with already pronounced differences in prevention, screening, and cancer outcomes, because, as Chen et al. have shown, it increases HPV vaccination among male adolescents across all racial and ethnic subgroups.[15] Medicaid expansion has had a positive effect on people diagnosed with cancer as well, demonstrating its value across the care continuum.[16] There are many documented benefits of Medicaid expansion on cancer prevention and control outcomes, including increased HPV vaccination coverage as shown by Chen et al.

However, the current political climate is directly in contrast with the scientific evidence showing that Medicaid expansion prevents HPV cancers in the future by increasing HPV vaccination today. Efforts to preserve Medicaid expansion and solidify the FPL at 200% are paramount for retaining hard-earned gains and expanding HPV vaccination coverage. According to recent Kaiser Family Foundation (KFF) estimates, policy changes targeting Medicaid expansion would reduce government spending but could also put access at risk for 20 million enrollees.[17] There are myriad reasons to preserve Medicaid expansion, and HPV cancer prevention represents one such advantage. Medicaid expansion prevents HPV cancers for everyone. In the absence of universal health care or a single-payer system in the United States, Medicaid and its expansion to cover as many people as possible must remain sacrosanct. The health of the nation depends on this. AJPH

CORRESPONDENCE

Correspondence should be sent to Heather M. Brandt, PhD, Director, HPV Cancer Prevention Program, St. Jude Children's Research Hospital, 262 Danny Thomas Place, Memphis, TN 38105 (e-mail: heather.brandt@stjude.org). Reprints can be ordered at https://www.ajph.org by clicking the "Reprints" link.

PUBLICATION INFORMATION

Full Citation: Brandt HM. Medicaid expansion prevents human papillomavirus cancers for everyone. *Am J Public Health*. 2025;115(9):1346–1348.

Acceptance Date: May 27, 2025.

DOI: https://doi.org/10.2105/AJPH.2025.308207

ORCID iD:

Heather M. Brandt https://orcid.org/0000-0003-1066-2879

ACKNOWLEDGMENTS

This publication was supported by the American Lebanese and Syrian Associated Charities (ALSAC) of St. Jude Children's Research Hospital.

CONFLICTS OF INTEREST

The author has no conflicts of interest to report.

REFERENCES

1. Gargano JW, Stefanos R, Dahl RM, HPV-IMPACT Working Group, et al. Trends in cervical precancers identified through population-based surveillance—Human Papillomavirus Vaccine Impact Monitoring Project, Five Sites, United States, 2008–2022. *MMWR Morb Mortal Wkly Rep*. 2025; 74(6):96–101. https://doi.org/10.15585/mmwr.mm7406a4
2. Hoff BM, Livingston MD 3rd, Thompson EL. The association between state Medicaid expansion and human papillomavirus vaccination. *Vaccine*. 2020;38(38):5963–5965. https://doi.org/10.1016/j.vaccine.2020.07.024
3. Churchill BF. Insurance coverage, provider contact, and take-up of the HPV vaccine. *Am J Health Econ*. 2021;7(2). https://doi.org/10.1086/713037
4. Hawkins SS, Horvath K, Cohen J, Pace LE, Baum CF. Associations between insurance-related affordable care act policy changes with HPV vaccine completion. *BMC Public Health*. 2021;

21(1):304. https://doi.org/10.1186/s12889-021-10328-4

5. Hawkins SS, Horvath K, Cohen J, Pace LE, Baum CF. Associations between ACA-related policies and a clinical recommendation with HPV vaccine initiation. *Cancer Causes Control.* 2021;32(7):783–790. https://doi.org/10.1007/s10552-021-01430-4
6. Chan JK, Mann AK, Lee D, et al. Human papillomavirus vaccination trends and disparities in the United States: who is getting left behind? *Sex Transm Dis.* 2021;48(10):714–719. https://doi.org/10.1097/OLQ.0000000000001410
7. Saxena K, Kathe N, Sardana P, Yao L, Chen YT, Brewer NT. HPV vaccine initiation at 9 or 10 years of age and better series completion by age 13 among privately and publicly insured children in the US. *Hum Vaccin Immunother.* 2023;19(1):2161253. https://doi.org/10.1080/21645515.2022.2161253
8. Agénor M, Unger ES, McConnell MA, et al. Affordable Care Act state Medicaid expansion and human papillomavirus vaccination among adolescent and young adult US women: a national study. *Health Serv Res.* 2023;58(4):792–799. https://doi.org/10.1111/1475-6773.14133
9. Ibrahim-Ojoawo A, Powe N, Rogers R, Learman K, Hefner H. A cross-sectional analysis of 2017–2022 National Immunization Survey: sociodemographic disparities associated with human papillomavirus vaccine initiation and completion series among US adolescents. *Cancer Control.* 2024;31:10732748241293674. https://doi.org/10.1177/10732748241293674
10. Gao MZ, Awonusi OO, Ramkumar SP, et al. The Affordable Care Act and change in human papillomavirus (HPV) vaccine uptake in the United States. *Vaccine.* 2025;50:126842. https://doi.org/10.1016/j.vaccine.2025.126842
11. Spencer JC, Calo WA, Brewer NT. Disparities and reverse disparities in HPV vaccination: a systematic review and meta-analysis. *Prev Med.* 2019;123:197–203. https://doi.org/10.1016/j.ypmed.2019.03.037
12. St. Jude Children's Research Hospital, HPV Cancer Prevention Program. Updated analysis of public policy decisions and factors driving HPV vaccination coverage in the United States. 2023. Available at: https://sjr-redesign.stjude.org/content/dam/research-redesign/centers-initiatives/hpv-cancer-prevention-program/fact-sheets/253601-hpv-vaccination-policy-summary-090523.pdf. Accessed May 10, 2025.
13. Pingali C, Yankey D, Chen M, et al. National vaccination coverage among adolescents aged 13–17 years—National Immunization Survey-Teen, United States, 2023. *MMWR Morb Mortal Wkly Rep.* 2024;73(33):708–714. https://doi.org/10.15585/mmwr.mm7333a1
14. Immunize.org. Meningococcal ACWY (MenACWY) vaccine requirements for secondary school. 2024. Available at: https://www.immunize.org/official-guidance/state-policies/vaccine-requirements/menacwy-school-2024. Accessed May 10, 2025.
15. Choi SK, Adams SA, Eberth JM, et al. Medicaid coverage expansion and implications for cancer disparities. *Am J Public Health.* 2015;105(suppl 5):S706–S712. https://doi.org/10.2105/AJPH.2015.302876
16. Hotca A, Bloom JR, Runnels J, et al. The impact of Medicaid expansion on patients with cancer in the United States: a review. *Curr Oncol.* 2023;30(7):6362–6373. https://doi.org/10.3390/curroncol30070469
17. Mathers J, Tolbert J, Chidambaram P, Cervantes S, Kaiser Family Foundation (KFF). 5 key facts about Medicaid expansion. 2025. Available at: https://www.kff.org/medicaid/issue-brief/5-key-facts-about-medicaid-expansion. Accessed May 10, 2025.

A Measure Aligned With Reproductive Justice, Human Rights, and Sexual Well-Being. . .? Yes Please, and Here's Why

Jenny A. Higgins, PhD, MPH, Diana N. Carvajal, MD, MPH, and Leigh Senderowicz, ScD, MPH

ABOUT THE AUTHORS

Jenny A. Higgins is with the Department of Obstetrics and Gynecology, Diane N. Carvajal is with the Department of Family Medicine and Community Health, and Leigh Senderowicz is with the Departments of Gender and Women's Studies and Obstetrics and Gynecology, University of Wisconsin-Madison.

See also Dehlendorf et al., p. 1463.

In our qualitative research and clinical care, we regularly talk with people about their sexual and reproductive lives. Whether interviewees in our studies or patients in our practice, few, if any, have a single domain that constitutes the entirety of their sexual and reproductive health and well-being. Nor do most consider their sexual bodies separately from their reproductive bodies. Rather, those we wish to serve through public health research and practice, just like public health and medical professionals, have complex, nuanced, and integrated desires to have healthy and well bodies, relationships, and communities. All of us want to be well and thrive more than we simply want to avoid potentially negative sexual and reproductive outcomes.

Yet, much of our research and practice in public health and medicine takes on a narrow, single-issue approach to sexuality and reproduction, with sexual health and reproductive health tending to run on parallel versus intersecting tracks in our field. We frequently use single, deficit-focused, and potentially irrelevant measures such as unintended pregnancy, contraceptive prevalence, use of long-acting reversible contraception (LARC), or rates of sexually transmitted infections to account for the sexual and reproductive health of a population.

In doing so, we have fashioned and perpetuated an unfortunate disconnect. On the one hand, many in our field now wish to adhere to a human rights framework that acknowledges the critical importance of sociopolitical context and antioppression for people's overall sexual and reproductive well-being. On the other hand, we are constricted in applying this framework given our narrow measurement of demographic and health indicators. To bridge this gap, we applaud the team efforts described by Dehlendorf et al. in this issue of *AJPH* (p. 1463) to develop a multidimensional measure of overall sexual and reproductive well-being (SRWB). In addition to the points made by the authors, we offer three rationales in favor of a more accurate, complete, and contextually relevant measurement approach to SRWB.

First, a more holistic, multilevel measure that assesses well-being is more equitable than single-domain measures that focus on negative outcomes. Single-domain measures such as "unintended pregnancy," for example, are often deficit-focused. As a result, research using these measures documents the worst outcomes in underresourced, socially marginalized communities, where policymakers and program professionals then disproportionately roll out interventions to address these "deficits." Examples include LARC-focused clinical guidelines, interventions, and public health campaigns that have dominated much of the sexual and reproductive health field for the last decade or more.[1] These efforts were, and continue to be, disproportionately targeted to people who experience the worst social marginalization and exclusion, especially women of color.[2,3] They have fueled coercion, community distrust, and an unnecessary (and sometimes unwelcome) focus on preventing pregnancy only.[4] Yet, when we attend to people's ability to thrive holistically and within the context of their lived experiences and personal desires—versus, say, whether their pregnancy was unintended, or whether they are using a LARC method—we can better understand and place responsibility on the inherently inequitable and oppressive sociopolitical structures, systems, and policies rather than on the "failings" of individuals.

A measure that focuses on overall sexual and reproductive well-being is also less likely to be used to justify coercive interventions. In contrast, as we have documented in our own work,[5,6] metrics such as LARC uptake can replicate systems of power and oppression that pressure some and not others to limit fertility, but often fail to provide the necessary, equitable resources and care to support healthy pregnancies, thriving infants, and overall "well" communities. But if we assess sexual and reproductive health and well-being holistically and comprehensively, we can focus less on which individuals most need changing or intervening, and more on the social structures, policies, and programs that must change drastically to improve health and well-being.

Second, a comprehensive, contextual measure of sexual and reproductive well-being will result in better science, which could inform more relevant and impactful policies and public health programs to ultimately improve overall health and well-being. Examples of mainstream measures that lack internal validity are hardly in short supply. The body of research that criticizes the demographic measure of unintended pregnancy, for example, for its failure to capture true meaning for pregnant people and useful information for programmers and policymakers, is now more robust than the research that led to the creation of this metric in the first place.[7,8] The percentage of people using a highly effective contraceptive method fails to tell us whether an individual wishes or prefers to use that method, let alone what the experience of accessing contraceptive care was like for them. Further, a reliance on LARC-use metrics disproportionately creates barriers to LARC removal for people who wish to discontinue those methods.[9,10] Yet, such measures are often used to direct the allocation of public health resources. Communities would be better served if such resources were instead used to improve outcomes based on comprehensive, carefully created, and validated measures with both scientific merit and community resonance.

Lastly, a measure that truly accounts for sexuality and sexual health alongside reproductive health will better reflect people's experiences with their bodies and their well-being. As the measure's name suggests, it's sexual and reproductive well-being, not sexual or reproductive health. For example, no one has sex just so they can use contraception. Rather, people use contraception for a variety of reasons, including the ability to have enjoyable sex without the risk of unwanted pregnancy. Yet, many programs, studies, and clinical guidelines ignore the ways that reproduction and sexuality are inextricably linked. And although public health scholars now recognize that reproduction is deeply stratified by power differentials, we often overlook how sexuality is, too. In a review of 47 studies from more than 22 countries, 44 indicated that study participants with more constrained socioeconomic conditions also reported poorer indicators of sexual well-being, especially sexual satisfaction and overall sexual functioning.[11] Sociopolitical, structural constraints affect sexual bodies, too.[12] Greater awareness of this fact, as well as a measure to assess sexual well-being and not only negative sexual outcomes, will improve and renew a commitment by public health and health services research to positive sexual health for all. Everyone deserves the basic human right of sexual well-being. Sexual flourishing and justice can and should coexist with reproductive flourishing and justice, in tandem with a broader human rights framework. An integrated SRWB measure will make this consolidation more possible.

We appreciate that a new measure may come with drawbacks. Any novel metric will require that we start from scratch in our ability to document trends over time. That said, replicability alone is an insufficient reason to continue using invalid, irrelevant, or harmful metrics. We also appreciate that the SRWB may be more aspirational and sweeping in its vision than more immediately addressable metrics. Such sweeping composite measures may be less helpful for program planning, policymaking, or other practical ends if they render us unable to pinpoint possible action steps. For example, if someone has a low SRWB score, we may be unable to discern whether that score is caused by contraceptive coercion, housing insecurity, or a host of other factors. But like the architects of the new SRWB measure, we owe it to our communities to move forward with a more relevant and comprehensive measure of well-being. Let's all work to accurately measure, and equitably address, people's ability to thrive in their sexual and reproductive lives. AJPH

CORRESPONDENCE

Correspondence should be sent to Jenny Higgins, 4245 Medical Sciences Center, 1300 University Ave, University of Wisconsin-Madison, Madison, WI 53706 (email: jenny.a.higgins@wisc.edu). Reprints can be ordered at http://www.ajph.org by clicking the "Reprints" link.

PUBLICATION INFORMATION

Full Citation: Higgins JA, Carvajal DN, Senderowicz L. A measure aligned with reproductive justice, human rights, and sexual well-being. . .? Yes please, and here's why. *Am J Public Health*. 2025;115(9): 1349–1351.

Acceptance Date: May 11, 2025.

DOI: https://doi.org/10.2105/AJPH.2025.308197

ORCID iDs:

Jenny A. Higgins https://orcid.org/0000-0002-1352-8416

Diana N. Carvajal https://orcid.org/0000-0002-6264-1861

Leigh Senderowicz https://orcid.org/0000-0002-6713-1473

CONTRIBUTORS

J. A. Higgins wrote the first draft. D. N. Carvajal and L. Senderowicz added important intellectual content and critically revised the initial material. All three authors reviewed subsequent drafts until reaching consensus on the final version.

ACKNOWLEDGMENTS

We thank the large, anonymous family foundation that provides support for the UW Collaborative for Reproductive Equity (https://core.wisc.edu).

CONFLICTS OF INTEREST

The authors have no conflicts of interest to report.

REFERENCES

1. Holt K, Reed R, Crear-Perry J, Scott C, Wulf S, Dehlendorf C. Beyond same-day long-acting reversible contraceptive access: a person-centered framework for advancing high-quality, equitable contraceptive care. *Am J Obstet Gynecol.* 2020; 222(4S):S878.e1–S878.e6. https://doi.org/10.1016/j.ajog.2019.11.1279
2. Brandi K, Fuentes L. The history of tiered-effectiveness contraceptive counseling and the importance of patient-centered family planning care. *Am J Obstet Gynecol.* 2020;222(4S):S873–S877. https://doi.org/10.1016/j.ajog.2019.11.1271
3. Carvajal DN, Gioia D, Mudafort ER, Brown PB, Barnet B. How can primary care physicians best support contraceptive decision making? A qualitative study exploring the perspectives of Baltimore Latinas. *Womens Health Issues.* 2017;27(2):158–166. https://doi.org/10.1016/j.whi.2016.09.015
4. Sznajder K, Carvajal DN, Sufrin C. Patient perceptions of immediate postpartum long-acting reversible contraception: a qualitative study. *Contraception.* 2020;101(1):21–25. https://doi.org/10.1016/j.contraception.2019.09.007
5. Senderowicz L, Sokol N, Pearson E, Francis J, Ulenga N, Bärnighausen T. The effect of a postpartum intrauterine device programme on choice of contraceptive method in Tanzania: a secondary analysis of a cluster-randomized trial. *Health Policy Plan.* 2023;38(1):38–48. https://doi.org/10.1093/heapol/czac094
6. Senderowicz L. "I was obligated to accept": a qualitative exploration of contraceptive coercion. *Soc Sci Med.* 2019;239:112531. https://doi.org/10.1016/j.socscimed.2019.112531
7. Santelli JS, Rochat R, Hatfield-Timajchy K, et al. The measurement and meaning of unintended pregnancy. *Perspect Sex Reprod Health.* 2003; 35(2):94–101. https://doi.org/10.1363/3509403
8. Potter JE, Stevenson AJ, Coleman-Minahan K, et al. Challenging unintended pregnancy as an indicator of reproductive autonomy. *Contraception.* 2019; 100(1):1–4. https://doi.org/10.1016/j.contraception.2019.02.005
9. Senderowicz L, Kolenda A. "She told me no, that you cannot change": understanding provider refusal to remove contraceptive implants. *SSM Qual Res Health.* 2022;2:100154. https://doi.org/10.1016/j.ssmqr.2022.100154
10. Manzer JL, Bell AV. The limitations of patient-centered care: the case of early long-acting reversible contraception (LARC) removal. *Soc Sci Med.* 2022;292:114632. https://doi.org/10.1016/j.socscimed.2021.114632
11. Higgins JA, Lands M, Ufot M, McClelland SI. Socioeconomics and erotic inequity: a theoretical overview and narrative review of associations between poverty, socioeconomic conditions, and sexual wellbeing. *J Sex Res.* 2022;59(8):940–956. https://doi.org/10.1080/00224499.2022.2044990
12. Higgins JA, Kramer R, Senderowicz L, Everett B, Turok DK, Sanders JN. Sex, poverty, and public health: connections between sexual wellbeing and economic resources among US reproductive health clients. *Perspect Sex Reprod Health.* 2022; 54(1):25–28. https://doi.org/10.1363/psrh.12189

Gun-Free Zones in Sensitive Places

Louis Klarevas, PhD

ABOUT THE AUTHOR

Louis Klarevas is with Teachers College, Columbia University, New York, NY.

See also Crifasi et al., p. 1472.

The Second Amendment of the US Constitution states, "A well regulated Militia, being necessary to the security of a free State, the right of the people to keep and bear Arms, shall not be infringed." In 2008, the US Supreme Court in *District of Columbia v Heller* held that, pursuant to the Second Amendment, individuals have a right to possess ("keep") ordinary arms "in common use" at their homes for the purpose of self-defense.[1] In 2022, in *New York State Pistol & Rifle Association v Bruen*, the Supreme Court expanded on the Second Amendment and held that individuals also have a right to carry ("bear") "commonly used arms in public subject to certain reasonable, well-defined restrictions."[2] As first raised in *Heller* and subsequently elaborated on in *Bruen*, a law "forbidding the carrying of firearms in 'sensitive places' such as schools and government buildings" is one such example of a restriction on the right to bear arms that is presumptively constitutional.[1,2]

The Supreme Court has vaguely defined "sensitive places" as locations "where arms carrying could be prohibited consistent with the Second Amendment."[2] Inevitably, a more comprehensive definition of sensitive places will be left to legislative bodies and lower courts. And, as the study by Crifasi et al. in this issue (p. 1472) correctly notes, the question of what is a sensitive place is likely to be affected by public perceptions of whether a particular location is one "where people enjoy a reasonable expectation of safety, where conflict is likely, or where the presence of guns is incompatible with the primary function of the place." Toward this end, opinion surveys on how the American people view a space, including how "they think about the presence of firearms in that space," will likely play a central role in helping governmental bodies in the process of delineating which places are sensitive.

In a way, sensitive places are akin to "gun-free zones," where the possession of personal firearms by private individuals is lawfully prohibited.[3] Although the prohibition of arms in certain sensitive places has a long historical tradition in the United States, the idea of explicitly designated gun-free zones only traces its roots to the mid-1980s.[3–4] In recent years, gun-free zones have become a focal point of public debate.[5] One analysis claims that as many as 92% of mass public shootings have occurred in gun-free zones, suggesting that such settings attract active shooters.[6] Another analysis, however, found that as few as 12% of high-fatality mass shootings have occurred in gun-free zones.[7] Obviously, even accounting for differences in how mass shootings are defined, there is a massive difference between 92% and 12%. At the very least, one of these policy analyses is way off the mark.

New scientific analyses have found no support for the idea that gun-free zones serve as magnets for gun violence, especially active and mass shootings. If anything, it appears that active shootings might be substantially less likely to occur in gun-free zones than in gun-allowing zones.[8] And looking beyond potential mass-casualty acts of violence, the latest evidence suggests that gun-free zones at schools and bars have protective effects against gun violence at these locations.[9–10] Equally important, there is little evidence to suggest, regardless of the scenario, that gun-allowing zones experience significantly less gun violence than gun-free zones.[8–10]

Although additional research on this topic is welcome, the emerging view suggests that gun-free zones appear to be fulfilling their legislative intent: they appear to be keeping people in such sensitive places relatively safer. Aware of these findings, legislative bodies may wish to identify additional sensitive places and statutorily define them as gun-free zones. As Crifasi et al. point out, public opinion surveys can play a critical role in guiding elected officials and their constituents on this important—and potentially life-saving—policy endeavor.

The American people, in general, seem to support restrictions on possessing firearms in a variety of sensitive places: public demonstrations and protests, sports stadiums, bars, restaurants, service settings, retail stores, places of worship, schools, college campuses, and government buildings. National surveys have consistently found plurality support—and, for most of these categories, majority support—for prohibiting the carrying of personal firearms at all of these types of places.[11,12] For most Americans, it seems that the risks of having firearms at most of these locations outweigh the benefits.

However, for each of these location categories, another consistent pattern is that non–gun owners expressed greater support for sensitive-place prohibitions than gun owners.[11,12] Although this is a significant finding, it is also one that requires nuance in terms of interpretation.

One of the most original findings in the study by Crifasi et al. is that, although gun owners generally exhibit lower support for sensitive-place prohibitions on the carrying of firearms, when compared with non–gun owners, gun owners should not be seen as a monolithic group. Indeed, in terms of race and ethnicity, non-Hispanic White and Hispanic gun owners tend to share similar views on sensitive-place restrictions, and they differ substantially from the views of Asian and non-Hispanic Black gun owners, with the latter two (especially non-Hispanic Black gun owners) expressing greater support for prohibitions than the former two. In terms of gun-owner support for sensitive-place prohibitions, a gap also exists between new gun owners (who purchased their first firearm in the three years or so prior to being surveyed) and more-established gun owners (who owned a firearm for more than three years prior to being surveyed). Compared with more-established gun owners, new gun owners express less support for sensitive-place restrictions, regardless of location.

But, arguably, the most important takeaway to emerge from this new survey research is that an individual's perception of firearm carrying appears to be more impactful than gun ownership. People who feel safer if more people can legally carry firearms, regardless of whether or not they personally own guns, tend to express the lowest support for sensitive-place prohibitions. This suggests that general attitudes on the utility of firearms for purposes of defending oneself and others are perhaps the strongest driver of political opposition toward gun-free zones.

Policymakers and researchers have an obligation not only to familiarize themselves with the latest science on the public-safety effects of firearm laws, but also to engage with the public about those effects. Thanks to research like that of Crifasi et al., the policy and scientific communities have a better understanding of how best to target the messaging on sensitive-place laws.

In the last few years, we have begun learning that gun-allowing zones do not fare better than gun-free zones. If anything, the latest evidence suggests that, for the most part, gun-free zones at sensitive places appear to experience less firearm violence than gun-allowing zones. It is incumbent on our elected officials and their constituents to be mindful of this valuable lesson. As a society, we need to remember that a better-informed public makes for a smarter public—and, in turn, a smarter public makes for a safer public. AJPH

CORRESPONDENCE

Correspondence should be sent to Louis Klarevas, 525 W. 120th St, Teachers College, Columbia University, New York, NY 10027 (email: ljk2149@tc.columbia.edu). Reprints can be ordered at https://www.ajph.org by clicking the "Reprints" link.

PUBLICATION INFORMATION

Full Citation: Klarevas L. Gun-free zones in sensitive places. *Am J Public Health*. 2025;115(9):1352–1353.

Acceptance Date: May 21, 2025.

DOI: https://doi.org/10.2105/AJPH.2025.308203

ORCID iD:
Louis Klarevas https://orcid.org/0009-0005-4341-7003

CONFLICTS OF INTEREST

The author has no conflicts of interest to report.

REFERENCES

1. *District of Columbia v Heller*, 554 US 570 (2008).
2. *New York State Pistol & Rifle Association v Bruen*, 597 US 1 (2022).
3. RAND. The effects of gun-free zones. July 16, 2024. Available at: https://www.rand.org/research/gun-policy/analysis/gun-free-zones.html. Accessed May 13, 2025.
4. Blocher J, Siegel RB. Guided by history: protecting the public sphere from weapons threats under *Bruen*. *NYU L Rev*. 2023;98:1795. Available at: https://nyulawreview.org/wp-content/uploads/2023/12/98-NYU-L-Rev-1795.pdf. Accessed May 13, 2025.
5. Shaw K. What is a "gun-free zone," and what's behind the movement to get rid of them? The Trace. March 16, 2017. Available at: https://www.thetrace.org/2017/03/gun-free-zone-facts. Accessed May 13, 2025.
6. Lott JR. Updated detailed information on mass public shootings from 1998 to 2024. Crime Prevention Research Center. January 2, 2025. Available at: https://crimeresearch.org/2025/01/updated-information-on-mass-public-shootings-from-1998-to-2024. Accessed May 13, 2025.
7. Klarevas L. *Rampage Nation: Securing America From Mass Shootings*. Amherst, NY: Prometheus; 2016.
8. Reeping PM, Morrison CN, Gobaud AN, Rajan S, Wiebe DJ, Branas CC. Gun-free zones and active shootings in the United States: a matched case–control study. *Lancet Reg Health Am*. 2024;37:100837. https://doi.org/10.1016/j.lana.2024.100837
9. Reeping PM, Gobaud AN, Morrison CN, Branas CC. The effect of gun-free school zones on crimes committed with a firearm in Saint Louis, Missouri. *J Urban Health*. 2023;100(6):1118–1127. https://doi.org/10.1007/s11524-023-00800-4
10. Reeping PM, Laqueur HS, Kagawa RMC. Gun free zones in alcohol-serving establishments and risk for firearm violence: a cross-sectional, geospatial study in Texas. *J Urban Health*. 2024. Online ahead of print. https://doi.org/10.1007/s11524-024-00928-x
11. Wolfson JA, Teret SP, Azrael D, Miller M. US public opinion on carrying firearms in public places. *Am J Public Health*. 2017;107(6):929–937. https://doi.org/10.2105/AJPH.2017.303712
12. Crifasi CK, Ward JA, McGinty EE, Barry CL, Webster DW. Public opinion on laws regulating public gun carrying. *Prev Med*. 2022;159:107067. https://doi.org/10.1016/j.ypmed.2022.107067

Did COVID-19 Slow Our Progress Toward Ending the HIV Epidemic?

Ank E. Nijhawan, MD, MPH, MSCS

ABOUT THE AUTHOR

Ank E. Nijhawan is a professor of Internal Medicine, Division of Infectious Diseases and Geographic Medicine at the University of Texas Southwestern Medical Center, Dallas.

See also Maierhofer et al., p. 1480.

In this issue of *AJPH*, Maierhofer et al. (p. 1480) report on HIV care outcomes among persons newly diagnosed with HIV in the state of North Carolina before and during the COVID-19 pandemic. In this fifth decade of the HIV epidemic, we need to continue to be vigilant in our efforts to End the HIV Epidemic (EHE)[1] and strive for improved outcomes for all people living with or at risk for HIV. Setting goals—such as reducing overall new infections by at least 90% by 2030 and achieving "95-95-95"[2]—is critical; however, the real work lies in measuring gaps in the HIV care continuum and implementing interventions to close those gaps.

VULNERABILITIES REVEALED IN THE HIV CARE SYSTEM

The COVID-19 pandemic was disruptive in many ways and exposed "cracks in the system,"[3] including in health care delivery for people with HIV (PWH). Many studies have identified disparities in outcomes among PWH, which were exacerbated by the COVID-19 pandemic, including greater visit reductions for African Americans at Ryan White facilities in the Deep South[4] and higher rates of viral nonsuppression after shelter-in-place orders, especially for unhoused individuals.[5] Other studies focused on the changes in health care delivery, with a large shift to telehealth visits, multimonth prescribing for antiretroviral therapy, and reducing the frequency of laboratory visits—innovations that many patients welcomed—though technology gaps and changes in payor mix may have worsened access to care for certain groups.[6] Identifying and understanding these vulnerabilities can help us fortify and improve HIV care and continue to move toward EHE goals.[7]

ADAPTATION OF HIV CARE DELIVERY IN NORTH CAROLINA

Using 4 years of comprehensive HIV surveillance data from across the state of North Carolina, Maierhofer et al. examined initial linkage to care (defined as first CD4 or HIV RNA within 30 days of diagnosis), stable HIV care linkage (defined as first CD4 or HIV RNA between 30 days and up to 150 days after linkage) and initial HIV viral suppression (defined as HIV RNA < 200 copies per milliliter of blood within 14 to 180 days of diagnosis). These outcomes were compared between three different time frames—before the pandemic, early pandemic, and late pandemic. The strength of this approach is that the research team was able to include data from 4402 newly diagnosed individuals, regardless of where in the state they received care. However, using laboratory results as a proxy for care engagement does not capture visit attendance (whether virtual or in-person), support services provided, or medication receipt, processes that were vulnerable during the COVID-19 pandemic.

A surprising finding from this study is that initial linkage to care, stable linkage to care, and initial HIV viral suppression did not show a notable decline (and initial linkage even increased) when comparing outcomes from during versus before the pandemic. Though early retention and viral suppression did not decrease, they also did not improve, and this in and of itself could be considered a setback for achieving EHE goals. However, in part, these findings also reflect the resilience of the HIV care system and its ability to rapidly adapt care delivery to COVID-19 restrictions. The Ryan White HIV/AIDS Program (RWHAP), a federally funded program that provides services to more than half of PWH in the United States, has shown improved virologic suppression (89.7% vs 65.9%) compared with the general population of PWH as well as over time, including spanning the COVID-19 pandemic with 89.7% versus 70% virologic suppression among RWHAP recipients in 2021 versus 2017.[8]

PERSISTENCE OF HIV-RELATED DISPARITIES DURING THE PANDEMIC

However, many of the disparities in the United States that predated the COVID-19 pandemic, including less favorable HIV-related outcomes for people living in the South, Black and Hispanic individuals, and gender and

AJPH September 2025, Vol. 115, No. 9

sexual minority groups,[9] persisted during the pandemic. In this study, lower stable linkage to HIV care was observed for Black, Hispanic, and transgender individuals. Furthermore, it has been demonstrated that HIV prevention services and HIV testing decreased during the early pandemic,[10] and it is possible that people who did present for HIV testing were more ill and in urgent need of care. This is supported by the higher HIV viral loads and lower CD4 counts at presentation for people newly diagnosed during the COVID-19 pandemic during this study.

Overall, this provocative article on linkage and initial viral suppression among people newly diagnosed with HIV in North Carolina between 2018 and 2022 underscores the critical role of epidemiology in EHE efforts. In this most recent decade of the HIV epidemic, health departments and HIV care systems have moved beyond the annual surveillance reporting role, not only to identify critical gaps in HIV care but also to provide solutions to closing these gaps. For example, "data to care" initiatives utilize state-level longitudinal HIV surveillance data to identify PWH who may be out of care (e.g., missing repeat HIV laboratory results > 6 months) and to direct community-based outreach efforts to re-engage individuals in care.[11] Similarly, though the findings from Maierhofer et al. highlight a resilient HIV care system in North Carolina, it is the persistent or worsening gaps among vulnerable groups they have identified that merit action.

A CALL TO ACTION

If we are to reach a 90% reduction in HIV incidence in the United States by 2030, an admittedly ambitious goal, we need to more aggressively apply lessons from past experience, continue to innovate, and not settle for stagnant results. As a country, we could have done more to apply what we knew from the early HIV epidemic to combat the stigma, misinformation, and disproportionate impact on marginalized groups from the COVID-19 pandemic. Currently, we must leverage what we learned from the innovative provision of HIV services during the COVID-19 pandemic, including what did and did not work, to prospectively improve health outcomes among all PWH. Ultimately, we need better integration of epidemiological, health services, and qualitative data across the entire spectrum of HIV care—prevention, diagnosis, linkage, retention in care, and virologic suppression—to comprehensively identify and address the continued gaps in achieving EHE targets. This type of data integration requires societal investment and collaboration between health departments, health systems, and academic institutions and can help us recognize, as Maierhofer et al. have highlighted, that stable outcome metrics actually signal a need for improvement.

The future of EHE is in jeopardy, as funding for the Centers for Disease Control and Prevention, local health departments, and HIV prevention efforts has not only been threatened but has already been withdrawn.[12] The implications for our care system for people living with HIV and those at risk for HIV will be devastating, with long-term consequences including increased incidence of HIV and increased mortality. Just as it is not sufficient to simply report on stagnant HIV surveillance data with persistent outcome disparities, we must act on this information. To protect and fortify our HIV care and public health system, as researchers, clinicians, and members of society, we must advocate legislative action not only to maintain but also to increase current support for HIV care and treatment. AJPH

CORRESPONDENCE

Correspondence should be sent to Dr. Ank Nijhawan, 5323 Harry Hines Blvd, Dallas, TX 75390 (e-mail: ank.nijhawan@utsouthwestern.edu). Reprints can be ordered at https://www.ajph.org by clicking the "Reprints" link.

PUBLICATION INFORMATION

Full Citation: Nijhawan AE. Did COVID-19 slow our progress toward ending the HIV epidemic? *Am J Public Health*. 2025;115(9):1354–1356.

Acceptance Date: May 10, 2025.

DOI: https://doi.org/10.2105/AJPH.2025.308198

ORCID iD:
Ank E. Nijhawan https://orcid.org/0000-0003-0522-4110

CONFLICTS OF INTEREST

The author reports no conflicts of interest.

REFERENCES

1. Fauci AS, Redfield RR, Sigounas G, Weahkee MD, Giroir BP. Ending the HIV Epidemic: a plan for the United States. *JAMA*. 2019;321(9):844–845. https://doi.org/10.1001/jama.2019.1343
2. Frescura L, Godfrey-Faussett P, Feizzadeh AA, on and behalf of the 2025 Testing Treatment Target Working Group, et al. Achieving the 95 95 95 targets for all: a pathway to ending AIDS. *PloS One*. 2022;17(8):e0272405. https://doi.org/10.1371/journal.pone.0272405
3. Tulenko K, Vervoort D. Cracks in the system: the effects of the coronavirus pandemic on public health systems. *Am Rev Public Adm*. 2020;50(6–7):455–466. https://doi.org/10.1177/0275074020941667
4. Li Z, Qiao S, Ning H, et al. Place visitation data reveals the geographic and racial disparities of COVID-19 impact on HIV service utilization in the Deep South. *AIDS Behav*. 2024;28(suppl 1):47–60. https://doi.org/10.1007/s10461-023-04163-4
5. Spinelli MA, Hickey MD, Glidden DV, et al. Viral suppression rates in a safety-net HIV clinic in San Francisco destabilized during COVID-19. *AIDS*. 2020;34(15):2328–2331. https://doi.org/10.1097/qad.0000000000002677
6. Dawson L, Kates J. Delivering HIV care and prevention in the COVID era: a national survey of Ryan White providers. KFF. December 16, 2020. Available at: https://www.kff.org/hivaids/issue-brief/delivering-hiv-care-prevention-in-the-covid-era-a-national-survey-of-ryan-white-providers. Accessed April 7, 2025.
7. Sullivan PS, Woodyatt CR, Kouzouian O, et al. America's HIV epidemic analysis dashboard: protocol for a data resource to support Ending the HIV Epidemic in the United States. *JMIR Public*

Health Surveill. 2022;8(2):e33522. https://doi.org/10.2196/33522

8. Ryan White Clinics for 340B Access. Value of Ryan White providers and impacts associated with resource reduction. Available at: https://rwc340b.org/wp-content/uploads/2023/10/RWC340B-White-Paper-Value-of-Ryan-White-Providers.pdf. Accessed April 7, 2025.
9. Sullivan PS, Satcher Johnson A, Pembleton ES, et al. Epidemiology of HIV in the USA: epidemic burden, inequities, contexts, and responses. *Lancet.* 2021;397(10279):1095–1106. https://doi.org/10.1016/S0140-6736(21)00395-0
10. Rao A, Rucinski K, Jarrett BA, et al. Perceived interruptions to HIV prevention and treatment services associated with COVID-19 for gay, bisexual, and other men who have sex with men in 20 countries. *J Acquir Immune Defic Syndr.* 2021;87(1):644–651. https://doi.org/10.1097/qai.0000000000002620
11. Sweeney P, DiNenno EA, Flores SA, et al. HIV data to care—using public health data to improve HIV care and prevention. *J Acquir Immune Defic Syndr.* 2019;82(suppl 1):S1–S5. https://doi.org/10.1097/qai.0000000000002059
12. Dawson L. Cutting HIV prevention funding at CDC: what would it mean? KFF. March 19, 2025. Available at: https://www.kff.org/quick-take/cutting-hiv-prevention-funding-at-cdc-what-would-it-mean. Accessed May 8, 2025.

Hidden in Plain Sight: The Case for Disaggregated HIV Data and Tailored Interventions for African Immigrants

Olihe Okoro, PhD, MPH

ABOUT THE AUTHOR

Olihe Okoro is an associate professor of Social and Administrative Pharmacy at the University of Minnesota, College of Pharmacy, Duluth.

See also Aidoo-Frimpong et al., p. 1490.

Ongoing global efforts to end the HIV epidemic as a public health threat by 2030 aim to reduce HIV incidence and AIDS-related mortality and establish sustainability in HIV response thereafter.[1] The Ending the HIV Epidemic in the US (EHE) initiative is a strategic response that anticipates a reduction of HIV incidence by 90% or more by 2030—prevention of approximately 250 000 new infections.[2] The EHE initiative leverages four pillars of evidence-based strategies: diagnosis, treatment, prevention, and response.[2]

UNDERSTANDING AFRICAN IMMIGRANT HIV DISPARITIES

In the United States, HIV disparities persist. Washington, DC; San Juan, Puerto Rico; and 48 counties account for more than 50% of HIV diagnoses, with an additional seven states that are disparately burdened by HIV incidence in their rural areas.[2] In addition, there are racial disparities, with Black individuals being the most disproportionately affected. Blacks/African Americans accounted for 37% of new cases (2018–2022) while constituting 12% of the US population.[3] This racial/ethnic statistic is inclusive of native-born US Blacks, Afro-Caribbeans, and Black immigrants born in their African countries of origin.

In this issue of *AJPH*, Aidoo-Frimpong et al. (p. 1490) highlight the detriments of aggregating HIV data, given the differences in historical, economic, and sociocultural contexts, with distinct aspects that make unique contributions to HIV risk and outcomes for each group, respectively. The authors make a case for disaggregating HIV data to inform interventions targeting African immigrants who have higher HIV incidence rates compared with native-born Blacks.[4]

There are unique sociocultural and structural underlying causes of high HIV incidence among African immigrants.[5,6] The authors also note a key difference: heterosexual transmission as the prevalent mode of HIV transmission among African immigrants versus male-to-male in the general population. The differences in drivers of HIV risk and facilitators of effective engagement in HIV prevention and care are collectively the imperative for the disaggregation of HIV data by race/ethnicity. The authors further recommend considering "country of origin" and even more granular demographic data to accommodate the heterogeneity of cultures, languages, and diasporic experiences within this population.

Aidoo-Frimpong et al. also present data that demonstrate significant representation of African immigrants in the EHE's jurisdictions of high priority. Resources deployed to these areas and strategies employed are aligned with the broad racial/ethnic categorization of Black/African American that does not distinguish African immigrants as a priority population. The distinct historical backgrounds, socioeconomic context, cultural norms and values, linguistic factors, and underlying impact of structural inequities (e.g., postcolonial trauma, systemic racism, and immigration policies) necessitate tailored interventions that are responsive to their unique needs.

CULTURAL AND STRUCTURAL CONSIDERATIONS

The authors outline cultural and structural barriers to health care utilization among African immigrants. For further context, it is important to keep in mind preimmigration health care utilization experiences that often influence health care–seeking behaviors in diaspora. The African continent consists largely of developing countries with poorly resourced health care delivery systems where acute (and often emergent) care is typically the sole focus because of limited resources and workforce shortages.[7] Patient health care

AJPH September 2025, Vol. 115, No. 9

expenses are mostly out of pocket; hence, health care seeking is typically prompted by debilitating symptoms that significantly impede functioning. These economic realities that have shaped health care–seeking behaviors in African countries likely carry over after immigration, compounded by economic challenges that immigrants are commonly confronted with when settling in the United States. These factors contribute to the likelihood of late-stage diagnosis of conditions like HIV that do not immediately present with symptoms—hence, the emphasis on HIV testing for early detection.

Addressing HIV disparities requires mobilization for HIV testing. Even when testing is freely available and accessible, there are cultural beliefs and norms that pose barriers to uptake in the African immigrant population, as outlined by the authors. Community-engaged approaches (e.g., strategic partnerships with community-based organizations) and organizational cultural competence (e.g., a racially/ethnically representative health care workforce, medical information in patient's preferred language and format) become critical in addressing these barriers.

A key consideration in HIV intervention efforts is the communal identity that centers self as connected and integral to community—a core value in African cultures.[8] While a strength in most regards, communal identity may also be a deterrent to testing, for fear of alienation if HIV positive. However, the same value can be leveraged to increase uptake of testing by HIV education that centers community values and promotes community health. Increased HIV literacy can thus foster community support for individuals living with HIV and enhance acceptability of HIV testing, care, and preexposure prophylaxis (PrEP). The authors describe how community-engaged efforts, especially when championed by community and faith-based leaders, have demonstrated effectiveness in increasing uptake of health care–related services such as HIV testing.

HIV care must be culturally responsive and linguistically appropriate. Communication in African cultures is very nuanced and contextual—markedly different from the Western world. Provider–patient concordance in HIV care will be beneficial for communicating diagnostic findings, initiating antiretroviral therapy (ART), and providing adherence counseling. The inclusion of African immigrants living with HIV in health care encounters as trained peer navigators and educators, where possible, should also be considered.[9]

Written information in a patient's preferred language, as recommended by the authors, may not be adequate. There may be a need to provide audio-recorded instructions. African immigrants with low English proficiency, while adept in speaking their own language(s), are often unable to read it. Ordinarily, this would not pose a problem, as they can have someone else read the instructions to them. However, because of stigma, African immigrants living with HIV are less likely to have disclosed their status to others in their social network,[10] limiting who they can approach to read the instructions for them. With the ubiquitous use of technology, audio files detailing ART instructions will be beneficial for patients with low English proficiency. This approach should only augment continuing patient education and adherence counseling facilitated by certified medical interpreters.

COMMUNITY-RESPONSIVE APPROACHES TO HIV PREVENTION

Additional areas to leverage are advances in HIV PrEP and evolving public health roles of pharmacists, which both hold great potential, barring issues of access and affordability. Advantages associated with injectable PrEP include increased adherence, reduced frequency of health care visits, minimal disruption of work schedules, and mitigation of privacy concerns and attendant stigma within family and community settings. The challenge remains that African immigrants have thus far not been prioritized as a distinct group for targeted HIV prevention with injectable PrEP.

To ensure uptake, it will be important to establish points of care for PrEP within easy reach. An innovative approach would be to utilize community pharmacies that are already in community spaces and frequently used by African immigrants for health needs. In most African countries, pharmacies are the entry points to health care, with the public accessing care in community pharmacies more than any other health care service facility.[11] Community pharmacists can be trained and, under collaborative practice agreement, provide HIV services including testing, PrEP, and care. Pharmacy-based efforts implemented with cultural sensitivity have the potential to significantly increase HIV testing, PrEP uptake, and ART adherence, with improved outcomes in this priority population.

Critical to ongoing efforts, as advanced by Aidoo-Frimpong et al., are the disaggregation of HIV data, dedication of specific funds, and adoption of community-engaged approaches to adequately address the unique challenges and needs of African immigrants. In prioritizing this population, intervention efforts must take into account their historical, sociocultural, and economic contexts, adopting strategies that are culturally and structurally responsive to achieve the desired outcomes. AJPH

CORRESPONDENCE

Correspondence should be sent to Olihe Okoro, University of Minnesota, College of Pharmacy, Duluth, 235 Life Science, 1110 Kirby Dr, Duluth, MN 55812-3003 (e-mail: ookoro@d.umn.edu). Reprints can be ordered at https://ajph.org by clicking the "Reprints" link.

PUBLICATION INFORMATION

Full Citation: Okoro O. Hidden in plain sight: the case for disaggregated HIV data and tailored interventions for African immigrants. *Am J Public Health*. 2025;115(9):1357–1359.

Acceptance Date: May 27, 2025.

DOI: https://doi.org/10.2105/AJPH.2025.308206

ORCID iD:
Olihe Okoro https://orcid.org/0000-0002-1598-4415

CONFLICTS OF INTEREST

The author has no conflicts of interest to declare.

REFERENCES

1. UNAIDS. Global HIV target setting for 2030. 2025. Available at: https://www.unaids.org/sites/default/files/2025-05/20250328_recommended_2030_HIV_targets_livedocument_en_13_May_2025.pdf. Accessed May 19, 2025.
2. US Department of Health and Human Services. About Ending the HIV Epidemic in the US. 2025. Available at: https://www.hiv.gov/federal-response/ending-the-hiv-epidemic/overview. Accessed May 20, 2025.
3. Centers for Disease Control and Prevention. HIV surveillance supplemental report: estimated HIV incidence and prevalence in the United States, 2018–2022. 2024. Available at: https://stacks.cdc.gov/view/cdc/156513. Accessed May 20, 2025.
4. Kerani RP, Lugg A, Berzins B, et al. Post-migration HIV acquisition among African immigrants in the US. *J Immigr Minor Health*. 2022;24(6):1459–1468. https://doi.org/10.1007/s10903-022-01356-2
5. Okoro ON, Whitson SO. Sexual health, HIV care and pre-exposure prophylaxis in the African immigrant population: a needs assessment. *J Immigr Minor Health*. 2020;22(1):134–144. https://doi.org/10.1007/s10903-019-00873-x
6. Okoro ON, Whitson SO. HIV risk and barriers to care for African-born immigrant women: a sociocultural outlook. *Int J Womens Health*. 2017;9:421–429. https://doi.org/10.2147/IJWH.S129355
7. Oleribe OO, Momoh J, Uzochukwu BS, et al. Identifying key challenges facing healthcare systems in Africa and potential solutions. *Int J Gen Med*. 2019;12:395–403. https://doi.org/10.2147/IJGM.S223882
8. Ochieng'-Odhiambo F. African philosophy of communalism. In: Imafidon E, Tshivhase M, Freter B, eds. *Handbook of African Philosophy*. Cham, Switzerland: Springer; 2023: 13–30. https://doi.org/10.1007/978-3-031-25149-8_21
9. Krulic T, Brown G, Bourne A. A scoping review of peer navigation programs for people living with HIV: form, function and effects. *AIDS Behav*. 2022;26(12):4034–4054. https://doi.org/10.1007/s10461-022-03729-y
10. Koku EF. Social networks and stigma: the experiences of African immigrants living with HIV in the United States. *Soc Sci Med*. 2021;281:114103. https://doi.org/10.1016/j.socscimed.2021.114103
11. Makole TJ. How pharmacists can help tackle antimicrobial resistance in the African region. *PLOS Blog, Speaking of Medicine and Health*. July 7, 2023. Available at: https://speakingofmedicine.plos.org/2023/07/07/how-pharmacists-can-help-tackle-antimicrobial-resistance-in-the-african-region. Accessed May 20, 2025.

Food Is Medicine: Prioritizing Equitable Implementation

Matthew J. Landry, PhD, RDN, and Kelseanna Hollis-Hansen, PhD, MPH

ABOUT THE AUTHORS

Matthew J. Landry is with the Joe C. Wen School of Population & Public Health, University of California, Irvine. Kelseanna Hollis-Hansen is with the UT Southwestern Medical Center, O'Donnell School of Public Health, and the Harold C. Simmons Comprehensive Cancer Center, Dallas, TX.

The Food Is Medicine (FIM) movement encompasses health care and community-based interventions that use food and nutrition to prevent, manage, and treat diet-related health conditions, ranging from produce prescriptions to medically tailored meals.[1] While the movement's goals are well-intended and have attracted significant investment,[2] we describe potential pitfalls and opportunities for improvement[3] in the execution of the top three tiers of the FIM pyramid (i.e., healthy food prescriptions, medically tailored groceries, and medically tailored meals).[1] One concern is that some populations—specifically, people living with a lower income and those experiencing food insecurity—may be inadvertently overlooked because of a lack of health insurance or health care access. Rather than suggesting we abandon health care–based FIM delivery, which would deny access to millions who could benefit through existing insurance coverage, we propose a dual approach that strengthens health care–based implementation while developing complementary pathways for those currently excluded.

CHALLENGES IN IMPLEMENTATION AND ACCESS

Health insurance plays a pivotal role in facilitating access to interventions like FIM. Unfortunately, many people living with a lower income, experiencing food insecurity, or both also lack sufficient health insurance coverage. In 2024, approximately 8.2% of Americans—representing more than 27 million people—lacked health insurance coverage, while millions more were underinsured, meaning their out-of-pocket costs were high relative to their income despite having insurance.[4]

Paradoxically, these groups could benefit most from FIM, given the movement's focus on the preventive and therapeutic properties of a well-balanced diet. Their potential exclusion based on a lack of sufficient health insurance coverage could exacerbate existing health disparities and perpetuate a cycle of poor health outcomes. Counties with the highest rates of food insecurity often have higher uninsured rates. Families experiencing food insecurity have been found to have 20% greater total health care expenditures than food-secure families.[5] If FIM programs are primarily implemented through the medical system or by medical referral, they could inadvertently widen disparities.[6] Communities with better health care infrastructure might benefit more, while underserved areas lag behind.[7,8] These challenges should not lead us to abandon health care–and insurance-based FIM delivery but instead simultaneously strengthen health care–based implementation while developing robust alternative access pathways.

POLICY AND SYSTEMS-LEVEL SOLUTIONS

Bipartisan support for nutrition-based health interventions exists, as evidenced by the recent formation of the Make America Healthy Again Caucus and Commission,[9] which prioritize FIM initiatives. Existing federal nutrition programs demonstrate the viability and impact of food-based health interventions. For instance, the US Department of Agriculture's (USDA's) Special Supplemental Nutrition Program for Women, Infants, and Children (WIC) effectively functions as the nation's first medically tailored grocery program, providing targeted nutritional support for pregnant women, infants, and young children. WIC's success in reducing anemia, maternal and child mortality, and low birthweight births, while improving fruit and vegetable consumption and cognitive development, illustrates how nutrition programs can generate both health improvements and health care cost savings.[10]

It is important to acknowledge potential funding tensions between emerging FIM programs and established federal nutrition assistance programs. These legacy programs already serve populations at nutritional risk without requiring health insurance coverage. While FIM initiatives primarily access funding through different mechanisms—namely Medicaid and Medicare state waivers and the tax-exempt status of supporting nonprofit organizations—they may still compete for limited federal resources.

To harness the benefits of FIM for underresourced populations requires addressing the underlying disparities that hinder people from accessing adequate health care services. Policymakers must consider ways to expand health insurance coverage that specifically includes FIM programs.[11] This includes efforts to enroll eligible people in Medicaid and close coverage gaps in states that have not adopted Medicaid expansion and the creation of affordable insurance options for those who do not qualify for public assistance but cannot afford comprehensive coverage through their workplace or the Health Insurance Marketplace. These efforts could involve subsidies for FIM-inclusive plans or federal mandates to include FIM coverage in basic insurance packages (e.g., Medicaid, Medicare, Indian Health Service, and Veterans Affairs coverage, and inclusion in state-defined essential health benefits). While policy changes can expand insurance coverage for FIM, a comprehensive approach must look beyond these solutions alone.

COMMUNITY-BASED IMPLEMENTATION STRATEGIES

FIM programming is complementary to, and does not replace, broader population health and community-based initiatives. Investing in local community programs can provide organizations with funding required to address specific needs of people experiencing food insecurity without health insurance. Federally qualified health centers (FQHCs), which already serve many uninsured and underinsured patients and maintain strong community connections, could be ideal sites for implementing FIM programs that bridge health care and community delivery approaches. Recipe4Health exemplifies an evidence-based FIM program that brings together FQHCs, community health coaches, farmers, and researchers to deliver programming shown to improve produce consumption, non–high-density lipoprotein (HDL) cholesterol, and mental health symptoms.[12,13] This model could be effectively scaled up nationally, facilitated by Medicaid expansion, Section 1115 waivers (which allow states to expand services to cover programs and tools that address nonmedical drivers of health, including food insecurity), and funding to provide training and infrastructure support to FQHCs and communities to work together.

Another useful approach is exemplified by FeedMore WNY (Western New York) and the Central Texas Food Bank, which are two food assistance organizations that repurpose food donations into nutritious prepared meals. These organizations also offer workforce development programs that train community members in culinary skills and report high rates of job placement at the program's end. Multilevel programs like these can address several nonmedical drivers of health concurrently. Instead of divesting resources away from community organizations, insurers, health systems, and providers interested in implementing FIM should prioritize partnering with and financially supporting existing initiatives.

To systematically encourage these partnerships, federal funding agencies (e.g., USDA, National Institutes of Health, Centers for Disease Control and Prevention) could require community partnerships as a condition of FIM program and research funding, creating financial incentives for health systems to invest in these collaborations. However, many community organizations need substantial support to build the infrastructure required for health care system participation, such as billing systems, documentation protocols, and quality monitoring processes. Funding for capacity building should be included to ensure community partners can successfully provide services both through traditional community channels and within health care system partnerships.

CULTURAL RESPONSIVENESS AND PROGRAM DESIGN

A one-size-fits-all approach is inadequate for FIM, given the diverse needs and dietary preferences of different communities, and current FIM programs may not deliver benefits equitably if they are not aligned with participant preferences. To maximize impact, FIM programs must be culturally responsive. This involves engaging community members and incorporating local cultural norms, food preferences, and socioenvironmental landscapes.[14] Like any pharmaceutical or medical device intervention, adherence is necessary. If foods provided in FIM programs are not desirable or provided where and how people want to receive them, people will not adhere. Collaborating with community organizations and members to conduct formative research could inform strategies to improve FIM recruitment, adherence, fidelity, and retention. For example, understanding where and how community members would like to receive FIM programming (e.g., pick-up location, home delivery), as well as their preferred cuisines, meals, and food items, is useful information that could improve long-term success.

ENSURING LONG-TERM PROGRAM SUSTAINABILITY

Current evidence suggests promising cost-effectiveness for specific FIM interventions (medically tailored meals and produce prescriptions).[11] However, this evidence base is still developing.[11,15] Additional quasi-experimental, randomized, and simulation research is needed to fully understand the economic and health impacts of FIM programs relative to existing nutrition assistance approaches. Health equity should remain a fundamental goal of the FIM movement. However, the demonstrated cost–effectiveness or cost–savings benefits of FIM programs would provide further compelling rationale for their expansion.

The optimal duration of FIM programs also has yet to be determined.[15] FIM programs often come with substantial costs that make long-term implementation prohibitive, particularly for underinsured and uninsured populations. If programs are time-limited, understanding how to taper them in a way that empowers participants to sustain behavioral changes is valuable. A well-designed tapering process could utilize step-down models that gradually transition participants across the FIM intervention spectrum. For example, participants might move from medically tailored meals to medically tailored groceries, and then to produce prescriptions, rather than ending support abruptly. This approach, while simultaneously increasing education and skill-building activities, could help enhance the effectiveness of the program and, more importantly, engender people to continue making healthful dietary choices independently even after the programming ends. For people who are underresourced, this tapering phase might also include additional programmatic components that enhance self-efficacy and address root causes of social and economic disparities (e.g., food resource coaching, providing budget-friendly meal planning workshops, or food assistance navigation).

CONCLUSION

The top three tiers of the FIM pyramid hold promise in promoting health and preventing diet-related chronic diseases, but reach must extend beyond those with established health care access. FIM access should not necessarily drive insurance expansion, but, instead, given the reality of our current health care system, FIM implementation must pursue both health care–based and community-based pathways to maximize reach, impact, and sustainability. Complementary community-based programs must be simultaneously developed and supported. When these approaches work in synergy—with health care reimbursements allowing community organizations to strategically redirect other resources to serve the uninsured and underinsured—FIM can achieve broader reach while maintaining sustainability. AJPH

CORRESPONDENCE

Correspondence should be sent to Matthew Landry, 856 Health Sciences Rd, Suite 3800, Irvine, CA 92697 (e-mail: landrymj@hs.uci.edu). Reprints can be ordered at https://ajph.org by clicking the "Reprints" link.

PUBLICATION INFORMATION

Full Citation: Landry MJ, Hollis-Hansen K. Food Is Medicine: prioritizing equitable implementation. *Am J Public Health*. 2025;115(9):1360–1363.

Acceptance Date: April 1, 2025.

DOI: https://doi.org/10.2105/AJPH.2025.308147

ORCID iDs:

Matthew J. Landry https://orcid.org/0000-0003-2285-7702

Kelseanna Hollis-Hansen https://orcid.org/0000-0002-0243-2830

CONTRIBUTORS

Both authors contributed equally to the conceptualization, drafting, and revisions of the editorial. The authors share first authorship.

CONFLICTS OF INTEREST

The authors report no conflicts of interest.

REFERENCES

1. Mozaffarian D, Blanck HM, Garfield KM, Wassung A, Petersen R. A Food is Medicine approach to achieve nutrition security and improve health. *Nat Med.* 2022;28(11):2238–2240. https://doi.org/10.1038/s41591-022-02027-3
2. Mozaffarian D, Andrés JR, Cousin E, Frist WH, Glickman DR. The White House Conference on Hunger, Nutrition and Health is an opportunity for transformational change. *Nat Food.* 2022;3(8):561–563. https://doi.org/10.1038/s43016-022-00568-x
3. Moran AJ, Roberto CA. A "Food Is Medicine" approach to disease prevention: limitations and alternatives. *JAMA.* 2023;330(23):2243–2244. https://doi.org/10.1001/jama.2023.24472
4. Office of the Assistant Secretary for Planning and Evaluation. *National Uninsured Rate at 8.2 Percent in the First Quarter of 2024 (Issue Brief No. HP-2024-17).* August 2024. Available at: https://aspe.hhs.gov/reports/national-uninsured-rate-first-quarter-2024. Accessed September 29, 2024.
5. Palakshappa D, Garg A, Peltz A, Wong CA, Cholera R, Berkowitz SA. Food insecurity was associated with greater family health care expenditures in the US, 2016–17: study examines the relationship between food insecurity and family health care expenditures. *Health Aff (Millwood).* 2023;42(1):44–52. https://doi.org/10.1377/hlthaff.2022.00414
6. Ford J, Sowden S, Olivera J, et al. Transforming health systems to reduce health inequalities. *Future Healthc J.* 2021;8(2):e204–e209. https://doi.org/10.7861/fhj.2021-0018
7. Lorenc T, Petticrew M, Welch V, Tugwell P. What types of interventions generate inequalities? Evidence from systematic reviews. *J Epidemiol Community Health.* 2013;67(2):190–193. https://doi.org/10.1136/jech-2012-201257

8. McGowan V, Buckner S, Mead R, et al. Examining the effectiveness of place-based interventions to improve public health and reduce health inequalities: an umbrella review. *BMC Public Health.* 2021;21(1):1888–1817. https://doi.org/10.1186/s12889-021-11852-z
9. The White House. Establishing the President's Make America Healthy Again Commission. February 13, 2025. Available at: https://www.whitehouse.gov/presidential-actions/2025/02/establishing-the-presidents-make-america-healthy-again-commission. Accessed January 17, 2025.
10. Caulfield LE, Bennett WL, Gross SM, et al. Maternal and child outcomes associated with the Special Supplemental Nutrition Program for Women, Infants, and Children (WIC). *Comparative Effectiveness Review.* April 2022;253. Agency for Healthcare Research and Quality. Report No.: 22-EHC019. Available at: https://www.ncbi.nlm.nih.gov/books/NBK579797. Accessed April 14, 2025.
11. Mozaffarian D, Aspry KE, Garfield K, ACC Prevention of Cardiovascular Disease Section Nutrition and Lifestyle Working Group and Disparities of Care Working Group, et al. "Food Is Medicine" strategies for nutrition security and cardiometabolic health equity: JACC state-of-the-art review. *J Am Coll Cardiol.* 2024;83(8):843–864. https://doi.org/10.1016/j.jacc.2023.12.023
12. Rosas LG, Chen S, Xiao L, et al. The effectiveness of Recipe4Health: a quasi-experimental evaluation. *Am J Prev Med.* 2024;68(2):377–390. https://doi.org/10.1016/j.amepre.2024.10.020
13. Thompson-Lastad A, Chiu DT, Ruvalcaba D, et al. Food as medicine, community as medicine: mental health effects of a social care intervention. *Health Serv Res.* 2025:e14431. https://doi.org/10.1111/1475-6773.14431
14. Landry MJ, Alford S, Singleton CR. Call for evaluation and reporting of the equity impact of culturally responsive nutrition interventions. *J Nutr Educ Behav.* 2022;54(2):97–98. https://doi.org/10.1016/j.jneb.2021.12.006
15. Volpp KG, Berkowitz SA, Sharma SV, American Heart Association, et al. Food is medicine: a presidential advisory from the American Heart Association. *Circulation.* 2023;148(18):1417–1439. https://doi.org/10.1161/cir.0000000000001182

School Nurses: An Upstream Investment for Achieving Menstrual Equity

Sadie Bergen, PhD, Erin D. Maughan, RN, PhD, MS, Molly Secor, RN, PhD, MS, Karen E. Johnson, RN, PhD, Robin Cogan, RN, MEd, NCSN, and Marni Sommer, RN, DrPH

ABOUT THE AUTHORS

Sadie Bergen is with Department of Medical Humanities and Ethics, Columbia University Irving Medical Center, New York, NY. Erin D. Maughan is with the George Mason University College of Public Health, Fairfax, VA. Molly Secor is with Montana State University Mark and Robyn Jones College of Nursing, Bozeman. Karen E. Johnson is with the University of Texas at Austin School of Nursing. Robin Cogan is with Rutgers School of Nursing and is a school nurse in the Camden City School District, NJ. Marni Sommer is with the Department of Sociomedical Sciences at Columbia University Mailman School of Public Health, New York, NY.

AJPH September 2025, Vol. 115, No. 9

Menstrual equity has emerged as an important public health issue, with a growing political coalition advocating improved access to menstrual products. In the September 2024 issue of *AJPH*, we described and analyzed the history of the role of school nurses in the US education system in relation to menstruation and its intersection with population health.[1] In recognition of School Nurse Day and Menstrual Hygiene Day—both of which took place in the month of May—we build on this work and make the case for honoring both occasions through investments in school nurse staffing and training as essential public health investments toward menstrual equity. Adequately staffed and trained, school nurses—who are often the only health care providers in the school setting—can fulfill the full scope of their role in menstrual health education and care, from identifying potential menstrual health disorders to dispelling the stigma still attached to menstruation.

Much attention has been placed on menstrual product access in schools. Recent policies have focused on tackling menstrual inequity in schools by guaranteeing menstrual products to students.[2,3] These policies, and the school nurse–led advocacy they have inspired, represent critical first steps toward menstrual equity. Building on these efforts, a comprehensive, justice-oriented approach to menstrual equity requires investing in school nurses as a vital aspect of the public health infrastructure that underlies school health. School nurses are crucial to achieving menstrual equity at multiple levels, as they can work both downstream on education and care in the school setting and upstream, crafting and advocating policies that create supportive environments for menstruating students.

A MULTILEVEL APPROACH TO MENSTRUAL EQUITY IN SCHOOLS

School nurses have an important role to play at the individual, downstream level in educating students, providing clinical menstruation-related care, and improving access to menstrual products in their schools. Nurses are well-positioned to provide information to students about the menstrual cycle and how to differentiate normal from abnormal experiences, and can refer to more advanced clinical care if needed. At the institutional level, the role of the school nurse touches upon every facet of the menstrual health needs of students and can ensure that they have access and appropriate referrals to care for intense bleeding, pain, or other menstrual disorders; access to menstrual products; and freedom from menstruation-related stigma and discrimination.[4,5] School nurses can also provide menstrual health education, both informally while delivering care and more formally in a health classroom. To provide proof of concept, grant funds should be made available to support systematic examinations of innovative school nursing and menstrual health programs that reflect this broad scope of practice.

However, recommendations that school nurses be more involved in school menstrual health neglect the deeper issue of a lack of public health infrastructure in schools in the form of adequate school nurse staffing. In spite of evidence connecting school nurse staffing and school nurse–led interventions with positive health and educational outcomes, models for school nurse staffing vary considerably across the United States, with about one third of schools lacking a full-time school nurse and significant disparities in school nurse employment between urban and rural schools.[6,7]

To combat this inequity, school districts must follow National Association of School Nurses' (NASN's) and American Academy of Pediatrics' (AAP's) recommendations to ensure that schools are adequately staffed with school nurses and that nurses are supported in practicing to their full scope of practice (including providing both supportive menstrual health–related clinical care and education to individual students, groups, or populations, and influencing policy).[8,9] School nurses are the natural public health workforce members who, given adequate capacity, can help contribute to the multipronged approach needed to expand effective strategies for achieving menstrual equity for students who menstruate.

Of course, safe school nurse staffing rests on adequate funding, which is far from assured in a country where school nurses must compete for space in education budgets. Funds for school nurses come from a range of sources, including local departments of education, health departments, grants, and Medicaid.[6] Funding adequate school nursing is an investment in a foundational public health aspect of the US education system. Thus, it is worth exploring creative solutions with public health agencies and lawmakers at the state and local level to stabilize funding shortages by braiding together funding sources, including local property or education taxes, direct state funding, and Medicaid reimbursements.[10,11]

The NASN School Nursing Practice Framework[12] clearly articulates a more comprehensive scope of practice that extends beyond the nurse's office and the classroom to improving population health more broadly within learning environments. This expansive framework suggests school nurses can serve as leaders in multidisciplinary spaces to address health equity and the social determinants of health. To that end, school nurses can address structural and cultural barriers to menstrual equity by developing policies to combat menstrual stigma through health education and the creation of school environments supportive of discussing and managing menstruation.[4] Upstream actions that take place at the structural, environmental, and policy level will be most effective in creating sustainable improvements, especially if they are developed in collaboration with other stakeholders, such as public health agencies, which can be a partner in policy development and a source of educational resources.

PRIORITIZING MENSTRUAL HEALTH EDUCATION

To be full participants in the menstrual equity movement, nurses need financial and educational resources to support training and curriculum development on menstrual education, as well as training on how to advocate policies that challenge ongoing stigma and delivery of menstrual education. School nurses can ensure that the movement evolves beyond product access to include comprehensive, research-informed educational standards that serve to reduce menstrual stigma and inequity.

There has been a historical silence surrounding menstrual health in mainstream American culture.[13,14] Despite the reality that menstruation is a natural physiology of the body, the topic too often remains taboo. School nurses can counter this stigma by advocating to ensure menstrual health education is prioritized, to promote healthy maturation and lifelong positive health outcomes. The negative health and well-being impacts of menstrual disorders, such as severe cramping, irregular periods, and endometriosis, should be addressed through education to improve health literacy and, ultimately, health outcomes across the life course.

To achieve true menstrual equity, we must incorporate menstrual health education into schools and even further upstream to ensure state standards for education and supportive environments. The latter would include policies that enable students to use bathrooms as needed, with menstrual products and discreet disposal in toilet stalls, sensitized and educated teachers and peers, and importantly, yet often overlooked, investing in adequate school nurse staffing, to alleviate young people's menstrual discomforts and support the provision of menstrual health learning.

The provision of menstrual education is uneven and inconsistent across the United States.[15–18] It is imperative that states and school districts incorporate research-informed, age-appropriate educational materials into their educational standards. At a minimum, this includes having adolescent-centered texts in school libraries and health classes, such as *A Girl's Guide to Puberty and Periods*, a book for 9- to 12-year-olds developed through participatory research with girls across the country to reflect their experiences and concerns, and the AAP's *You-ology: A Puberty Guide for EVERY Body*, an educational resource that is inclusive of transgender and nonbinary students who menstruate.[19,20] School nurses, if provided with office space for students to seek out rest and pain relief from menstrual-related symptoms, could also stock these or other puberty-content books in their waiting areas, serving to both educate and support students.

In May 2023, the District of Columbia released new standards for menstrual health education in schools, demonstrating strong leadership in moving beyond simply providing period products. These standards were developed with feedback from school health educators and health care providers.[21] In explaining the new mandated menstrual health curriculum, the state superintendent said that new standards like these should "reflect the dynamism of education, that reflect what students should be learning in age-appropriate ways, and for us to grapple with topics and frame them out to our community in service of our children."[22] This legislative effort can serve as a model for other states, and may indicate a shift toward a more expansive vision of menstrual equity that also includes education and clinical support.[23] School nurses, if sufficiently staffed and trained, could serve an important role in both providing this education to students and as a resource for additional menstrual health questions that arise.

State standards for menstrual health education help strengthen an upstream approach, as do other approaches such as the April 2024 Title IX legislation, which incorporates menstruation-related discrimination into the definition of sex discrimination, explicitly highlighting the deleterious impact of menstruation-related stigma in the school environment.[24(p1248)] Supportive environments for students include policies that allow students to access the bathroom as needed, the availability of clinical care, and spaces to rest for those experiencing intense menstrual pain or disorders.

UPSTREAM ADVOCACY AND COLLABORATION

School nurses are well poised to lead these efforts with the support of professional health and education organizations. The NASN should work with other equity-minded organizations (e.g., American Public Health Association, American Nurses Association) to develop advocacy and policy statements to support nurses in this work. The NASN's ongoing advocacy for school nurse staffing and comprehensive health education in schools, as well as its engagement with the issue of period poverty, provide a firm basis for the organization to take a strong stance on the interrelated issue of menstrual health equity in schools. The NASN has a platform to draw strong connections between the need for investment in school nursing and menstrual equity as mutually reinforcing aims.

School nurses have clearly been engaged in the work of menstruation education and menstrual care for more than a century.[1] What is missing from the landscape of menstrual health education in the United States is not school nurses' involvement but, rather, sufficient school nurse staffing, a commitment to supporting this work through dedicated curricular resources, pedagogical training, and paid effort that reflects their full scope of practice beyond the school nurses' office. For our country to achieve menstrual equity, we must look expansively at the upstream barriers to menstrual health and invest in the menstrual health education and school nursing infrastructure needed to support student health. AJPH

CORRESPONDENCE

Correspondence should be sent to Sadie Bergen, PhD, Department of Medical Humanities and Ethics, Columbia University Irving Medical Center, 630 W 168th St, PH15E-1525, New York, NY 10032 (e-mail: srb2161@columbia.edu). Reprints can be ordered at https://www.ajph.org by clicking the "Reprints" link.

PUBLICATION INFORMATION

Full Citation: Bergen S, Maughan ED, Secor M, Johnson KE, Cogan R, Sommer M. School nurses: an upstream investment for achieving menstrual equity. *Am J Public Health*. 2025;115(9):1364–1367.

Acceptance Date: April 25, 2025.

DOI: https://doi.org/10.2105/AJPH.2025.308183

ORCID iDs:

Sadie Bergen https://orcid.org/0000-0002-3939-7645

Molly Secor https://orcid.org/0000-0002-2360-4080

Marni Sommer https://orcid.org/0000-0001-7442-9270

CONTRIBUTORS

All authors contributed equally to this editorial.

CONFLICTS OF INTEREST

The authors report no conflicts of interest.

REFERENCES

1. Bergen S, Maughan ED, Johnson KE, Cogan R, Secor M, Sommer M. The history of US menstrual health, school nurses, and the future of menstrual health equity. *Am J Public Health*. 2024;114(9):903–908. https://doi.org/10.2105/AJPH.2024.307705
2. Pereda D, Mahuna S. Period poverty: how school nurses can support menstrual health and hygiene. *NASN Sch Nurse*. 2025;40(1):38–45. https://doi.org/10.1177/1942602X241268540
3. Francis L, Meraj S, Konduru D, Perrin EM. An update on state legislation supporting menstrual hygiene products in US schools: a legislative review, policy report, and recommendations for school nurse leadership. *J Sch Nurs*. 2023;39(6): 536–541. https://doi.org/10.1177/105984052 21131012
4. LeBlanc SS. School nurses and menstrual communication: destigmatizing the stigma among adolescents. *Womens Health (Lond)*. 2024;20: 17455057241247793. https://doi.org/10.1177/17455057241247793
5. Hennegan J, Winkler IT, Bobel C, et al. Menstrual health: a definition for policy, practice, and research. *Sex Reprod Health Matters*. 2021;29(1): 1911618–1911638. https://doi.org/10.1080/26410397.2021.1911618
6. Willgerodt MA, Tanner A, McCabe E, Jameson B, Brock D. Public school nurses in the United States: National School Nurse Workforce Study 2.0. *J Sch Nurs*. 2024;40(5):468–481. https://doi.org/10.1177/10598405241253565

7. Best NC, Oppewal S, Travers D. Exploring school nurse interventions and health and education outcomes: an integrative review. *J Sch Nurs.* 2018;34(1):14–27. https://doi.org/10.1177/1059840517745359
8. National Association of School Nurses. Position statement: School nurse workload: staffing for safe care. Available at: https://www.nasn.org/nasn-resources/professional-practice-documents/position-statements/ps-workload. Accessed April 17, 2025.
9. Holmes BW, Sheetz A, Allison M, Council on School Health, et al. Role of the school nurse in providing school health services. *Pediatrics.* 2016;137(6):e20160852. https://doi.org/10.1542/peds.2016-0852
10. McCabe EM, Jameson BE, Maughan ED. Nursing partnerships are crucial for bridging education and public health. *Public Health Nurs.* 2025;42(2):992–995. https://doi.org/10.1111/phn.13527
11. The Center for School Health Innovation & Quality. *School Nurse Staffing and Funding in Northeastern Pennsylvania.* 2023. Available at: https://mosestaylorfoundation.org/wp-content/uploads/2023/11/School-Nurse-Executive-Summary-Rep-1123-update-2.pdf. Accessed April 20, 2025.
12. Tanner A, Griffin R, Stanislo KJ, et al. A contemporary framework update for today's school nursing landscape: introducing the School Nursing Practice Framework. *NASN School Nurse.* 2024;39(3):140–147. https://doi.org/10.1177/1942602X241241092
13. Brumberg JJ. "Something happens to girls": menarche and the emergence of the modern American hygienic imperative. *J Hist Sex.* 1993;4(1):99–127.
14. Freidenfelds L. *The Modern Period: Menstruation in Twentieth-Century America.* Baltimore, MD: Johns Hopkins University Press; 2009.
15. Sebert Kuhlmann A, Hunter E, Wall LL, Boyko M, Teni MT. State standards for menstrual hygiene education in US schools. *J Sch Health.* 2022;92(4):418–420. https://doi.org/10.1111/josh.13135
16. Crockett LJ, Deardorff J, Johnson M, Irwin C, Petersen AC. Puberty education in a global context: knowledge gaps, opportunities, and implications for policy. *J Res Adolesc.* 2019;29(1):177–195. https://doi.org/10.1111/jora.12452
17. Weresh MH. Deconstructing the curse: menstrual education and the stigma of shame. *Women's Rts L Rep.* 2021;43(1/2):1–42.
18. Bhoda K, Burgoa S, Zerrouki Y, et al. Examining menstrual health and hygiene educational initiatives for American middle and high school menstruating students: a scoping review. *J Pediatr Adolesc Gynecol.* 2024;37(5):465–476. https://doi.org/10.1016/j.jpag.2024.06.004
19. Sommer M, Hagstrom C, Schmitt M, Gruer C. *A Girl's Guide to Puberty and Periods.* New York, NY: Ingram-Spark; 2022.
20. Holmes M, Hutchison T, Lowe K. *You-Ology: A Puberty Guide for Every Body.* Itasca, IL: American Academy of Pediatrics; 2022. https://doi.org/10.1542/9781610025720
21. Mitchell AS. Menstrual health education standards draft process. DC Office of the State Superintendent of Education. 2023. Available at: https://osse.dc.gov/page/menstrual-health-education-standards-draft-process. Accessed April 17, 2025.
22. Lumpkin L. D.C. kids will get new menstrual health education next year, a first in the country. *Washington Post.* June 21, 2023. Available at: https://www.washingtonpost.com/education/2023/06/21/dc-schools-menstrual-health-standards-curriculum. Accessed April 20, 2025.
23. Office of the State Superintendent of Education. DC menstrual health education standards. 2023. Available at: https://osse.dc.gov/sites/default/files/dc/sites/osse/page_content/attachments/WNS_MenstrualEduStandards_051923.pdf. Accessed November 15, 2023.
24. Department of Education Office for Civil Rights. Nondiscrimination on the Basis of Sex in Education Programs or Activities Receiving Federal Financial Assistance. 2024. Available at: https://www.federalregister.gov/documents/2024/04/29/2024-07915/nondiscrimination-on-the-basis-of-sex-in-education-programs-or-activities-receiving-federal. Accessed May 21, 2025.

The FDA Acts to Eliminate Asbestos in Talc: A Half-Century–Long Struggle

Gerald Markowitz, PhD, and David Rosner, PhD, MPH

ABOUT THE AUTHORS

Gerald Markowitz is with John Jay College and the Graduate Center, CUNY, New York, NY. David Rosner is with the Mailman School of Public Health, Columbia University, New York, NY.

Since the 1920s, reports of talc deposits being contaminated with asbestos have appeared,[1] and beginning in the 1930s, there have been reports that asbestos in talc deposits caused disease among miners and millers. In the 1960s, researchers discovered the presence of asbestos-contaminated cosmetic talc, and in the early 1970s, the Food and Drug Administration (FDA) sought to regulate various products, including baby and body powders, to eliminate the threat of asbestos-related diseases in consumers.[2] The industry successfully stymied these efforts for more than half a century. Finally, in late December 2024, the FDA issued a new proposed regulation on testing for asbestos in talc that, if adopted, would be a tremendous public health victory, assuring consumers that talc is asbestos-free. But, because of the new administration's deregulatory efforts and continued resistance from some talc manufacturers, it will take continued public pressure for this proposal to have any chance of being adopted.

BACKGROUND

In 2019, we published "'Nondetected': The Politics of Measurement of Asbestos in Talc, 1971–1976," in this journal's pages. The article traced the efforts of the members of the Cosmetic, Toiletry, and Fragrance Association (CTFA), the trade association for the manufacturers of cosmetic talc in the United States, to stifle a stringent federal regulation and to promote self-regulation and specifically their own methodology for the detection of asbestos in talc. A struggle between federal officials and the cosmetics industry ensued. This struggle was to control the methodology of measurement of asbestos that emerged in light of the discovery in the late 1960s by Lewis Cralley of the National Institute of Occupational Safety and Health (NIOSH), and early 1970s by Seymour Lewin of New York University,[3] of the presence of asbestos fibers in a variety of off-the-shelf talcum powder products. This issue of whether asbestos was present in these products had taken on significant importance in light of the passage of the Occupational Safety and Health Act of 1970 and the establishment of NIOSH, which had concluded in 1972 that there was no safe level of exposure to asbestos that would guarantee protection against cancer. Our article documented that the cosmetic industry was successful in getting the government to accept the industry's own method for determining the presence of asbestos in talc, the "J4-1" methodology, that the industry privately acknowledged was not "accurate, reliable and practical" [emphasis in the original].[4] Yet this voluntary methodology has been used by the industry until the present day.

In the absence of any public pressure, the industry engaged in prolonged scientific, political, and legal battles to stymie the FDA's efforts at regulation. In an internal memo to G. Mennen, president of the Mennen Company, the company's representative to the CTFA told of the discussions he had had with the acting head of the Department of Cosmetics at the FDA in which it became clear that the "FDA is reluctant to take any legal action in any problems with industry. They have neither the money nor manpower to pursue matters so that they will have airtight cases in scientific matters."[5]

In recent years, the inadequacy of the voluntary standard has been made apparent by the growing recognition that the asbestos in talc is responsible for ovarian cancer among women and mesothelioma deaths among men and women who have been exposed to talc in their homes or on the job. Lawsuits have proliferated that have held a variety of talc manufacturers liable for billions of dollars. In 2023, Johnson & Johnson, one of the nation's largest cosmetics and health–related companies, filed for bankruptcy for the second time, proposing a $6.5 billion fund to settle more than 40 000 lawsuits over allegations that asbestos in their talc products caused ovarian and other cancers.[6] These lawsuits and the public attention they have garnered have transformed the social and political environment, finally leading the Congress and the FDA to act on behalf of consumers rather than industry. This history played a role in these cases. Juries learned of what the cosmetic industry knew as early as the 1970s of the potential contamination with asbestos of baby powders, body powders, cosmetics, and other personal care products and the companies' efforts to stymie regulation and held the companies accountable.

In 2022, Congress passed new legislation that required the FDA to establish "standardized testing methods for detecting and identifying asbestos in talc-containing cosmetic products"[7] to address the failure of the FDA to do so in the 1970s. The FDA itself had recently tested for asbestos in 52 products, confirming its presence in nine, including body powders, face powders, eye shadows, blushes, bronzers, and face makeup. As a result, in December 2024, it issued a proposed federal rule to ensure that talc had no asbestos in it. It has now been placed in the *Federal Register* and is awaiting comments before the FDA finally decides whether to adopt it. In their proposed rule, the FDA specifically criticized that "CTFA method J4-1" for having "long-recognized short comings in specificity and sensitivity compared with electron microscopy-based methods," which they were proposing to use under the new federal rule. [7]

One shortcoming of the industry's longstanding method they noted was that it was "intended only to test for asbestiform amphibole minerals and not for chrysotile asbestos. On review of the protocol, we did not find it to have any utility to test for chrysotile or detect chrysotile with adequate sensitivity."[8] Another shortcoming of their methodology was that the x-ray diffraction analysis they depended upon had a nominal limit of detection of amphibole of 0.5% by weight. They noted that this was a major problem because that meant, as we identified in our earlier article, there could be "billions of asbestos fibers per gram of talc."[7]

Even in the 1970s, the CTFA understood that their method would not assure the absence of asbestos from their products, and, therefore, they adopted terminology to specifically obscure this fact. Rather than guarantee to the public and regulators that their cosmetic talc was free of any asbestos, they adopted ambiguous language; the asbestos was "nondetected" by their testing as a way to assuage public anxiety over the possible dangers of baby and body powders and cosmetics, which were the profit centers for member companies. They had adopted a methodology that could not identify small amounts of asbestos and then hid behind imprecision. One representative to the CTFA said privately that using an insensitive method would allow manufacturers to claim that asbestos had not been detected but was not right to do as it might lead to "serious breaks in communication between the buyer and the seller," who might falsely believe that powder they were using on their babies and themselves was truly asbestos-free.[9] In sum, the J4-1 method "absent any additional microscopic analysis, can lead to false-negative results for talc containing chrysotile asbestos at any level or amphibole asbestos at levels below 0.5%."[7]

CONTEMPORARY DISCUSSION

The FDA has acted on the information that NIOSH had developed 50 years ago: "asbestos at any level in talc-containing cosmetic products may render these products injurious to users."[7] Their new standard, relying on their microscopy methods, could detect one asbestos particle, whether chrysotile or amphibole, per 0.1 microgram of talc. This means that any asbestos detected in even the smallest measures of talc essentially assures the banning of tainted talc in the consumer market.[7]

In the 1970s, when the FDA first tried to establish methodologies that would largely eliminate asbestos from cosmetics, the industry, through the CTFA, mobilized an army of lobbyists, public relations personnel, and scientists to fight their efforts. In the intervening decades, as attention to the problem of asbestos-tainted cosmetic products has grown, industry itself began to wean itself from talc, leading to a weakening of opposition to regulation. Finally, as a result of lawsuits, growing public awareness of the role of industry in creating environmental dangers, and the resulting consumer activism around asbestos, Congress and the FDA began to act. But the public health community should be aware that the new administration may undo this victory as part of its antiregulatory agenda. Consumer advocates and the public health community may need to mobilize once again to counter what may be enormous pressure from a wounded, if weakened, industry.

We are proud that the history of this issue that we published 6 years ago has been noted in the proposed rule by the FDA. It is a tribute to *AJPH* on its 115th anniversary that its leadership understands the importance of history as well. For more than half a century, *AJPH* has supported historical research with some of the most prominent historians in the country represented in its pages because its editors have understood that history is more than just nostalgia and can provide context, insights, and forewarning of vital issues in public health to come as well as practical help in educating the public. Since the eminent historian George Rosen first began the "Public Health: Then and Now" column, some of the most prominent historians in the country have taken over its helm, including Barbara Rosenkrantz, Ted Brown, and, today, Marian Moser Jones. They all have understood the importance of history for public health practitioners, and we are proud to have been published in the *AJPH* pages. As we face an uncertain future where we see powerful forces gathering in the political arena to deny the reality of climate change and the usefulness of vaccination, and efforts to limit Medicare and Medicaid funding, unbiased scientific research, and support of universities through limitations of indirect costs and institutional support, looking back is proscriptive, not nostalgia. AJPH

CORRESPONDENCE

Correspondence should be sent to David Rosner, Department of Sociomedical Sciences, Mailman School of Public Health, 722 W 168th St, Room 935, New York, NY 10032 (e-mail: dr289@cumc.columbia.edu). Reprints can be ordered at https://ajph.org by clicking the "Reprints" link.

PUBLICATION INFORMATION

Full Citation: Markowitz G, Rosner D. The FDA acts to eliminate asbestos in talc: a half-century–long struggle. *Am J Public Health*. 2025;115(9):1368–1370.

Acceptance Date: April 27, 2025.

DOI: https://doi.org/10.2105/AJPH.2025.308180

ORCID iD:
David Rosner https://orcid.org/0000-0002-0127-6987

CONTRIBUTORS

The authors contributed equally to all aspects of this work.

CONFLICTS OF INTEREST

The authors have participated as expert witnesses in asbestos–talc lawsuits on behalf of plaintiffs.

REFERENCES

1. Newland D, Cushing H. *New York State Museum Bulletin: Geology of the Gouverneur Quadrangle.* Albany, NY: The State University of New York. 1925;259:81.
2. Dreessen W. Effects of certain silicate dusts on the lungs. *J Industrial Hyg.* 1933;15:66–78.
3. Rosner D, Markowitz G, Chowkwanyun M. 'Nondetected': the politics of measurement of asbestos in talc, 1971–1976. *Am J Public Health.* 2019;109(7):969–974. https://doi.org/10.2105/AJPH.2019.305085
4. CFTA Task Force on Round Robin Testing of Consumer Talcum Products for Asbestiform Amphibole Minerals. Minutes, May 17, 1977. Available at: https://cdn.toxicdocs.org/Mx/MxRLgx1X6b9z7D59NGKKenwV/MxRLgx1X6b9z7D59NGKKenwV.pdf. Accessed February 25, 2019.
5. H.P. Schwartz to G. Mennen, et al., January 18th, 1973. Available at: https://cdn.toxicdocs.org/zo/zoQjL87oyxvjNQ5D6LY3znQE0/zoQjL87oyxvjNQ5D6LY3znQE0.pdf. Accessed June 8, 2025.
6. Edward Moreno J. Johnson & Johnson proposes $6.5 billion in new talc settlement offer. *New York Times.* May 1, 2024: B4. Available at: https://www.nytimes.com/2024/05/01/business/johnson-johnson-talc-settlement.html. Accessed June 8, 2025.
7. Food and Drug Administration. Testing Methods for Detecting and Identifying Asbestos in Talc-Containing Cosmetic Products. 21 CFR Part 730, [Docket No. FDA-,2023-N-4225] RIN 0910-AI82. Available at: https://www.federalregister.gov/documents/2024/12/27/2024-30544/testing-methods-for-detecting-and-identifying-asbestos-in-talc-containing-cosmetic-products. Accessed June 8, 2025.
8. US Food and Drug Administration. Executive Summary, Preliminary Recommendations on Testing Methods for Asbestos in Talc and Consumer Products Containing Talc. January 6, 2020. Available at: https://www.fda.gov/media/134005/download. Accessed June 8, 2025.
9. Harold D. Stanley to R.E. Norwood, "Minutes of the CTFA Talc Subcommittee meeting," July 2, 1976. Available at: https://cdn.toxicdocs.org/zb/zb02zbxnMgamYQzjoGgY1DMb6/zb02zbxnMgamYQzjoGgY1DMb6.pdf. Accessed June 8, 2025.

Is Your Home Making You Sick? Health Risks Associated With Black Mold in Air Vents

Osmari B. Novoa, MPH

ABOUT THE AUTHOR

Osmari B. Novoa is a doctoral candidate and graduate research assistant at Robert Stempel College of Public Health and Social Work in the Department of Health Promotion and Disease Prevention, Florida International University, Miami.

Black mold is a type of fungus that may cause the immune system to react, typically appearing dark green or black.[1–3] While there are various types of black mold, the term usually refers to *Stachybotrys chartarum*. It is a highly toxic species of mold and can often manifest as dark spots, which may appear scattered or, in more severe cases, clustered and densely packed.[2,3]

Air vents provide an ideal environment for black mold growth, posing a particular challenge for homeowners, as spores can easily circulate throughout the home via the heating, ventilation, and air conditioning (HVAC) system.[3,4] The majority of mold issues can be visually identified; however, mold that is hidden inside vents or ducts may not be noticeable until individuals begin to experience symptoms often associated with mold.[3] When air vents are not cleaned regularly, accumulated dust can serve as an ideal food source for mold growth.[3,4] In addition, neglected air ducts with leaks or other structural issues can create damp conditions that promote black mold proliferation.[3,4]

Exposure to black mold can trigger immune responses, particularly in individuals with allergies to mold spores or microbial volatile organic compounds (mVOCs).[1,2] Common symptoms include sneezing, coughing, nasal congestion, and eye irritation.[1,2] Even individuals without known allergies may experience mild symptoms from exposure to mVOCs.[1,2] While black mold exposure is unlikely to cause severe illness in most healthy individuals, it can exacerbate asthma symptoms.[1,2]

Specifically, individuals with mold allergies may react to any type of mold, and despite its reputation, black mold is not inherently more dangerous than other mold species.[1,2] Symptoms caused by black mold can be treated with various treatments such as nasal irrigation, antihistamine medications, nasal corticosteroids, decongestants, leukotriene receptor antagonists, and asthma inhalers.[1,2] In addition, people with weakened immune systems—whether because of immunodeficiency disorders or medications that suppress immune function—may be more vulnerable to developing fungal infections (mycoses) in the respiratory tract or other parts of the body.[1,2]

The US Environmental Protection Agency (EPA) outlines a straightforward step-by-step process for treating and removing black mold.[5] The most important step in mold control is addressing moisture, as mold cannot thrive without it. Mold on hard surfaces can be scrubbed off using soap or detergent and water, but the area must be thoroughly dried afterward.[5] Any sources of moisture, such as plumbing leaks or water damage, should be addressed as soon as possible. Mold-infested porous or absorbent materials, like ceiling tiles or carpet, should be discarded, as they are often difficult to clean completely.[5]

The EPA advises wearing proper protective gear when cleaning areas affected by mold.[6] To reduce exposure to

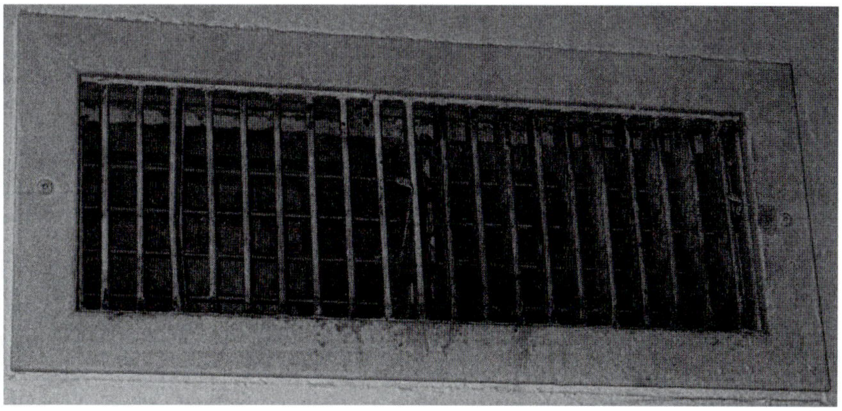

FIGURE 1— Black Mold Growing in a Central Heating and Cooling Intake Duct

AJPH September 2025, Vol. 115, No. 9

airborne mold particles, using an N95 respirator may be necessary. Long gloves that reach the middle of the forearm are recommended to protect the skin, and direct contact with mold or contaminated items should be avoided.[6] In addition, safety goggles without ventilation holes are suggested to protect the eyes from mold spores and debris.[6]

There are several effective strategies to help prevent mold from spreading within a home. Humidity levels should be maintained at or below 50% throughout the day.[7] Using an air conditioner or dehumidifier can assist in keeping humidity under control.[7] Proper airflow is essential, so ensuring that indoor air circulates freely is important.[7] Exhaust fans that vent to the outside should be used in kitchens and bathrooms, and clothes dryers should also vent outdoors. Bathrooms should be cleaned regularly with mold-killing products.[7] Carpets and upholstered furniture that have been soaked and cannot be dried quickly should be removed or replaced. Finally, carpet should be avoided in moisture-prone areas such as bathrooms and basements.[7] Implementing these measures can help maintain healthy indoor air quality and reduce potential asthma triggers and mild symptoms caused by mold exposure. AJPH

CORRESPONDENCE

Correspondence should be sent to Osmari B. Novoa, 8200 Cleary Blvd Apt 2012, Plantation, FL 33324 (e-mail: onovoa@fiu.edu). Reprints can be ordered at https://www.ajph.org by clicking the "Reprints" link.

PUBLICATION INFORMATION

Full Citation: Novoa OB. Is your home making you sick? Health risks associated with black mold in air vents. *Am J Public Health*. 2025;115(9):1371–1372.

Acceptance Date: April 22, 2025.

DOI: https://doi.org/10.2105/AJPH.2025.308178

ORCID iD:
Osmari B. Novoa https://orcid.org/0000-0002-8240-9090

CONFLICTS OF INTEREST

The author does not have any potential or actual conflicts of interest from funding or affiliation-related activities to report.

HUMAN PARTICIPANT PROTECTION

Institutional review board approval was not required because of the use of publicly available information regarding black mold exposure.

REFERENCES

1. Cleveland Clinic. Black mold exposure: Symptoms, risks & treatment. January 7, 2025. Available at: https://my.clevelandclinic.org/health/diseases/24862-black-mold. Accessed March 16, 2025.
2. Caceres V. Black mold illness: Symptoms and treatment. *US News and World Report*. January 10, 2025. Available at: https://health.usnews.com/wellness/articles/black-mold-illness. Accessed March 16, 2025.
3. Green Orchard Group. Signs of black mold in air vents & should you be worried? December 9, 2022. Available at: https://greenorchardgroup.com/signs-of-black-mold-in-air-vents. Accessed March 16, 2025.
4. Green VJ. Mold in air vents: harmful, or nothing to worry about? ABC Home & Commercial Services. February 19, 2020. Available at: https://blog.abchomeandcommercial.com/mold-in-air-vents-harmful. Accessed April 15, 2025.
5. Environmental Protection Agency. What are the basic mold cleanup steps? August 20, 2019. Available at: https://19january2021snapshot.epa.gov/mold/what-are-basic-mold-cleanup-steps_.html. Accessed April 15, 2025.
6. Environmental Protection Agency. A brief guide to mold, moisture and your home. November 23, 2020. Available at: https://19january2021snapshot.epa.gov/mold/brief-guide-mold-moisture-and-your-home_.html#tab-4. Accessed April 15, 2025.
7. Centers for Disease Control and Prevention. Mold. Available at: https://www.cdc.gov/mold-health/about/index.html. Accessed April 15, 2025.

Classical Syndromes in Occupational Medicine: Dimethylaminopropionitrile

Excerpted from: James P. Keogh, "Classical Syndromes in Occupational Medicine: Dimethylaminopropionitrile," *American Journal of Industrial Medicine* 4, no. 3 (1983): 479–481, https://doi.org/10.1002/ajim.4700040309

Dimethylaminopropionitrile (DMAPN), used as a catalyst in the manufacture of polyurethane, caused outbreaks of urinary retention, impotence, and peripheral neuropathy in exposed workers in 1978. Symptomatic workers at two plants were studied, leading to the recognition of DMAPN as the cause of these problems and to the restriction of its use in the United States.

In March of 1978, a 28-year-old man presented at Baltimore City Hospitals with a history of several months of difficult voiding. He noted decreased urge to void and decreased stream. He reported he could go for many hours without the sensation of a full bladder and then have to empty his bladder by manual pressure on his suprapubic area. Most interestingly, he reported that four of five coworkers on his shift at a local polyurethane plant were similarly affected.

Inquiries to the Maryland Occupational Safety and Health Administration (MOSH) revealed that the agency had conducted an inspection of the plant some months before, but only toluene diisocyanate (TDI) had been sampled for. The symptoms of urinary retention had apparently not been focused on by the inspectors, who had no medical training. Ventilation and skin protection were virtually nonexistent, and workers also complained of respiratory difficulties, skin irritation, blurring vision, nausea, and a host of other symptoms.

By happy coincidence, MOSH had just hired its first nurse epidemiologist, who immediately began a systematic investigation of symptoms. Many of the colors and catalysts were purchased as trade name products and MOSH began to contact manufacturers to compile all of the ingredients. MOSH learned from coworkers about a former employee, who was among the first to be affected, who was hospitalized for evaluation at The Johns Hopkins Hospital.

This patient, the most severely affected from this plant, had begun to have urinary retention in the fall. He had been seen by a urologist, who documented a neurogenic bladder, and was subsequently seen by a neurologist who, at that time, found no other abnormalities on examination and proposed no further work-up. The patient said he told both physicians that coworkers were similarly affected, but that no interest was shown.

Several months later at a family gathering he told his story to a distant relative who was a family physician in a rural area of Pennsylvania. This doctor immediately recognized the nature and importance of the problem, initiated the referral that brought the patient to Hopkins, and wrote to Federal OSHA. After traveling through bureaucratic channels, the letter arrived a few weeks later, after the investigation was well underway.

The staff at Hopkins had questioned the plant management, who claimed that no other workers were ill, producing some initial confusion. When it was realized that other physicians might be seeing affected workers and be misled by such denials, the need for an organized multidisciplinary investigation became apparent. A meeting of MOSH staff and physicians from Baltimore City and Hopkins hospital was arranged.

In planning the clinical investigation, The Maryland group contacted colleagues across the country and discussed their suspicions about DMAPN. None had heard of a similar syndrome, but many offered suggestions as to how to proceed. Two days later, Dr. David Wegman at Harvard called back to report similar symptoms at a polyurethane plant in Massachusetts. Workers there had gone to an emergency room as a group, demanding appropriate treatment. When health authorities contacted Dr. Wegman, he was quickly able to identify that the offending catalyst was the only chemical besides TDI that the Maryland and Massachusetts plants had in common.

The epidemic in Massachusetts had also been going on for some months: OSHA inspectors there had also been called in; because of their lack of medical background, they thought the symptoms might be from epidemic urinary infections and spent some time looking for bacterial contamination of drinking water and beverages.

With the recognition of a previously undescribed syndrome of urinary retention occurring in two polyurethane plants sharing one common chemical exposure, preventive action was taken.

Dr. Eula Bingham, then Assistant Secretary of Labor and Director of OSHA,[1] sent OSHA inspectors into every polyurethane plant that had purchased the catalyst to warn management and workers. The manufacturer voluntarily withdrew the product.

Once use of the catalyst ceased, no new cases occurred in the plant and symptoms began to abate in most workers. AJPH

James P. Keogh, MD: Advocate for Bringing Environmental Medicine to Worker Protection

Eric Persaud, DrPH, MEA

In 1978, a 28-year-old man who was experiencing bladder issues saw a physician at Baltimore City Hospital in Maryland. The physician was James (Jim) P. Keogh. The man, who had to empty his bladder by manually pressing on his lower abdomen, worked at a local polyurethane plant. He was among four of the five people on his shift at the plant experiencing similar health issues. Other workers suffered from impotence, insomnia, irritability, muscle weakness, and paresthesia—a tingling or numbness in a body part.

Dimethylaminopropionitrile (DMAPN) had been introduced as a catalyst in the manufacturing of polyurethane at the worker's plant. The patient had been moving and stacking foam containing this substance and it had touched his skin. He also inhaled DMAPN while processing it when it was a warm foam and it was still giving off vapors.

Previous inspections of the plant never sampled for DMAPN and did not focus on the urinary retention symptoms of the workers. Plant management did not provide the workers with skin protection or proper ventilation.

The patient had been experiencing urinary retention symptoms for months before he was seen by Keogh. Yet, when the patient had seen his urologist and neurologist when he first exhibited symptoms, neither doctor offered follow-up and both brushed off the patient's remark that other co-workers were experiencing similar symptoms. It was not until months later at a family gathering that a distant relative, who was also a family doctor, heard of his health issues and recognized the problem and possible connections to work.

Keogh and his colleagues then notified the federal Occupational Safety and Health Administration, or OSHA, and referred the patient to the Johns Hopkins Hospital. When the staff realized physicians were being misled by plant management denials that other workers were ill, they arranged a meeting with the Baltimore City Hospital. At this meeting, epidemiologists and physicians, including Keogh, helped identify DMAPN as the likely source of the epidemic. Days later, a group of workers from another polyurethane plant, this time in Massachusetts, went to an emergency room demanding treatment.

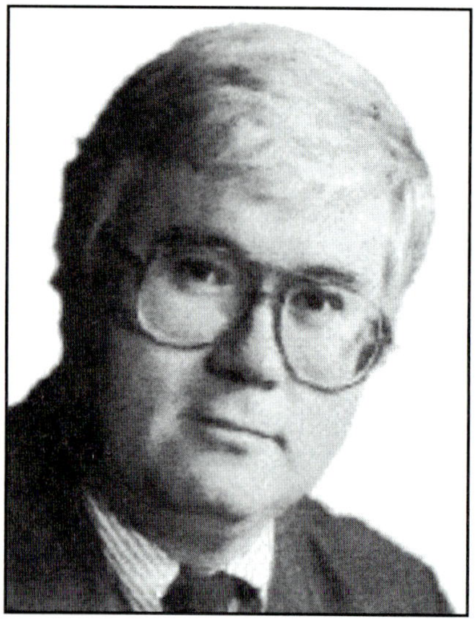

FIGURE 1— James P. Keogh, MD (1949–1999)

Source. Julie Tisdale-Pardi, "Recognizing Exemplary Science and Service." Available at: https://blogs.cdc.gov/niosh-science-blog/2021/05/20/awards (accessed June 6, 2025).

This epidemic in Massachusetts was not new; it had been ongoing for months, and OSHA inspectors believed the illness originated from bacterial contamination. Keogh again spearheaded studies and determined that DMAPN, indeed, had caused the urinary retention epidemic.

Eula Bingham, director of OSHA (1977–1981), was able to take action and had inspectors go to all polyurethane plants that used DMAPN and alert the workers and management. The manufacturers withdrew the product, and the plant stopped using the catalyst containing DMAPN. No new cases emerged, and the epidemic was ended through Keogh's efforts.

It was through Keogh's leadership that everyone was pulled together to address workers who had been exposed at a polyurethane manufacturing plant and were experiencing difficulty urinating.[1,2] This example of the importance of practitioners listening to patients and their perspectives underscores James P. Keogh's mission to champion occupational health and safety.

Born in 1949 in Washington, DC, James P. Keogh graduated from Johns Hopkins University in 1970 and from the University of Maryland School of Medicine in 1974.[3] He trained at Baltimore City Hospitals, where he eventually founded and directed the occupational and environmental health program.

In the late 1960s, during residency, Keogh worked in a nitroglycerin plant that produced explosives and medicinals (Debra S. Wertheimer, oral communication, March 24, 2025).[4] He worked as an unpaid intern under Anthony Mazzocchi, a prominent labor leader of the Oil, Chemical and Atomic Workers International Union. Keogh was the first doctor to intern for Mazzocchi, volunteering his services for the plant in Pennsylvania. The local union reported that the workers at the plant were dying of heart attacks, but only on the weekends. Keogh discovered that the workers were being exposed to nitroglycerin during the work week, reducing their blood pressure. When the weekend came and the workers were off shift, their blood pressure skyrocketed back up and caused heart attacks. Keogh witnessed some workers adding nitroglycerin to the brims of their hats on Fridays so that they were exposed over the weekend to reduce the risk of a heart attack. The workers were aware nitroglycerin could induce heart disease; however, the plant management did not recognize or act on the risk.[5] This experience played a central role in Keogh's life by highlighting the importance of listening to workers.

Keogh's work was far reaching. He worked to address the rights of those who developed lung cancer from asbestos exposure, first noting the high occurrence while reviewing the retirement benefits of United Steelworkers Local 2610.[3] His ability to recognize that these workers were being injured with the manufacturer's knowledge led him to set up medical screenings.

Other major aspects of Keogh's career include addressing the health effects of depleted uranium among Gulf War veterans and performing studies on repetitive strain injuries related to work.[6,7] Keogh's work played a pivotal role in the inclusion of construction workers in the occupational safety and health lead standard in Maryland.[7,8] His activism contributed to improved working conditions, decreased illnesses, and legal compensation for victims. Known for standing up for workers, he famously quipped, "If you poison your boss a little bit each day it's called murder; if your boss poisons you a little each day it's called a Threshold Limit Value."[3]

Keogh passed away in June 1999 at the age of 49 from gallbladder cancer.[9] Even when in the hospital, he mentored medical students, encouraging them to ask about patients' work history and to advocate for workers' rights (Debra S. Wertheimer, oral communication, March 24, 2025). This was a time when few primary care physicians were knowledgeable about occupational and environmental health. "Physicians may treat an illness without realizing its environmental cause" and "there isn't too much else out there" said Keogh in 1996 about how physicians were treating symptoms without focusing on the causes and the need for curricula to address this gap.[10] Yet, Keogh, an inaugural recipient of awards by the National Institute of Environmental Health Sciences to address environmental and occupational medical curricula in 1990, continuously worked to innovate and improve the training and education of students.[11] From the use of videos in curriculum,[12] including worker participation in the production of occupational health education materials,[13] to small-group, problem-based learning,[11] Keogh was on the forefront of occupational health and safety training and education. A steward of active mentorship, Keogh once said, "We found that students can learn technical content and problem-solving skills by participating in an active learning experience. . . . This approach helps with the curricular goal of creating lifelong learners."[11(p150–151)] His goal was not just to train physicians but to educate them "enough to play a positive role in the community."[10]

Keogh's legacy lives on in the empowerment and education of advocates, including having the National Institute of Occupational Safety and Health's Outstanding Service award named in his honor.[8] The American Public Health Association's (APHA's) Occupational Health and Safety section has a memorial scholarship dedicated to James P. Keogh that funds and supports students and workers to participate in the annual APHA conference.[14] Keogh was posthumously awarded the APHA Occupational Health and Safety Alice Hamilton lifetime achievement award for a career dedicated to improving workers' lives. Remembered not just as a physician and advocate for public health but also as an educator and mentor, this continued legacy of training future generations truly encapsulates Keogh's legacy of being an outspoken advocate for the rights of workers. AJPH

ABOUT THE AUTHOR

Eric Persaud is a member of the Occupational Health and Safety Section of the American Public Health Association.

CORRESPONDENCE

Correspondence should be sent to Eric Persaud, 109-03 103 Ave, Queens, NY, 11419 (e-mail: epersau01@gmail.com). Reprints can be ordered at http://www.ajph.org by clicking the "Reprints" link.

PUBLICATION INFORMATION

Full Citation: Persaud E. James P. Keogh, MD: advocate for bringing environmental medicine to worker protection. *Am J Public Health*. 2025; 115(9):1373–1376.

Acceptance Date: June 6, 2025.

DOI: https://doi.org/10.2105/AJPH.2025.308215

ORCID iD:

Eric Persaud https://orcid.org/0000-0003-4577-7975

ACKNOWLEDGMENTS

The author thanks Jim's wife of 23 years, Debra S. Wertheimer, MD, for her loving review and support.

CONFLICTS OF INTEREST

The author has no conflicts of interest to disclose.

ENDNOTES

1. James P Keogh, "Classical Syndromes in Occupational Medicine. Dimethylaminopropionitrile," *American Journal of Industrial Medicine* 4, no. 3 (1983): 479–489. https://doi.org/10.1002/ajim.4700040309
2. James P. Keogh, Alan Pestronk, Debra Wertheimer, and R. Moreland, "An Epidemic of Urinary Retention Caused by Dimethylaminopropionitrile," *JAMA* 243, no. 8 (1980): 746–749. https://doi.org/10.1001/jama.1980.03300340022013
3. Baltimore Sun, "James P. Keogh, 49, Doctor Who Exposed Occupational Hazards," June 17, 1999. Available at: https://www.baltimoresun.com/1999/06/17/james-p-keogh-49-doctor-who-exposed-occupational-hazards (accessed March 7, 2025).
4. Les Leopold, *The Man Who Hated Work and Loved Labor: The Life and Times of Tony Mazzocchi* (White River Junction, VT: Chelsea Green Publishing, 2007).
5. James P. Keogh, "Nitroglycerin Induced Heart Disease," *Journal of Occupational Medicine* 21, no. 3 (1979): 153.
6. Melissa A. McDiarmid, James P. Keogh, Frank J. Hooper, et al. "Health Effects of Depleted Uranium on Exposed Gulf War Veterans," *Environmental Research* 82, no. 2 (2000): 168–180. https://doi.org/10.1006/enrs.1999.4012
7. James P. Keogh, Iman Nuwayhid, Janice L. Gordon, and Patricia W. Gucer. "The Impact of Occupational Injury on Injured Worker and Family: Outcomes of Upper Extremity Cumulative Trauma Disorders in Maryland Workers," *American Journal of Industrial Medicine* 38, no. 5 (2000): 498–506. https://doi.org/10.1002/1097-0274(200011)38:5<498::AID-AJIM2>3.0.CO;2-I
8. Julie Tisdale-Pardi, "Recognizing Exemplary Science and Service." Available at: https://blogs.cdc.gov/niosh-science-blog/2021/05/20/awards (accessed March 9, 2025).
9. Maryland Medical Alumni, "In Memorium." Available at: https://www.medicalalumni.org/bulletin/fall1999/memorium.html (accessed March 9, 2025).
10. J. Wakefield, "Healing Environmental Harm: Is There a Doctor in the House?" *Environmental Health Perspectives* 104, no. 2 (1996): 150–153. https://doi.org/10.1289/ehp.96104150
11. "Training Doctors in Environmental and Occupational Medicine," *Environmental Health Perspectives* 102, no. 2 (1994): 150–151. https://doi.org/10.1289/ehp.102-1567206
12. James P. Keogh and Janie Gordon, "Using Video to Bring Patients Into the Curriculum," *Journal of Occupational and Environmental Medicine* 38, no. 4 (1996): 418. https://doi.org/10.1097/00043764-199604000-00029
13. Debra L. Roter, Rima E. Rudd, James Keogh, and Betty Robinson. "Worker Produced Health Education Material for the Construction Trades," *International Quarterly of Community Health Education* 7, no. 2 (1986): 109–121. https://doi.org/10.2190/fjpl-n1rh-829q-pqrj
14. American Public Health Association, "Occupational Health and Safety Section Awards." Available at: https://www.apha.org/apha-communities/member-sections/occupational-health-and-safety/awards (accessed April 1, 2025).

Adolescents' Mental Health: Disparities, Prevention Strategies, and Future Directions

Tanya Telfair LeBlanc, PhD, MS, Jihong Liu, ScD, Hua He, PhD, and Michelle Livings, PhD, MPH

ABOUT THE AUTHORS

All authors are AJPH *associate editors. Jihong Liu is with the Department of Epidemiology and Biostatistics, University of South Carolina, Columbia. Hua He is with the Department of Epidemiology and the Department of Biostatistics and Data Science, Tulane University, New Orleans, LA. Michelle Livings is with the Department of Health Sciences, Rutgers University, Camden, NJ.*

See also Adolescent Mental Health, pp. 1379–1453.

Adolescence can be a challenging stage of life. Although most adolescents have reached a degree of social and emotional maturity by 16 years, their brains are still developing, and they often lack the life experiences and judgment needed to make the best choices for their lives. Adolescence is also the period in which a number of potential dangers become important to consider, including sensation seeking, risk-taking behaviors, and negative peer influence. How children experience adolescence has changed as social and family organization structures have yielded to emerging economic pressures, making the transition to adulthood more difficult. Today's adolescents face a range of contemporary challenges, including academic pressure, exposure to violence (e.g., mass killings in schools, violence against racialized minorities), the burden of adult responsibilities in families, and pervasive access to technology and social media (which may include bigoted, violent, and sexualized content). Many also struggle with social isolation and diminished opportunities to build effective and appropriate social skills. Challenges that adolescents encounter are not distributed equally across racial, socioeconomic, and geographic groups.

The COVID-19 pandemic further exacerbated these alarming trends. According to a 2021 report from the Centers for Disease Control and Prevention, more than 4 in 10 (42%) high school students felt persistently sad or hopeless. Nearly one third (29%) experienced poor mental health, more than one in five (22%) seriously considered attempting suicide, and 1 in 10 (10%) attempted suicide (http://bit.ly/44rsXfS).

The collection of seven articles in this issue of *AJPH* represents the culmination of a year-long search for research, programmatic, or editorial contributions focusing on adolescent mental health.

RESEARCH ARTICLES

In a groundbreaking study titled "Authenticity, Racial Discrimination, Depression, and Suicidal Ideation Among Young Black Men, United States, 2024" (p. 1417), Boyd et al. explored a concept called "authenticity," defined as "the perception that one's behavior is self-authored, internally motivated, and aligned with how individuals view themselves." Authenticity may work as a buffer between racial discrimination and depressive symptoms and suicidal ideation. Therefore, it is a protective factor for mental health among Black/African American males aged 18 to 24 years.

Jackson et al., in "Persistent Sadness, Violence, and Bullying and Associations With Screen Time Among New York City Public High School Students, 2021" (p. 1397), analyzed data from the New York City Youth Risk Behavior Survey, a school-based health and behavior assessment administered among a diverse sample of public school students in grades 9 through 12. Persistent feelings of hopelessness and sadness in relation to violence-related experiences, in-school bullying, and cyberbullying were associated with emotional distress for both male and female students. Elevated screen time was associated with a higher prevalence of sadness and hopelessness only among female students.

To examine associations between adolescent dating violence and suicide planning among girls and differences by race/ethnicity, Sharpless et al. (p. 1388), in "Adolescent Dating Violence and Suicide Planning Among Girls in US High Schools: An Intracategorical Intersectional Analysis by Race and Ethnicity," used data from the 2021 Youth Risk Behavior Survey, a cross-sectional, nationally representative study of 9th through 12th grade adolescents from US high schools (n = 3886). Any form of adolescent dating violence increased the odds of suicide planning among girls, with stronger impacts for Latina girls experiencing sexual adolescent dating violence.

Ssewamala et al., in "Cost-Effectiveness of an Economic Empowerment and Family Intervention on Mental Health Among School-Going Adolescent Girls in Uganda, 2017–2022" (p. 1408), conducted a cost-effectiveness study of a combination intervention designed to reduce sexual risk-taking and improve mental health among disadvantaged adolescent girls aged 14 to 17 years in southern Uganda, where new HIV infections are highly concentrated among individuals aged 15 to 24 years. The three-arm, randomized controlled trial compared the effectiveness of (1) a combination intervention that included a savings-led economic empowerment program (using youth development accounts) and a family strengthening approach (multiple family group), (2) youth development accounts alone, and (3) the standard health and sex education (usual care). The combination intervention led to a statistically significant improvement in mental health outcomes (i.e., depressive symptoms, hopelessness, self-concept) at both 12 and 24 months into the intervention, relative to usual care. It was also more cost-effective than the other approaches.

Komro et al., in "Primary Prevention of Drug Overdoses in Rural Low-Resource and Tribal Communities: A Cluster Randomized Trial" (p. 1508), examined the effectiveness of an intervention designed with input from tribal behavioral health experts. The program targeted rural and Native American high school students aged 16 to 18 years in northeastern Oklahoma, with the goal of reducing substance use among adolescents. The intervention was shown to be effective in reducing the escalation of various forms of substance use, including alcohol use, binge drinking, cannabis use, and prescription opioid misuse.

OPINIONS AND PRACTICE

Tucker et al., in "Sibling Aggression and Abuse: Invisible and Widespread Public Health Problems" (p. 1383), highlight complex dynamics and close, intense relationships in families, which may mask bullying and abuse patterns among siblings in a household, causing physical or emotional harm to the recipient child. The authors suggest that sibling aggression and abuse measures should be included in the Adverse Childhood Experiences inventory, which practitioners use to assess family trauma and decision-making regarding follow-up care.

Mulkey et al., in "Wellness Coaching in a Summer Internship Program to Address the Mental Health Pandemic Among College Students, 2022–2023" (p. 1379), describe the integration of a mental health support and wellness component into a 10-week public health career summer internship program for students aged 18 to 24 years. This enhancement was developed in response to recent emerging mental health concerns observed during the previous program implementation. The added mental health support and wellness component included coaching, workshops, consultation, and access to other resources, which are all aimed at reducing depression and anxiety among internship participants.

Importantly, some of the studies presented in this special section highlight sex disparities in adolescents' experiences, which is well supported by research, including findings from the Pew Research Center's recent report (https://bit.ly/4lOeH6u). We hope to see continued investigations that shed light on the chasm between boys and girls, which appears to be widening in education and career outcomes, aspirations, and even "worldviews" that may contribute to mental health impairment. In addition, we encourage further exploration into the deeper origins of adolescent mental illness, such as issues of family resources, composition, organization, fluidity, relationships, and trauma, similar to those suggested by Tucker et al. in this special section. Looking further upstream, we acknowledge that mental health challenges in adolescence often have roots in economic and social challenges experienced in early childhood. Ensuring that families with younger children receive the support required for a stable and nurturing environment may be a critical factor in preventing long-term mental health problems. AJPH

CORRESPONDENCE

Correspondence should be sent to Tanya Telfair LeBlanc, associate editor with the *American Journal of Public Health*, 800 I St, NW, Washington, DC 20001 (e-mail: ttantelfair@gmail.com). Reprints can be ordered at https://www.ajph.org by clicking the "Reprints" link.

PUBLICATION INFORMATION

Full Citation: LeBlanc TT, Liu J, He H, Livings M. Adolescents' mental health: disparities, prevention strategies, and future directions. *Am J Public Health*. 2025;115(9):1377–1378.

Acceptance Date: June 21, 2025.

DOI: https://doi.org/10.2105/AJPH.2025.308235

ORCID iDs:

Jihong Liu https://orcid.org/0000-0001-8685-3036

Michelle Livings https://orcid.org/0000-0002-8529-1614

CONTRIBUTORS

T. T. LeBlanc wrote the editorial. J. Liu, H. He, and M. Livings reviewed the text. All authors participated in the editorial processes for the special section.

ACKNOWLEDGMENTS

We heartfully thank Alfredo Morabia for his collegial leadership and the opportunity to advance the science of adolescent mental health in a special section.

CONFLICTS OF INTEREST

The authors have no conflicts of interest to declare.

Wellness Coaching in a Summer Internship Program to Address the Mental Health Pandemic Among College Students, 2022–2023

Sadé Mulkey, DSW, MPH, LMSW, Christopher Knaub, MSGH, Mishelle Rodriguez, PhD, Dana Thomas, MPH, Hallie Williams, Mariya Bahrenburg, and Paul J. Fleming, PhD, MPH

See also Adolescent Mental Health, pp. 1377–1453.

In this article, we describe and present evaluation data for an innovative initiative and approach that integrate a wellness program into a summer pathway program for underrepresented undergraduate students in public health to address the students' mental health needs. This collaborative partnership and integrated wellness approach provide opportunities for summer programs at academic institutions to creatively address the needs of the students they serve. (*Am J Public Health*. 2025;115(9):1379–1382. https://doi.org/10.2105/AJPH.2025.308014)

AJPH September 2025, Vol. 115, No. 9

Current undergraduate students will become the future public health workforce, and it is vital to support their positive mental health as part of their professional development.

INTERVENTION AND IMPLEMENTATION

Funded by the Centers for Disease Control and Prevention, the Future Public Health Leaders Program (FPHLP) at the University of Michigan is a 10-week summer public health program designed to increase underrepresented college students' awareness of and interest in public health careers. Several years ago, FPHLP identified growing concerns regarding the mental health of the students that paralleled national trends on college campuses, including increases in mental health issues, distress related to the COVID-19 pandemic and societal-level trauma (e.g., school shootings, deaths caused by police brutality), and other identity- and achievement-related difficulties (e.g., imposter syndrome, burnout).

Students attending summer programs outside their home institution are considered guests and often cannot access their host or home institutions' medical and behavioral health services. To address the increasing mental health needs of summer students and bridge gaps in access to services, FPHLP developed programming aimed at fostering students' mental health growth and development.

In 2020, FPHLP hired a mental health counseling and consulting organization (Collaborative ChangeMakers) to design and implement a wellness program tailored to FPHLP's needs. The program aimed to (1) train FPHLP staff and partners to handle mental health concerns, (2) provide students with positive experiences related to mental health, (3) reduce stigma and isolation associated with mental health issues, (4) help students understand the importance of mental health in all aspects of life and professional development, and (5) equip students with knowledge and skills to manage mental health challenges and enhance their personal and professional effectiveness.

In 2021, FPHLP integrated the wellness program into its 10-week curriculum. The program consists of several components, as follows (Box 1).

1. Wellness coaching: Collaborative ChangeMakers staff members offer confidential, individual coaching sessions that address students' goals and concerns through support and problem solving. These sessions equip students with awareness, knowledge, and skills to address their mental health needs and meet their goals (Box 2).
2. Small-group wellness workshops: These psychoeducational, interactive, and experiential workshops

BOX 1— Wellness Coaching Intervention Design

Intervention Type	Details
Individual sessions	• One on one • Optional • Self-initiated
Group sessions	• Small groups/ cluster meetings • Mandatory
Wellness video library	• Preestablished online modules • Self-paced • Recommended
Ongoing consultation	• Staff consultation and support as needed

allow students to practice skills, apply concepts, and relate to and learn from each other to reduce mental health stigma and increase social support. The small groups (eight people) promote personal sharing. Students suggest workshop topics (e.g., stress and burnout, imposter syndrome, perfectionism, and boundaries).

3. Wellness video library: This library provides 18 videos on current mental health and professional wellness topics for self-paced learning. Each topic includes activities for reflection and practice.
4. Ongoing consultation: FPHLP staff and partners receive ongoing consultation to address emerging student concerns. On-site and on-call mental health professionals promptly address acute distress, offer mediation, and consult on interpersonal and group dynamics among students.

PLACE, TIME, AND PERSONS

FPHLP participants are college-aged students or emerging adults (18–24 years old) readying themselves for graduate programs and careers in public health within a rigorous summer program. As noted, FPHLP exists within the University of Michigan, a highly competitive, predominantly White institution. FPHLP participants have diverse lived experiences from across the United States and its territories. The wellness program was launched with these factors in mind, grounded in a sociocultural and developmental lens that addresses different socioeconomic backgrounds, intersecting social identities, and experiences of varying levels of systemic oppression.

PURPOSE

Undergraduates represent the future public health workforce. Building their coping and resilience skills to address their own emergent mental health needs is critical for robust, responsive, and effective public health institutions. The percentages of undergraduate students who meet the criteria for major depression, overall depression, and anxiety disorder have increased dramatically in the past 10 years.[1] However, in 2024, only 46% of respondents who screened positive for depression or anxiety received counseling or therapy.[1]

In addition, students of color are more likely to experience severe symptoms of depression, anxiety, and suicidal ideation than their non-Hispanic White counterparts.[2] Summer programs such as FPHLP that are designed to support and prepare underrepresented students for public health work are uniquely positioned to address mental health and normalize caring for one's mental health as part of professional development. This advanced preparation assists them in developing positive and healthy habits that ready them for their future careers in public health. Since COVID-19, 56% of public health workers have reported at least one symptom of posttraumatic stress disorder, and one in five employees rate their mental health as poor or fair.[3] Equipping students with awareness, knowledge, and skills to navigate mental health challenges builds their readiness for the workforce, and academic institutions and summer programs can facilitate this process. Taking a proactive, preventive approach is essential.[4]

The demand for student mental health resources is rising, but traditional systems—focused on therapy and medication—are overwhelmed and lack sufficient resources.[5,6] To address this gap, wellness coaching provides a student-centered approach that establishes individual goals achieved through self-accountability under the guidance of a trained professional.[7] A pilot project at a large urban university showed that students who participated

BOX 2— Wellness Coaching Process

Wellness Coaching Steps	Specific Tasks
Step 1: define goal(s)	Make sure goals are clear and right sized
Step 2: explore	Understand person, context, and contributing factors
Step 3: inform	Equip with knowledge related to goals
Step 4: establish strategies	Equip with tools and plan of action
Step 5: refine and maintain	Check progress, identify obstacles, and adjust plan
Step 6: conclude	Review progress and provide resources for further development

in wellness coaching had increased motivation, confidence, and ability to overcome barriers in their academic pursuits.[8] Findings were similar for FPHLP programs implemented in the summers of 2022 and 2023.

EVALUATION

In 2022, 38.6% of the 43 enrolled students received 36 sessions of individual coaching throughout the summer program, and, in 2023, 27.5% of the 29 students enrolled requested individual services (representing 11 sessions). Students who sought individual coaching sessions expressed mental health challenges in areas consistent with national college student data: anxiety, stress, and depression.[9] In a 2022 precoaching survey of 17 students, 80% indicated that they had experienced some level of trauma.

Thirty-eight percent of students self-identified as having a preexisting mental health diagnosis, and 61% stated that they had eating concerns. Fifty-five percent of students reported significant symptoms of depression on the Depression, Anxiety, and Stress Scales-21, with 45% reporting moderate to extremely severe symptoms. Sixty percent (60%) reported symptoms of anxiety (with 55% reporting moderate to extremely severe symptoms), and 65% reported symptoms of stress (with 30% reporting moderate to severe symptoms). These data suggest that there are significant mental health needs among our student population.

All students participated in small group sessions, and 93% of responses to the 2022 feedback survey indicated that students were highly or moderately satisfied with small group discussions. Eighty-nine percent of respondents reported that small group discussions helped them feel less alone or isolated in dealing with stressors or difficulties, and 86% reported that they learned practical skills to help them cope with stress and improve their well-being.

In 2023, more group sessions were integrated into the curriculum to address students' time constraints in attending individual sessions. This change increased the benefit of programming for all students. Ninety-six percent of 2023 respondents expressed satisfaction with small group discussion sessions, 92% indicated that small group discussions helped them feel less alone or isolated in dealing with stressors or difficulties, and 80% reported that they learned practical skills to help them cope with stress and improve their well-being. These high satisfaction levels suggest that the students positively evaluated this approach of providing mental health support. The findings also provide preliminary support for the effectiveness of this approach in reducing stigma and isolation related to mental health concerns and equipping students with skills to address these concerns as they navigate their educational goals.

PUBLIC HEALTH SIGNIFICANCE

Public health professionals are experiencing alarming rates of burnout and vicarious trauma.[3] The type of intervention described here (linking positive mental health with professional wellness) is essential for the future of the field. Education on and practice of positive mental health as part of professional development (professional wellness) are important for retaining and matriculating students and professionals.

By implementing wellness coaching into its curriculum, FPHLP assists students in developing skills and knowledge to reduce the risk of potential mental health crises and engaging in practices that support positive mental health. Reducing the severity of mental distress and equipping students with wellness skills and strategies through psychoeducation are important in increasing their academic potential and aiding in their growth as public health professionals.[5–7]

The initiative outlined here highlights the importance of innovative approaches to meet the modern-day needs of students. The mental health needs of college students—and the future public health workforce—are a public health emergency, and academic institutions have a responsibility to respond. Integrated mental health education and support are powerful tools, among many, that can begin to assist in building resilient students. As educational institutions and programs evolve to meet the changing needs of diverse student populations, expanded program offerings that include wellness coaching will become increasingly evident. Shifting societal demands, increased globalization, and technological advancements require us to move beyond traditional curriculum approaches and expand offerings so that they meet the comprehensive needs of the students we serve and the complexities of the changing workforce. AJPH

ABOUT THE AUTHORS

Sadé Mulkey, Christopher Knaub, Dana Thomas, Hallie Williams, Mariya Bahrenburg, and Paul J. Fleming are with the University of Michigan, Ann Arbor. Mishelle Rodriguez is with Collaborative ChangeMakers, Ann Arbor, MI.

CORRESPONDENCE

Correspondence should be sent to Sadé Mulkey, DSW, MPH, LMSW, 1415 Washington Heights, Suite 2700, Ann Arbor, MI 48109 (e-mail: richsade@umich.edu). Reprints can be ordered at https://www.ajph.org by clicking the "Reprints" link.

PUBLICATION INFORMATION

Full Citation: Mulkey S, Knaub C, Rodriguez M, et al. Wellness coaching in a summer internship program to address the mental health pandemic among college students, 2022–2023. *Am J Public Health*. 2025;115(9):1379–1382.

Acceptance Date: January 2, 2025.

DOI: https://doi.org/10.2105/AJPH.2025.308014

ORCID iDs:

Sadé Mulkey https://orcid.org/0009-0007-5543-1886

Dana Thomas https://orcid.org/0000-0003-1112-1943

Mariya Bahrenburg https://orcid.org/0009-0001-7029-9680

Paul J. Fleming https://orcid.org/0000-0001-9150-1254

CONTRIBUTORS

All of the authors contributed to writing, editing, and revising the article.

ACKNOWLEDGMENTS

The Future Public Health Leaders Program is funded by the Centers for Disease Control and Prevention as part of the John R. Lewis Scholars program (grant NU50CD300861).

Note. The findings, content, and conclusions of this article are those of the authors and do not necessarily represent the views or opinions of the funder.

CONFLICTS OF INTEREST

The authors have no financial conflicts of interest to disclose.

HUMAN PARTICIPANT PROTECTION

The data we collected were not used as part of a research study, and therefore institutional review board approval was not required. All data were anonymous and did not include personal identifiers.

REFERENCES

1. Healthy Minds Network. Healthy Minds Study among Colleges and Universities, 2014–2024. Available at: https://healthymindsnetwork.org/research/data-for-researchers. Accessed March 20, 2024.
2. Kodish T, Lau AS, Gong-Guy E, et al. Enhancing racial/ethnic equity in college student mental health through innovative screening and treatment. *Adm Policy Ment Health*. 2022;49(2):267–282. https://doi.org/10.1007/s10488-021-01163-1
3. de Beaumont Foundation. The impact of the COVID-19 pandemic: rising stress and burnout in public health. Available at: https://debeaumont.org/wp-content/uploads/dlm_uploads/2022/03/Stress-and-Burnout-Brief_final.pdf. Accessed March 20, 2024.
4. Fusar-Poli P, Correll CU, Arango C, Berk M, Patel V, Ioannidis JP. Preventive psychiatry: a blueprint for improving the mental health of young people. *World Psychiatry*. 2021;20(2):200–221. https://doi.org/10.1002/wps.20869
5. Gallagher RP. Thirty years of the national survey of counseling center directors: a personal account. *J Coll Stud Psychother*. 2012;26(3):172–184. https://doi.org/10.1080/87568225.2012.685852
6. Mowbray CT, Megivern D, Mandiberg JM, et al. Campus mental health services: recommendations for change. *Am J Orthopsychiatry*. 2006;76(2):226–237. https://doi.org/10.1037/0002-9432.76.2.226
7. Wolever RQ, Simmons LA, Sforzo GA, et al. A systematic review of the literature on health and wellness coaching: defining a key behavioral intervention in healthcare. *Glob Adv Health Med*. 2013;2(4):38–57. https://doi.org/10.7453/gahmj.2013.042
8. Bleck J, DeBate R, Garcia J, Gatto A. A pilot evaluation of a university health and wellness coaching program for college students. *Health Educ Behav*. 2023;50(5):613–621. https://doi.org/10.1177/10901981221131267
9. American College Health Association. Undergraduate Student Reference Group data report. Available at: https://www.acha.org/NCHA/ACHA-NCHA_Data/Publications_and_Reports/NCHA/Data/Reports_ACHA-NCHAIII.aspx. Accessed March 20, 2024.

Sibling Aggression and Abuse: Invisible and Widespread Public Health Problems

Corinna Jenkins Tucker, PhD, Tanya Rouleau Whitworth, PhD, and Nathan H. Perkins, PhD

ABOUT THE AUTHORS

Corinna Jenkins Tucker and Tanya Rouleau Whitworth are with the Sibling Aggression and Abuse Research and Advocacy Initiative, Crimes against Children Research Center, University of New Hampshire, Durham. Nathan H. Perkins is with the School of Social Work, Loyola University Chicago, Chicago, IL.

See also Adolescent Mental Health, pp. 1377–1453.

Sibling aggression and abuse are largely overlooked public health problems. The invisibility of these harmful sibling dynamics is partly driven by the tendency to mislabel such behaviors as rivalry, which is considered temporary and harmless. As such, the nature and impact of these behaviors and public attention to them are minimized or dismissed.[1,2] This perception, along with the shame and stigma associated with incidents of family violence, has made addressing this public health issue challenging.

Visibility is needed, however, because sibling aggression and abuse are the most common forms of family violence[3] and are consistently associated with mental and physical health problems and familial and extrafamilial relationship difficulties in adolescence.[4,5] Screenings and evidence-based interventions aimed at identifying and responding to sibling aggression and abuse can improve the adolescent population's health, relationship functioning, and social skills such as emotion regulation and conflict management and resolution; they can also have a positive impact on society's functioning.

Sibling aggression and abuse are prevalent in the United States and are more common than caregiver neglect and abuse or peer assault.[3] Sibling aggression, one-sided or mutual competition for or protests about caregivers' attention or favor,[6] is different from rivalry, although in extreme cases rivalry can lead to aggressive behavior. The definition of sibling aggression includes minor and severe physical assault (without or with an injury or use of a weapon), psychological aggression (e.g., threats, belittling, isolation), and property violence (e.g., forcibly taking or damaging personal items). The extent of the emotional and physical impact of such behaviors on the harmed sibling is related to their severity.[2]

US Census Bureau data show that approximately 80% of US children have siblings.[7] The only US nationally representative study of harmful sibling dynamics showed that they are a frequent occurrence: 37.6% of children one month to 17 years of age who lived with a sibling were victimized in the past year by their sibling in one or more incidents of physical, psychological, or property aggression.[8] This study also revealed sociodemographic variations in frequency: relative to their counterparts, sibling victimization is more commonly reported by White children, boys, and children whose parents have some college education. Although sibling victimization peaks in childhood at 46.1%, 35.7% and 27.6% of adolescents 10 to 13 and 14 to 17 years of age, respectively, were victimized by a sibling in the past year. The most commonly reported form of sibling victimization was physical assault (31.4% among adolescents 10–13 years old and 23.1% among adolescents 14–17 years old).

Many incidents of sibling victimization are minor, but some are severe or abusive. Although both aggressive and abusive sibling behaviors cause harm and should be prevented and stopped, sibling abuse is distinguished by one sibling demonstrating power and control over the other on the basis of age, gender, physical size, cognitive ability, or parental favoritism.[1,5] Sibling abuse is characterized by a single incident or repetition of behaviors that include a high risk of serious physical or emotional harm to a sibling.[1,9]

Notably, 4.9% of adolescents 10 to 13 years of age and 6.9% of adolescents 14 to 17 years of age in the study just described reported that the incidents of sibling victimization they experienced included an injury or a weapon.[8] In another study, 62% of adolescents who experienced sibling victimization that included injury or use of a weapon reported being afraid of their sibling, and this finding was consistent according to gender, ethnicity, and level of parental education.[2] Adolescent sibling aggression and abuse co-occur with many family problems, including intimate partner violence, child maltreatment, problematic parenting, and adverse events such as job loss, divorce, and family illness.[4,10] This may reflect a family atmosphere of poor emotion regulation and violence. Unfortunately, these family difficulties often take precedence over adolescent sibling aggression and abuse, leaving victims ignored and, in some cases, poly-victimized.

In light of this research, it is clear that to adequately address adolescents' mental health needs, a public health approach is needed to identify and respond to sibling aggression and abuse. Public health practitioners are likely aware that, as with survivors of other forms of family violence, adolescents and their parents may not be comfortable identifying harmful sibling behaviors as abuse. Furthermore, practitioners generally receive little or no training on sibling aggression and abuse.[11] However, given the importance of sibling relationships to adolescents' mental health and the prevalence of sibling aggression and abuse, identification of these incidents and destigmatization of this form of family violence are paramount to enhance the adolescent population's health. One study showed that even a single harmful sibling incident in the past year is associated with mental health distress.[12] Reducing the prevalence of sibling aggression and abuse could lower incidents of family violence, increase help seeking, and have a positive societal impact on adolescents' mental health.

DIRECT IMPACTS ON ADOLESCENT MENTAL HEALTH

The unique characteristics of sibling relationships, including frequent contact and emotional intensity, make them especially salient for adolescent mental health.[6] Whereas sibling warmth and support are positively associated with well-being, sibling aggression and abuse are linked to a variety of mental health challenges in adolescence, including distress,[5,12] depression,[13] low self-esteem,[13] anxiety,[14] and psychotic disorders.[15] Sibling victimization, especially when it is chronic or severe, can cause fear and lead an adolescent to feel unsafe at home.[2] The negative effects of sibling aggression and abuse on mental health are independent of the impacts of co-occurring family problems such as parental child maltreatment and witnessing of family violence.[12,14,15] Most research has focused on mental health associations with sibling victimization, but there is also evidence that sibling aggressors experience mental health challenges.[15]

Importantly, research incorporating longitudinal data shows that whether sibling victimization increases, decreases, or persists over time is also linked to adolescent mental health. In one study, chronic sibling victimization that persisted across two time points was linked to more severe forms of victimization and greater mental health distress in adolescence.[5] Another study showed that adolescents who reported decreasing sibling victimization from age 11 years to age 14 years had levels of depressive symptoms, life satisfaction, and self-esteem similar to those of adolescents who reported consistently low levels of sibling victimization.[13] This line of research suggests that taking a public health approach to prevention and intervention programs aimed at reducing sibling aggression and abuse could lead to improvements in mental health for large numbers of adolescents.

Harmful sibling dynamics and their associated effects in adolescence can persist into adulthood. Some of the challenges reported by adult survivors include depression, anxiety, low self-esteem, eating disorders, posttraumatic stress disorder, and difficulty forming close and trusting relationships with others.[1] Far from being a temporary annoyance, aggressive and abusive sibling dynamics in adolescence can lead to lasting harm and likely have a significant impact on the adult population's mental health.

INDIRECT IMPACTS ON ADOLESCENT MENTAL HEALTH

In addition to direct impacts of sibling aggression and abuse on adolescent mental health, there are indirect pathways through which sibling aggression likely affects mental health. One pathway is its connection to other forms of peer aggression, including dating violence and bullying, both of which have known links to mental health challenges in adolescence.[16,17] Involvement in sibling aggression, especially as the aggressor, is associated with the occurrence of dating violence.[18]

In addition, there is a consistent positive association between sibling aggression and being the aggressor in or victim of peer bullying.[19,20] A longitudinal analysis of US nationally representative data revealed that chronic sibling victimization more than doubled the risk of peer victimization.[20] Sibling aggressors also have an increased likelihood of being involved in peer bullying as victims, aggressors, or both.[19] At least one study has linked sibling victimization to cyberbullying victimization.[21]

This accumulated evidence suggests that, through social learning processes, aggression learned in sibling relationships can spill over into other relationships. Thus, reducing sibling aggression could lead to decreases in significant societal problems such as peer bullying and dating violence and consequently improve the adolescent population's mental health.

The lack of parental validation and support experienced by many young people victimized by their siblings is another possible indirect pathway from sibling aggression and abuse to adolescent mental health challenges. Common parental responses, even to more severe forms of sibling abuse, include minimizing, ignoring, and blaming the victim.[22] These invalidating responses may come about from parents unfairly favoring the harming sibling while simultaneously labeling the disfavored harmed child as having problematic qualities (e.g., a difficult personality). These responses can happen when sibling victimization co-occurs with parental child maltreatment, or they can reflect the broader cultural invisibility of sibling aggression and abuse. When adolescents' experiences of sibling victimization are accompanied by the apparent unwillingness or inability of their parents to protect and support them, this represents additional victimization and can amplify their feelings of worthlessness, hopelessness, and despair.[1]

The COVID-19 pandemic and lockdown may also have exacerbated adolescent mental health challenges through sibling aggression and abuse. One study revealed a higher prevalence of sibling aggression and abuse during the pandemic than before the pandemic.[23] Another showed that children and adolescents with special educational needs and disabilities were more likely to be victims of sibling aggression and abuse as the COVID-19 lockdown progressed than when it began.[24] The negative effects of the COVID-19 pandemic and lockdown on adolescent mental health have been well documented,[25] and sibling aggression and abuse likely served as a connecting variable between COVID-19 and adolescent mental health challenges. Furthermore, it is likely that during the pandemic, adolescent aggressors in and victims of sibling aggression and abuse experienced mental health challenges, thereby potentially perpetuating a recursive cycle of such behaviors.

ADVERSE CHILDHOOD EXPERIENCES

Public health practitioners often use an adverse childhood experience (ACE) inventory to assess trauma and decisions about care. ACEs represent a list of experiences such as abuse, neglect, violence, and household dysfunction occurring before the age of 18 years that have a cumulative impact on mental and physical health over the life span and lead to significant public health costs. An ACE can be a single incident or occur over an extended period, leading to chronic stress and inflammation. Traditional ACE inventories have not explicitly included sibling aggression and abuse, missing an important source of trauma among adolescents. Given the pervasive mislabeling of sibling aggression as rivalry and a lack of practitioner training, this source of trauma is likely missed without explicit screening for harmful sibling experiences, thus limiting responsive approaches to adolescent mental health. Multiple scholars have called for sibling aggression and abuse to be considered ACEs to enhance the identification of this form of trauma and the development of innovative response strategies.[5,11]

Notably, sibling aggression and abuse have associations with mental health that are similar to (and sometimes larger than) associations involving traditional ACEs, including child maltreatment, sexual victimization, and witnessing of family and community violence.[12] Incidents of adolescent sibling aggression and abuse are stressful and can be trauma inducing, particularly for harmed siblings, depleting their emotional and physical resources and creating vulnerability to a range of health issues. In addition, for some adolescents, sibling aggression and abuse can be chronic and persistent.[5]

To help alleviate the public health costs of adolescents' trauma and chronic stress from exposure to sibling aggression and abuse, ACE inventories should be broadened to include sibling aggression and abuse explicitly. With greater awareness and recognition, sibling aggression and abuse are likely to be prioritized and considered part of comprehensive support for adolescents' mental health and their experiences with all forms of family violence. As with any ACE, however, it will be critical to develop evidence-based responses to healing the trauma of sibling aggression and abuse.

IMPLICATIONS FOR PRACTITIONERS

When sibling aggression and abuse are conceptualized as public health concerns, the need for practitioner involvement in preventing and intervening in instances of sibling aggression and abuse to address adolescents' mental health is readily apparent. On the basis of findings from their research on the association between sibling aggression and child and adolescent mental health, Tucker et al. noted that "the public should treat sibling aggression as potentially harmful and something not to be dismissed as normal, minor, or even beneficial."[12(p84)]

It is time for public health initiatives to address sibling aggression and abuse to prevent this form of family violence and improve adolescent mental health. A social awareness campaign aimed at a range of providers in different disciplines could be enacted to distinguish sibling rivalry from aggression and abuse and appropriately label the latter behaviors as family violence. Public health practitioners also need to receive training on identifying and responding to sibling aggression and abuse so that these behaviors are no longer overlooked. Currently, few organizations offer such training (an exception is the Sibling Aggression and Abuse Research and Advocacy Initiative), and the topic is generally absent from undergraduate and graduate curricula and continuing education requirements. Thus, expanding the capacity to offer education and training is essential and will have a positive societal impact.

Despite efforts to call sibling aggression and abuse an issue warranting consideration in family and public health,[1,5] prevention and intervention strategies remain scarce, and sibling aggression and abuse are rarely perceived as encompassed within family violence. Developing evidence-based strategies to create a shared understanding of and accessible approaches to communication and conflict management should be prioritized. These strategies could then be infused into existing parent education, antibullying, and dating violence programs to strengthen adolescent mental health. Furthermore, public health practitioners should consider expanding the focus of mental health and social services agencies, hospitals, and community centers to include sibling aggression and abuse.[1] This endeavor could begin with screening for sibling aggression and abuse as part of ACE inventories. Public health practitioners are likely to be first responders to incidents in which adolescents are harmed by siblings, thus giving them the unique opportunity to provide parent education and, if needed, a referral for abuse.

CONCLUSION

Given the prevalence of sibling aggression and abuse and their connections to mental health challenges in adolescence, efforts toward public education, interventions, and policy regarding sibling aggression and abuse are not only warranted but necessary for addressing this pervasive form of family violence that affects the adolescent population's mental health. With greater awareness, training, and evidence-based responses, societal perceptions that keep sibling aggression and abuse hidden will evolve with benefits for adolescents, their mental health, and their familial and extrafamilial relationships. AJPH

CORRESPONDENCE

Correspondence should be sent to Corinna Jenkins Tucker, PhD, Sibling Aggression and Abuse Research and Advocacy Initiative, Crimes against Children Research Center, 125 McConnell Hall, University of New Hampshire, Durham, NH 03824 (e-mail: cjtucker@unh.edu). Reprints can be ordered at https://www.ajph.org by clicking the "Reprints" link.

PUBLICATION INFORMATION

Full Citation: Tucker CJ, Whitworth TR, Perkins NH. Sibling aggression and abuse: invisible and widespread public health problems. *Am J Public Health*. 2025;115(9):1383–1387.

Acceptance Date: December 10, 2024.

DOI: https://doi.org/10.2105/AJPH.2024.307983

ORCID iDs:

Corinna Jenkins Tucker https://orcid.org/0000-0002-0786-523X

Tanya Rouleau Whitworth https://orcid.org/0000-0003-0629-1059

Nathan H. Perkins https://orcid.org/0000-0003-1209-8466

CONTRIBUTORS

C. Jenkins Tucker contributed to article conceptualization, was the primary writer, proofread the article, and was responsible for the final version. T. Rouleau Whitworth contributed to article conceptualization, wrote sections of the article, and proofread the article. N. H. Perkins contributed to article conceptualization, section writing, and proofreading.

ACKNOWLEDGMENTS

Corinna Jenkins Tucker and Tanya Rouleau Whitworth thank the Louis and Anne Abrons Foundation for its generous support.

CONFLICTS OF INTEREST

The authors have no potential conflicts of interest to declare.

REFERENCES

1. Perkins NH, Meyers A. The manifestation of physical and emotional sibling abuse across the lifespan and the need for social work intervention. *J Fam Soc Work*. 2020;23(4):338–356. https://doi.org/10.1080/10522158.2020.1799894
2. Tucker CJ, Finkelhor D, Turner H. Emerging ideas: is sibling aggression as scary as peer aggression in childhood and adolescence? *Fam Relat*. 2023;72(5):3023–3028. https://doi.org/10.1111/fare.12844
3. Finkelhor D, Turner HA, Shattuck A, Hamby SL. Prevalence of childhood exposure to violence, crime, and abuse: results from the National Survey of Children's Exposure to Violence. *JAMA Pediatr*. 2015;169(8):746–754. https://doi.org/10.1001/jamapediatrics.2015.0676
4. Tucker CJ, Finkelhor D, Turner H. Family predictors of sibling versus peer victimization. *J Fam Psychol*. 2020;34(2):186–195. https://doi.org/10.1037/fam0000592
5. Tucker CJ, Finkelhor D, Turner H. Patterns of sibling aggression and mental health in childhood and adolescence. *J Fam Trauma Child Custody Child Dev*. 2024;21(1):2–21. https://doi.org/10.1080/26904586.2023.2234369
6. McHale SM, Updegraff KA, Whiteman SD. Sibling relationships. In: Peterson GW, Bush KR, eds. *Handbook of Marriage and the Family*. Springer; 2013:329–351.
7. Knop B. More children live with half siblings than previously thought. Available at: https://www.census.gov/library/stories/2020/01/more-children-live-with-half-siblings-than-previously-thought.html. Accessed December 20, 2024.

8. Tucker CJ, Finkelhor D, Shattuck AM, Turner H. Prevalence and correlates of sibling victimization types. *Child Abuse Negl*. 2013;37(4):213–223. https://doi.org/10.1016/j.chiabu.2013.01.006
9. Caffaro JV. *Sibling Abuse Trauma: Assessment and Intervention Strategies for Children, Families, and Adults*. 2nd ed. Routledge; 2014. https://doi.org/10.4324/9781315808369
10. Tucker CJ, Finkelhor D, Turner H. Family adversity's role in the onset and termination of childhood sibling victimization. *Psychol Violence*. 2018;8(1):10–18. https://doi.org/10.1037/vio0000087
11. Perkins NH, Shadik JA, Cales MA, Ortiz SP. MSW students' experiences with ACEs and capacity to address sibling violence: a pilot study. *Soc Work Educ*. 2023;42(3):302–317. https://doi.org/10.1080/02615479.2021.1967311
12. Tucker CJ, Finkelhor D, Turner H, Shattuck A. Association of sibling aggression with child and adolescent mental health. *Pediatrics*. 2013;132(1):79–84. https://doi.org/10.1542/peds.2012-3801
13. Sharpe H, Fink E, Duffy F, Patalay P. Changes in peer and sibling victimization in early adolescence: longitudinal associations with multiple indices of mental health in a prospective birth cohort study. *Eur Child Adolesc Psychiatry*. 2022;31(5):737–746. https://doi.org/10.1007/s00787-020-01708-z
14. Renner LM, Schwab-Reese LM, Coppola EC, Boel-Studt S. The contribution of interpersonal violence victimization types to psychological distress among youth. *Child Abuse Negl*. 2020;106:104493. https://doi.org/10.1016/j.chiabu.2020.104493
15. Dantchev S, Zammit S, Wolke D. Sibling bullying in middle childhood and psychotic disorder at 18 years: a prospective cohort study. *Psychol Med*. 2018;48(14):2321–2328. https://doi.org/10.1017/S0033291717003841
16. Piolanti A, Waller F, Schmid IE, Foran HM. Long-term adverse outcomes associated with teen dating violence: a systematic review. *Pediatrics*. 2023;151(6):e2022059654. https://doi.org/10.1542/peds.2022-059654
17. Schneider SK, O'Donnell L, Stueve A, Coulter RWS. Cyberbullying, school bullying, and psychological distress: a regional census of high school students. *Am J Public Health*. 2012;102(1):171–177. https://doi.org/10.2105/AJPH.2011.300308
18. Rothman EF, Johnson RM, Azrael D, Hall DM, Weinberg J. Perpetration of physical assault against dating partners, peers, and siblings among a locally representative sample of high school students in Boston, Massachusetts. *Arch Pediatr Adolesc Med*. 2010;164(12):1118–1124. https://doi.org/10.1001/archpediatrics.2010.229
19. Tippett N, Wolke D. Aggression between siblings: associations with the home environment and peer bullying. *Aggress Behav*. 2015;41(1):14–24. https://doi.org/10.1002/ab.21557
20. Tucker CJ, Finkelhor D, Turner H. Patterns of sibling victimization as predictors of peer victimization in childhood and adolescence. *J Fam Violence*. 2019;34(8):745–755. https://doi.org/10.1007/s10896-018-0021-1
21. Dantchev S, Zemp M. Sibling, peer, and cyber bullying among children and adolescents: co-occurrence and implications for their adjustment. *Front Psychol*. 2021;12:761276. https://doi.org/10.3389/fpsyg.2021.761276
22. Elliott K, Fitz-Gibbon K, Maher J. Sibling violence: understanding experiences, impacts, and the need for nuanced responses. *Br J Sociol*. 2020;71(1):168–182. https://doi.org/10.1111/1468-4446.12712
23. Borualogo IS, Casas F. Sibling bullying, school bullying, and children's subjective well-being before and during the COVID-19 pandemic in Indonesia. *Child Indic Res*. 2023;16(3):1203–1232. https://doi.org/10.1007/s12187-023-10013-5
24. Toseeb U. Sibling conflict during COVID-19 in families with special educational needs and disabilities. *Br J Educ Psychol*. 2022;92(1):319–339. https://doi.org/10.1111/bjep.12451
25. Panchal U, Salazar De Pablo G, Franco M, et al. The impact of COVID-19 lockdown on child and adolescent mental health: systematic review. *Eur Child Adolesc Psychiatry*. 2023;32(7):1151–1177. https://doi.org/10.1007/s00787-021-01856-w

Adolescent Dating Violence and Suicide Planning Among Girls in US High Schools: An Intracategorical Intersectional Analysis by Race and Ethnicity

Laurel Sharpless, MPH, Kiara Alvarez, PhD, Trace Kershaw, PhD, and Tiara C. Willie, PhD, MA

See also Adolescent Mental Health, pp. 1377–1453.

Objectives. To examine associations between adolescent dating violence (ADV) and suicide planning among girls and differences by race/ethnicity.

Methods. Data were from the 2021 Youth Risk Behavior Survey (YRBS), a cross-sectional, nationally representative study of 9th- to 12th-grade adolescents from US high schools (n = 3886). We used weighted logistic regression to examine associations between ADV and suicide planning and assess moderation by race/ethnicity.

Results. Compared with girls who did not experience any ADV, girls who experienced both physical and sexual ADV had increased odds of making a suicide plan (adjusted odds ratio [AOR] = 5.35; 95% confidence interval [CI] = 3.27, 8.74), and the effect size was stronger than for experiencing either type of ADV alone. The relationship between sexual ADV and suicide planning was exacerbated for Latina girls (AOR = 6.36; 95% CI = 3.96, 10.19) compared with White girls (AOR = 2.51; 95% CI = 1.45, 4.35).

Conclusions. Experiencing any form of ADV is associated with increased odds of suicide planning among girls, with stronger impacts for Latina girls experiencing only sexual ADV.

Public Health Implications. Prevention of suicide planning for Latina girls who experience sexual ADV may be strengthened by integrating contextually tailored suicide prevention into prevention programs addressing healthy relationships and prevention of sexual violence. (*Am J Public Health*. 2025;115(9): 1388–1396. https://doi.org/10.2105/AJPH.2025.308043)

AJPH September 2025, Vol. 115, No. 9

Adolescent dating violence (ADV) and death by suicide are co-occurring epidemics among adolescent girls. Although national estimates have varied in the past decade, recent nationally representative data suggest that approximately 10% of adolescent girls attending high school have experienced past-year physical ADV and 15% have experienced past-year sexual ADV.[1] Moreover, in the past decade, death by suicide has increased and is currently the second leading cause of premature death among early adolescents and the third leading cause among older adolescents.[2] ADV experiences can result in negative mental health outcomes. Girls who experience physical, sexual, or both forms of ADV have a higher risk of suicide behaviors, such as suicide ideation, suicide planning, or suicide attempt, than girls without these experiences.[3–5] Moreover, girls who experience both types of ADV have a higher risk of suicide behaviors than those experiencing either physical or sexual ADV alone.[5]

Suicide planning is a critical but understudied part of the suicide continuum.[3] Protocols for suicide screening classify suicide planning as a key risk factor for attempting suicide.[6] For example, research shows that approximately 72% of those who make a suicide plan progress to attempting suicide.[7] Furthermore, data from the World Health Organization's World Mental Health Survey Initiative suggest that individuals in the United States who reported ever having had suicide ideation along with a suicide plan had a 54.5% probability of attempting suicide; by contrast, the probability of attempting suicide was 19.9% among individuals who reported ever having had suicide ideation but did not make a suicide plan.[8] Suicide planning is a particularly relevant stage for prevention among girls who experience physical, sexual, or both forms of ADV. Nationally representative data from 2013 suggest that girls who have experienced past-year physical or sexual ADV are 2 times more likely to make a suicide plan than girls without these experiences, and girls who experience both forms of ADV are 3.8 times more likely.[5] Although limited, prior research suggests that suicide planning may occur as a consequence of ADV through feelings of burdensomeness and thwarted belongingness.[9]

Burgeoning research has focused on ethnoracial disparities in suicide behaviors among adolescents. Latinx adolescents had higher rates of suicide attempts resulting in injury compared with White adolescents in 2021.[10] Furthermore, trends from 2001 to 2017 among non-Latinx Black adolescents showed a significant increase in suicide ideation, plans, and attempts that required medical treatment.[11] Gender disparities in suicide behaviors also exist among adolescents. A systematic review showed that girls aged 12 to 24 years have a greater lifetime prevalence and 12-month incidence of suicide attempts compared with boys in the same age group,[12] although boys have higher rates of suicide deaths.[12] However, the intersection of race/ethnicity and gender has implications for suicide behaviors among adolescents. For example, longitudinal data from 1991 to 2017 showed a significant upward trend in suicide ideation, plans, and attempts among Black girls. Moreover, these data showed significant quadratic trends in suicide ideation and plans among White, Black, and Latina girls.[13]

Despite growing research in this field, little is known about how the impact of physical, sexual, or both forms of ADV on suicide planning differs by race/ethnicity among adolescent girls. An intersectionality theoretical framework can be applied to contextualize how suicide planning may vary among ADV girl survivors, considering their intersecting social positions of race/ethnicity and gender. Intersectionality posits that social identities, such as race/ethnicity and gender, intersect at the individual level to reflect and embody interlocking systems of power and oppression, such as racism and sexism at a structural level.[14–16] These interlocking systems of power and oppression are embedded in policies, cultural norms and practices, and beliefs that compound and reinforce each other to produce health inequities across intersectional groups.[17] Black and Latina adolescent girls who reported ever experiencing gendered racial discrimination had 2.7 times greater odds of experiencing severe ADV than Black and Latina adolescent girls who did not report gendered racial discrimination.[18] Black and Latina ADV girl survivors may uniquely experience racism and sexism, which may influence their experiences of physical or sexual ADV and increase their risk for suicide planning. These factors may also reduce their access to and quality of services for ADV and its comorbid mental health conditions.[17] Therefore, understanding disparities in suicide planning by race/ethnicity among girls who have experienced physical, sexual, or both forms of ADV is important for identifying and tailoring a vital suicide prevention point.

In this study, we aimed to address this research gap by using an intracategorical intersectional approach[19] to examine associations between exposure to physical ADV only, sexual ADV only, both physical and sexual ADV, and suicide planning among adolescent girls, in addition to the moderating effects of race/ethnicity. We hypothesized that adolescent girls who solely experience physical or sexual ADV, or both forms of ADV, will be more likely to make a suicide plan than adolescent girls who do not experience ADV, with girls who experience both types of ADV having the strongest effect. We further hypothesized that these relationships will be moderated by race/ethnicity, such that the association between ADV and suicide planning will be stronger for Latina and non-Latina Black adolescent girls than for non-Latina White girls.

METHODS

For this secondary analysis, we used data from the 2021 National Youth Risk Behavior Survey (YRBS), a nationally representative, cross-sectional study conducted biennially among adolescents aged 14 to 18 years.[20] This survey used a 3-stage cluster sampling design among adolescents in the 9th through 12th grade who attended public and private high schools in the 50 US states and the District of Columbia, and it inquired about various health-related behaviors, including physical and sexual ADV and suicide planning. Participation in the YRBS was anonymous and voluntary, and parental permission was obtained. Students directly recorded their responses in a self-administered, computer-scannable questionnaire. More details about the development and implementation of the 2021 National YRBS are published elsewhere.[20]

For the 2021 National YRBS, 17 508 questionnaires were completed across 152 schools. Of the completed questionnaires, 276 failed quality control, leaving 17 232 usable questionnaires. The school response rate was 72.7%, and the student response rate was 79.1%.[20] The analytic sample used for the present study was restricted to complete data for all variables used in analyses (n = 3886).

Measures

The YRBS assessed grade using the question, "In what grade are you in?" Responses were made into an ordinal variable ranging from 0 (9th grade) to 3 (12th grade).

The YRBS assessed sexual identity using the question, "Which of the following best describes you?" We made response options into a categorical variable of 1 (heterosexual), 2 (gay, lesbian, or bisexual), and 3 (other, questioning) and dummy coded categories with heterosexual as reference.

The YRBS assessed race/ethnicity using the following questions: "Are you Hispanic or Latino?" with response options of yes or no, and "What is your race?" with response options of American Indian or Alaska Native, Asian, Black or African American, Native Hawaiian or Other Pacific Islander, and White, where more than 1 option can be chosen. We made these questions into a categorical variable: 1 (non-Latina White), 2 (non-Latina Black), or 3 (Latina, including Latina multiple race) and dummy coded categories with non-Latina White as reference. We removed Asian, Native Hawaiian or Other Pacific Islander, American Indian or Alaskan Native, and non-Latina multiple race responses from the analysis given that, if combined into a heterogeneous single category to yield sufficient sample size for analysis, results related to this category would be uninterpretable.

The YRBS assessed adolescent dating violence using the physical ADV question, "During the past 12 months, how many times did someone you were dating or going out with physically hurt you on purpose? (Count such things as being hit, slammed into something, or injured with an object or weapon.)" and the sexual ADV question, "During the past 12 months, how many times did someone you were dating or going out with force you to do sexual things that you did not want to do? (Count such things as kissing, touching, or being physically forced to have sexual intercourse.)" Response options for both questions ranged from 0 times to 6 or more times and were dichotomized as exposure (1 = $\geq$1 times) or no exposure (0 = 0 times) given the skewed nature of responses to both questions. These dichotomized responses to the questions were then made into a 4-level composite variable of having experienced physical ADV only, sexual ADV only, both physical and sexual ADV, and no ADV and dummy coded with no ADV as reference. According to the YRBS study design, adolescents who reported having not dated or gone out with someone in the past 12 months were excluded from this variable.[5] Test–retest reliabilities for physical ADV (κ = 0.64; P = .78) and sexual ADV (κ = 0.88; P = .99) indicate substantial agreement.[21]

The YRBS assessed suicide planning using the question, "During the past 12 months, did you make a plan about how you would attempt suicide?" We coded response options into a binary variable as 1 (yes) and 0 (no). Test–retest reliability for suicide planning (κ = 0.81, P = .87) indicates strong agreement.[21]

Data Analyses

We calculated unweighted sociodemographic frequencies and weighted percentages for adolescent girls with different ethnoracial identities and the overall sample. We used weighted logistic regression to examine unadjusted associations between ADV type and suicide planning. We then adjusted models for grade, race/ethnicity, and sexual identity. We did not adjust for age in the models because of multicollinearity between age and grade. We then stratified these adjusted models by race/ethnicity to assess prevalence of suicide planning within each intersectional group of girls. Lastly, we assessed race/ethnicity as a potential moderator by adding ADV type × race/ethnicity interaction terms to adjusted models for each ethnoracial group except for the referent group (White girls) to provide intracategorical comparisons. Consistent with the approach indicated by Aiken et al.,[22] significant interactions were followed up by simple slopes to determine the nature of significance. All analyses included stratification and clustering (primary sampling unit) variables to account for the complex sampling design used in the YRBS. We used model coefficients, denoted as odds ratios, adjusted odds ratios, 95% confidence intervals, and P value less than .05, to determine significance. We conducted all analyses using SAS statistical software.

TABLE 1— Frequencies, Weighted Percentages, and Differences by Race/Ethnicity of Adolescent Girls: United States, Youth Risk Behavior Survey, 2021

	Total (n = 3886)		Latina (n = 812; 27.2%)		Non-Latina Black (n = 610; 13.7%)		Non-Latina White (n = 2464; 59.1%)			
	No.[a]	% (95% CI)[b]	No.[a]	% (95% CI)[b]	No.[a]	% (95% CI)[b]	No.[a]	% (95% CI)[b]	χ^2	*P*
Adolescent dating violence (ADV)									40.4	< .01
Physical ADV only	223	5.5 (4.3, 6.6)	46	4.7 (2.8, 6.5)	33	6.0 (3.3, 8.6)	144	5.7 (4.3, 7.1)		
Sexual ADV only	317	8.9 (7.5, 10.3)	71	9.1 (6.3, 12.0)	19	3.3 (1.0, 5.7)	227	10.0 (7.8, 12.2)		
Both physical and sexual	165	4.6 (3.6, 5.6)	44	4.8 (3.1, 6.6)	13	1.7 (0.8, 2.5)	108	5.2 (3.8, 6.6)		
No ADV	3181	81.1 (79.4, 82.8)	651	81.4 (78.7, 84.0)	545	89.0 (85.0, 93.0)	1985	79.1 (76.9, 81.4)		
Suicide plan									1.3	.7
Yes	1026	27.2 (25.3, 29.1)	223	28.6 (25.1, 32.1)	167	26.6 (21.1, 32.2)	636	26.7 (24.2, 29.3)		
No	2860	72.8 (70.9, 74.7)	589	71.4 (67.9, 74.9)	443	73.4 (67.8, 78.9)	1828	73.3 (70.7, 75.8)		
Grade									27.4	.03
9th	847	21.8 (19.2, 24.4)	173	25.5 (21.2, 29.8)	164	25.2 (19.7, 30.7)	510	19.3 (16.4, 22.3)		
10th	1027	25.0 (22.8, 27.3)	198	22.8 (20.0, 25.6)	166	25.4 (20.3, 30.5)	663	26.0 (22.6, 29.4)		
11th	993	26.8 (24.7, 28.9)	219	27.0 (24.3, 29.8)	142	27.8 (22.9, 32.6)	632	26.5 (22.9, 30.1)		
12th	1019	26.3 (24.0, 28.7)	222	24.7 (22.0, 27.4)	138	21.6 (16.4, 26.8)	659	28.1 (24.7, 31.6)		
Sexual identity									25.1	.02
Gay, lesbian, or bisexual	889	25.0 (22.5, 27.4)	176	21.8 (17.2, 26.3)	166	30.6 (25.0, 36.1)	547	25.2 (21.4, 29.0)		
Other, questioning	378	9.9 (8.5, 11.4)	83	10.7 (8.5, 12.9)	71	12.7 (8.9, 16.6)	224	9.0 (7.2, 10.7)		
Heterosexual	2619	65.1 (62.3, 67.8)	553	67.5 (63.7, 71.4)	373	56.7 (50.6, 62.7)	1693	65.9 (62.0, 69.7)		

Note. CI = confidence interval.
[a]Counts are unweighted.
[b]Percentages are weighted. Percentages are rounded to the nearest tenth and may not equal 100.

TABLE 2— Associations Between Type of Adolescent Dating Violence (ADV), Race/Ethnicity, and Suicide Plan Among Adolescent Girls: United States, Youth Risk Behavior Survey, 2021

	Unadjusted OR (95% CI)	AOR (95% CI)
ADV		
Physical ADV only	3.78 (2.36, 6.07)	3.39 (1.97, 5.82)
Sexual ADV only	3.74 (2.73, 5.13)	3.35 (2.30, 4.89)
Both physical and sexual ADV	6.88 (4.37, 10.83)	5.35 (3.27, 8.74)
No ADV (Ref)	1	1
Grade	0.87 (0.82, 0.93)	0.79 (0.72, 0.86)
Race/ethnicity		
Latina	1.11 (0.94, 1.31)	1.17 (0.94, 1.44)
Non-Latina Black	1.08 (0.84, 1.38)	1.01 (0.67, 1.51)
Non-Latina White (Ref)	1	1
Sexual identity		
Gay, lesbian, or bisexual	3.95 (3.31, 4.70)	3.72 (3.05, 4.54)
Other, questioning	2.82 (2.34, 3.40)	3.17 (2.46, 4.10)
Heterosexual (Ref)	1	1

Note. AOR = adjusted odds ratio; CI = confidence interval; OR = odds ratio. Analyses are weighted.

RESULTS

Table 1 displays unweighted frequencies and weighted percentages of sociodemographic characteristics of the overall sample of 3886 adolescent girls. Of these girls, 223 reported solely experiencing physical ADV, 317 reported only experiencing sexual ADV, 165 reported experiencing both physical and sexual ADV, and 3181 reported no ADV exposure in the past year. More than half of the girls self-identified as non-Latina White (59.1%), followed by Latina (27.2%) and non-Latina Black (13.7%). Nearly two thirds of the girls self-identified as heterosexual (65.1%), and nearly one third were in the 12th grade (26.3%).

Chi-square analyses showed a significant difference between race/ethnicity and ADV type ($\chi^2 = 40.4$; $P < .01$), grade ($\chi^2 = 27.4$; $P = .03$), and sexual identity ($\chi^2 = 25.1$; $P = .02$).

Multivariable Associations

We examined weighted unadjusted and adjusted associations between ADV type and suicide planning (Table 2). Unadjusted results showed that girls who experienced only physical ADV had 3.78 times the odds of making a suicide plan (95% confidence interval [CI] = 2.36, 6.07), girls who experienced only sexual ADV had 3.74 times the odds of making a suicide plan (95% CI = 2.73, 5.13), and girls who experienced both physical and sexual ADV had 6.88 times the odds of making a suicide plan than girls who did not experience ADV (95% CI = 4.37, 10.83).

After we controlled for covariates, girls who experienced only physical ADV had 3.39 times the odds of making a suicide plan (95% CI = 1.97, 5.82), girls who experienced only sexual ADV had 3.35 times the odds of making a suicide plan (95% CI = 2.30, 4.89), and girls who experienced both physical and sexual ADV had 5.35 times the odds of making a suicide plan than girls who did not experience ADV (95% CI = 3.27, 8.74). These findings supported our hypotheses.

Stratified Models by Race/Ethnicity

We examined weighted adjusted associations between ADV type and suicide planning, stratified by race/ethnicity (Table 3). Among White girls, those who experienced only physical ADV had 3.83 times the odds of making a suicide

TABLE 3— Adjusted Associations Between Adolescent Dating Violence (ADV) and Suicide Plan Among Adolescent Girls, Stratified by Race/Ethnicity: United States, Youth Risk Behavior Survey, 2021

	Suicide Plan, AOR (95% CI)		
	Latina	Non-Latina Black	Non-Latina White
Physical ADV only	1.89 (0.59, 6.07)	4.00 (2.11, 7.59)	3.83 (2.07, 7.10)
Sexual ADV only	6.16 (3.82, 9.91)	3.68 (0.86, 15.80)	2.50 (1.40, 4.46)
Both physical and sexual ADV	5.23 (1.71, 15.98)	7.60 (1.59, 36.27)	5.10 (3.05, 8.54)
No ADV (Ref)	1	1	1

Note. AOR = adjusted odds ratio; CI = confidence interval. Analyses are weighted.

AJPH September 2025, Vol. 115, No. 9

plan (95% CI = 2.07, 7.10), those who experienced only sexual ADV had 2.50 times the odds of making a suicide plan (95% CI = 1.40, 4.46), and those who experienced both physical and sexual ADV had 5.10 times the odds of making a suicide plan than girls who did not experience ADV, adjusting for covariates (95% CI = 3.05, 8.54).

Among Black girls, those who experienced only physical ADV had 4.00 times the odds of making a suicide plan (95% CI = 2.11, 7.59), and those who experienced both physical and sexual ADV had 7.60 times the odds of making a suicide plan than girls without ADV experiences, adjusting for covariates (95% CI = 1.59, 36.27).

Among Latina girls, those who experienced only sexual ADV had 6.16 times the odds of making a suicide plan (95% CI = 3.82, 9.91), and those who experienced both physical and sexual ADV had 5.23 times the odds of making a suicide plan than girls without ADV experiences, adjusting for covariates (95% CI = 1.71, 15.98).

Interaction Models by Race/Ethnicity

The sexual ADV only × Latina interaction was significantly associated with suicide planning (B [SE] = 0.93 [0.36]; *P* = .02). Examining simple slopes showed that among Latina girls, those who solely experienced sexual ADV had 6.36 times the odds of making a suicide plan than those who did not experience ADV (95% CI = 3.96, 10.19), whereas among White girls, those who experienced only sexual ADV had 2.51 times the odds of making a suicide plan than those who did not experience ADV (95% CI = 1.45, 4.35; Figure 1). This finding supported our hypothesis.

DISCUSSION

The current study examined relationships between physical, sexual, and both types of ADV and suicide planning in addition to assessing race/ethnicity as a moderator. Our study adds to a growing body of literature suggesting that adolescent girls who experience either physical or sexual ADV or both forms of ADV are more likely to make a suicide plan than girls without ADV experiences. Our findings also showed that experiencing both physical and sexual ADV had the greatest impact on making a suicide plan, which is consistent with literature supporting the impact of cumulative effects of ADV on suicide behaviors.[5] To our knowledge, this study, which used 2021 National YRBS data, is one of the first to examine how race/ethnicity moderates the relationship between physical, sexual, or both forms of ADV and suicide planning among a sample exclusively composed of girls.

Stratification by race/ethnicity revealed distinct patterns in the prevalence of suicide planning among girls with ADV experiences. Among White girls, those who only experienced physical or sexual ADV or both were more likely to make a suicide plan compared with those without ADV experiences. Among Black girls, those who only experienced physical ADV or both physical and sexual ADV were more likely to make a suicide plan compared with those without ADV experiences. Among Latina girls, those who only experienced sexual ADV or both forms of ADV were more likely to make a suicide plan compared with those without ADV experiences. Across all groups of girls except for Latina girls, the findings suggested there was a greater impact among girls experiencing both physical and sexual ADV than among girls experiencing only 1 type of ADV. For Latina girls, the strongest effect was observed among those who only experienced sexual ADV.

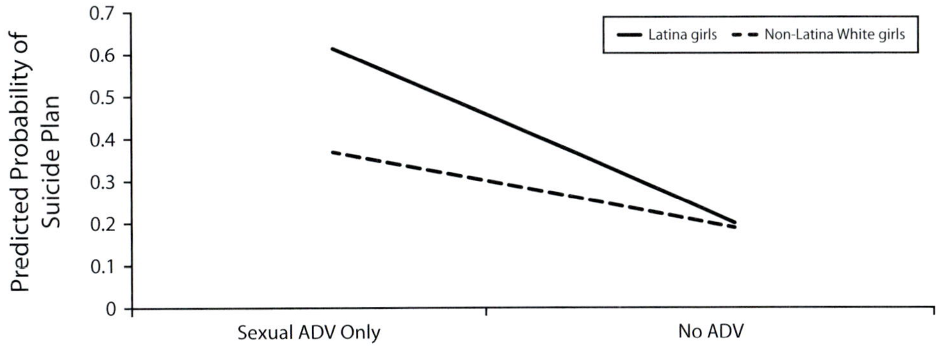

FIGURE 1— Moderation of Latina (vs Non-Latina White) Identity on the Adjusted Association Between Sexual Adolescent Dating Violence (ADV) Only and Making a Suicide Plan Among Adolescent Girls: United States, Youth Risk Behavior Survey, 2021

We also assessed moderation by race/ethnicity, which adds to the pattern of stratification findings among Latina girls. Specifically, our results suggest that race/ethnicity moderates the relationship between sexual ADV only and suicide planning among girls, such that the link is exacerbated for Latina girls compared with White girls. One possible explanation for this finding is the structural gendered racism that this intersectional group may experience based on their social positions of ethnicity and gender. For example, Latina girls are hypersexualized by the media, but simultaneously may feel pressured to uphold the traditional values of *marianismo*, particularly female virtue and chastity.[23] Therefore, these gendered racial characteristics typically ascribed to Latina girls can shape patterns of ADV, increase susceptibility to sexual ADV, and legitimize victim-blaming,[23] potentially prompting the formation of a suicide plan. These stereotypes that disenfranchise Latina girls who experience sexual ADV may be perpetuated by key settings for suicide prevention, such as schools and juvenile justice systems.[24] For example, schools are the most common formal help-seeking resource for Latina ADV girl survivors, but the majority of survivors seek out help informally from friends.[25,26] Schools may conform to cultural stereotypes[27] and accept sexual ADV behaviors toward Latina girls, thereby fostering an environment where these girls are less likely to be heard or protected. Additionally, qualitative data show that Latina ADV survivors fear seeking help from the police, who are agents of the juvenile justice system, because of anticipated harmful treatment,[25] which may limit their options for protection and accountability. However, if Latina girls do seek justice via the juvenile justice system for sexual ADV, they may be less likely to be believed because of these pervasive stereotypes. These experiences may be compounded for Latina ADV girl survivors who experience structural xenophobia, an additional dimension of structural gendered racism, based on their immigration status.[24,28] Despite the potential for harm, schools have been identified as a protective factor for Latina ADV girl survivors by providing healthy activities that foster social support.[23] School-based restorative justice, a survivor-centered justice approach focused on repairing harm between the survivor and the person who caused harm, has gained traction as a practice with the potential to disrupt structural gendered racism by schools and juvenile justice systems if practiced equitably, offering a potential source of social support, healing, and accountability that may be protective of mental health.[29,30] School-based restorative justice has also been associated with greater academic success, school safety, and school connectedness.[30] Future research should focus on how school-based restorative justice specifically affects Latina sexual ADV girl survivors and their suicide planning behaviors.

We also found that self-identifying as Black did not significantly moderate the association between ADV type and suicide planning among adolescent girls. There are a few potential explanations for this finding. First, the 2021 YRBS data yielded a limited sample size of Black girls who experienced physical, sexual, or both forms of ADV (n = 65). Future research can combine waves of YRBS data to build a sufficient sample size for all subgroup analyses. An additional potential explanation is that research using national and population-representative data has shown that Black adolescents are not exhibiting typical precursors to attempting suicide, such as suicide planning, but have increased in rates of attempts.[31–33] Moreover, prior research suggests that for Black adolescents, suicide planning and suicide attempts do not always occur in a linear fashion.[34] A possible explanation may be high exposure to trauma and violence in their socio-structural context, prompting a more direct path between suicide ideation to suicide.[35] Therefore, it is possible that suicide planning is not capturing the full scope of the suicide continuum for this intersectional group of girls.

Limitations

There are several limitations that should be considered. This is a cross-sectional study, so we cannot infer causality with our study findings. Our exposure and outcome were measured during the same timeframe, so we are unable to disentangle temporality because of the artifact of measurement. Future research should use longitudinal data to establish temporality between ADV and suicide planning across diverse girls. Students may not have responded to ADV and suicide planning questions, biasing results toward the null. Given the timeframe of the survey, study findings should be considered within the context of the COVID-19 pandemic. We chose not to examine suicide attempts in this study because of lack of power. Future research can combine multiple waves of national YRBS data to gain power to detect effects among this population. Our sample consists of girls in schools. Therefore, findings may not generalize to and do not include girls who may not be in school because of incarceration or dropping out. This may be a particularly relevant group to examine in future research. The 2021 National YRBS did not include questions about gender identity, limiting our ability to distinguish experiences of cisgender girls from those of transgender or nonbinary youths. Our analysis also excludes girls outside the 3 ethnoracial groups used because of low sample size. Future work should use a more inclusive sample of ADV girl survivors. Our article focuses on racism and sexism; future work should include other axes of identity and power like heterosexism, ableism, and classism. Because of the YRBS study design, we cannot speak to direct experiences of immigration, nativity, and xenophobia among Latina girls, but this information could have helped inform our findings and potential intervention points given that Latina girls specifically experience greater levels of sexual ADV.[23]

Public Health Implications

Experiencing ADV is associated with increased odds of suicide planning among adolescent girls, with notable impacts for Latina girls experiencing only sexual ADV. Potential suicide planning prevention for Latina girls who solely experience sexual ADV may be strengthened by integrating contextually tailored suicide prevention into prevention programs that address healthy relationships and prevention of sexual violence. AJPH

ABOUT THE AUTHORS

Laurel Sharpless is with the Department of Health Behavior, Gillings School of Global Public Health, University of North Carolina, Chapel Hill. Kiara Alvarez is with the Department of Health, Behavior, and Society, Johns Hopkins Bloomberg School of Public Health, Baltimore, MD. Trace Kershaw is with the Department of Social and Behavioral Sciences, Yale School of Public Health, New Haven, CT. Tiara C. Willie is with the Department of Mental Health, Johns Hopkins Bloomberg School of Public Health.

CORRESPONDENCE

Correspondence should be sent to Tiara C. Willie, PhD, MA, Department of Mental Health, Johns Hopkins Bloomberg School of Public Health, 624 N. Broadway, 8th Floor, Baltimore, MD 21205 (e-mail: twillie2@jhu.edu). Reprints can be ordered at https://www.ajph.org by clicking the "Reprints" link.

PUBLICATION INFORMATION

Full Citation: Sharpless L, Alvarez K, Kershaw T, Willie TC. Adolescent dating violence and suicide planning among girls in US high schools: an intra-categorical intersectional analysis by race and ethnicity. *Am J Public Health*. 2025;115(9): 1388–1396.

Acceptance Date: January 24, 2025.

DOI: https://doi.org/10.2105/AJPH.2025.308043

ORCID iDs:

Laurel Sharpless https://orcid.org/0000-0003-4264-8553

Tiara C. Willie https://orcid.org/0000-0003-2848-7212

CONTRIBUTORS

L. Sharpless analyzed the data and wrote the initial drafts of the manuscript. L. Sharpless, T. Kershaw, and T. C. Willie conceptualized the study. L. Sharpless, K. Alvarez, and T. C. Willie contributed to data interpretation. All authors reviewed, revised, and approved the final article.

ACKNOWLEDGMENTS

L. Sharpless was supported by the National Institute of Mental Health via F31MH138053. T. C. Willie was supported by the National Institute on Minority Health and Health Disparities (K01MD015005 and L32MD016555) and the National Institute on Drug Abuse (R25-DA035692). The funding bodies did not play a role in the study's design, data analysis, or data interpretation, or the writing of this article.

We thank those who participated in the study.

CONFLICTS OF INTEREST

The authors declare that they have no conflicts of interest.

HUMAN PARTICIPANT PROTECTION

This study was reviewed by the University of North Carolina at Chapel Hill institutional review board (#24-2387) and determined to be exempt from further review. All human participants in the parent study conducted by the Centers for Disease Control and Prevention were subject to local parental permission procedures.

REFERENCES

1. Clayton HB, Kilmer G, DeGue S, et al. Dating violence, sexual violence, and bullying victimization among high school students—Youth Risk Behavior Survey, United States, 2021. *MMWR Suppl*. 2023;72(1):66–74. https://doi.org/10.15585/mmwr.su7201a8
2. Curtin S, Garnett M. *Suicide and Homicide Death Rates Among Youth and Young Adults Aged 10–24: United States, 2001–2021*. Hyattsville, MD: National Center for Health Statistics; 2023. https://doi.org/10.15620/cdc:128423
3. Baiden P, Mengo C, Small E. History of physical teen dating violence and its association with suicidal behaviors among adolescent high school students: results from the 2015 Youth Risk Behavior Survey. *J Interpers Violence*. 2021; 36(17–18):NP9526–NP9547. https://doi.org/10.1177/0886260519860087
4. Fix RL, Nava N, Rodriguez R. Disparities in adolescent dating violence and associated internalizing and externalizing mental health symptoms by gender, race/ethnicity, and sexual orientation. *J Interpers Violence*. 2022;37(17–18): NP15130–NP15152. https://doi.org/10.1177/0886260521997944
5. Vagi KJ, Olsen EO, Basile KC, Vivolo-Kantor AM. Teen dating violence (physical and sexual) among US high school students. *JAMA Pediatr*. 2015;169(5): 474–482. https://doi.org/10.1001/jamapediatrics.2014.3577
6. Bryan CJ, Corso KA, Neal-Walden TA, Rudd MD. Managing suicide risk in primary care: practice recommendations for behavioral health consultants. *Prof Psychol Res Pr*. 2009;40(2):148–155. https://doi.org/10.1037/a0011141
7. Kessler RC, Borges G, Walters EE. Prevalence of and risk factors for lifetime suicide attempts in the National Comorbidity Survey. *Arch Gen Psychiatry*. 1999;56(7):617–626. https://doi.org/10.1001/archpsyc.56.7.617
8. Nock MK, Borges G, Bromet EJ, et al. Cross-national prevalence and risk factors for suicidal ideation, plans, and attempts. *Br J Psychiatry*. 2008;192(2):98–105. https://doi.org/10.1192/bjp.bp.107.040113
9. Nahapetyan L, Orpinas P, Song X, Holland K. Longitudinal association of suicidal ideation and physical dating violence among high school students. *J Youth Adolesc*. 2014;43(4): 629–640. https://doi.org/10.1007/s10964-013-0006-6
10. Gaylor EM, Krause KH, Welder LE, et al. Suicidal thoughts and behaviors among high school students—Youth Risk Behavior Survey, United States, 2021. *MMWR Suppl*. 2023;72(1):45–54. https://doi.org/10.15585/mmwr.su7201a6
11. Price JH, Khubchandani J. The changing characteristics of African-American adolescent suicides, 2001–2017. *J Community Health*. 2019;44(4): 756–763. https://doi.org/10.1007/s10900-019-00678-x
12. Miranda-Mendizabal A, Castellví P, Parés-Badell O, et al. Gender differences in suicidal behavior in adolescents and young adults: systematic review and meta-analysis of longitudinal studies. *Int J Public Health*. 2019;64(2):265–283. https://doi.org/10.1007/s00038-018-1196-1
13. Lindsey MA, Sheftall AH, Xiao Y, Joe S. Trends of suicidal behaviors among high school students in the United States: 1991–2017. *Pediatrics*. 2019; 144(5):e20191187. https://doi.org/10.1542/peds.2019-1187
14. Bowleg L. The problem with the phrase women and minorities: intersectionality—an important theoretical framework for public health. *Am J*

Public Health. 2012;102(7):1267–1273. https://doi.org/10.2105/AJPH.2012.300750

15. Collins PH, Bilge S. *Intersectionality*. Hoboken, NJ: John Wiley & Sons; 2020.
16. Crenshaw KW. Mapping the margins: intersectionality, identity politics, and violence against women of color. *Stanford Law Rev*. 1991;43(6):1241–1299. https://doi.org/10.2307/1229039
17. Forrest LN, Beccia AL, Exten C, Gehman S, Ansell EB. Intersectional prevalence of suicide ideation, plan, and attempt based on gender, sexual orientation, race and ethnicity, and rurality. *JAMA Psychiatry*. 2023;80(10):1037–1046. https://doi.org/10.1001/jamapsychiatry.2023.2295
18. Roberts L, Tamene M, Orta OR. The intersectionality of racial and gender discrimination among teens exposed to dating violence. *Ethn Dis*. 2018;28(suppl 1):253–260. https://doi.org/10.18865/ed.28.S1.253
19. McCall L. The complexity of intersectionality. *Signs (Chic)*. 2005;30(3):1771–1800. https://doi.org/10.1086/426800
20. Mpofu JJ, Underwood JM, Thornton JE, et al. Overview and methods for the Youth Risk Behavior Surveillance System—United States, 2021. *MMWR Suppl*. 2023;72(1):1–12. https://doi.org/10.15585/mmwr.su7201a1
21. Jones SE, Brener ND, Queen B, et al. Reliability of the 2021 National Youth Risk Behavior Survey Questionnaire. *Am J Health Promot*. 2024;38(6):843–851. https://doi.org/10.1177/08901171241239735
22. Aiken LS, West SG, Reno RR. *Multiple Regression: Testing and Interpreting Interactions*. Newbury Park, CA: Sage; 1991.
23. Robinson LE, Valido A, Rivas-Koehl M, Espelage DL, Aguilar T, Wyman P. Protective factors for multiple forms of interpersonal violence experienced by adolescent Latinas. *J Lat Psychol*. 2024;12(3):211–227. https://doi.org/10.1037/lat0000249
24. Alvarez K, Polanco-Roman L, Breslow AS, Molock S. Structural racism and suicide prevention for ethnoracially minoritized youth: a conceptual framework and illustration across systems. *Am J Psychiatry*. 2022;179(6):422–433. https://doi.org/10.1176/appi.ajp.21101001
25. Gonzalez-Guarda RM, Ferranti D, Halstead V, Ilias VM. Experiences with dating violence and help seeking among Hispanic females in their late adolescence. *Issues Ment Health Nurs*. 2016;37(4):229–238. https://doi.org/10.3109/01612840.2016.1141341
26. Sabina C, Cuevas CA, Rodriguez RM. Who to turn to? Help-seeking in response to teen dating violence among Latinos. *Psychol Violence*. 2014;4(3):348–362. https://doi.org/10.1037/a0035037
27. Cala VC, Soriano-Ayala E. Cultural dimensions of immigrant teen dating violence: a qualitative metasynthesis. *Aggress Violent Behav*. 2021;58:101555. https://doi.org/10.1016/j.avb.2021.101555
28. Samari G, Wurtz HM, Abularrage TF, Sharif MZ. Structural gendered racism as conceptualized by immigrant women in the United States. *Soc Sci Med*. 2024;351:116396. https://doi.org/10.1016/j.socscimed.2023.116396
29. Schiff M. Can restorative justice disrupt the "school-to-prison pipeline"? *Contemp Justice Rev*. 2018;21(2):121–139. https://doi.org/10.1080/10282580.2018.1455509
30. Todić J, Cubbin C, Armour M, Rountree M, González T. Reframing school-based restorative justice as a structural population health intervention. *Health Place*. 2020;62:102289. https://doi.org/10.1016/j.healthplace.2020.102289
31. Baiden P, Onyeaka HK, Aneni K, et al. Racial/ethnic differences in adolescents' non-response to suicide attempt: findings from the Youth Risk Behavior Survey, 2015–2019. *J Psychiatr Res*. 2023;166:115–121. https://doi.org/10.1016/j.jpsychires.2023.09.015
32. Kernan AR, Jones MS, Lehmann PS, Meldrum RC. The intersection of race, ethnicity, and gender and the prevalence of suicidal thoughts and behaviors. *Prev Med Rep*. 2023;36:102426. https://doi.org/10.1016/j.pmedr.2023.102426
33. Romanelli M, Sheftall AH, Irsheid SB, Lindsey MA, Grogan TM. Factors associated with distinct patterns of suicidal thoughts, suicide plans, and suicide attempts among US adolescents. *Prev Sci*. 2022;23(1):73–84. https://doi.org/10.1007/s11121-021-01295-8
34. Richardson SC, Gunn LH. Factors associated with suicide risk behavior outcomes among black middle school adolescents. *J Am Acad Child Adolesc Psychiatry*. 2024;63(12):1215–1224. https://doi.org/10.1016/j.jaac.2024.03.019
35. Lee CS, Wong YJ. Racial/ethnic and gender differences in the antecedents of youth suicide. *Cultur Divers Ethnic Minor Psychol*. 2020;26(4):532–543. https://doi.org/10.1037/cdp0000326

Persistent Sadness, Violence, and Bullying and Associations With Screen Time Among New York City Public High School Students, 2021

Jaynisha Jackson, MS, Meghan Hamwey, PhD, MPH, Nicole Stratton, MPH, and Ashwin Vasan, MD, PhD, ScM

See also Adolescent Mental Health, pp. 1377–1453.

Objectives. To explore the association between persistent feelings of sadness or hopelessness and violence-related experiences, in-school bullying, cyberbullying, and screen time.

Methods. We used data from the 2021 New York City Youth Risk Behavior Survey. Overall and sex-stratified bivariate and logistic regression models were constructed to examine the relationship of persistent feelings of sadness or hopelessness with violence-related experiences, in-school bullying, cyberbullying, and elevated screen time usage.

Results. Persistent feelings of sadness or hopelessness were associated with violence-related experiences, in-school bullying, and cyberbullying among both male and female students, with the prevalence being higher among female students. There was an association between elevated screen time and persistent feelings of sadness and hopelessness only among female students (adjusted odds ratio [AOR] = 1.87; 95% confidence interval [CI] = 1.20, 2.90).

Conclusions. Sex-based differences existed in the association between persistent feelings of sadness or hopelessness and violence-related experiences, in-school bullying, cyberbullying, and elevated screen time. There is a need for interventions, programs, and resources promoting violence- and bullying-free environments and addressing the potential negative effects of screen time. (*Am J Public Health.* 2025;115(9):1397–1407. https://doi.org/10.2105/AJPH.2025.308051)

AJPH September 2025, Vol. 115, No. 9

Mental health encompasses our emotional and psychological well-being and affects the lives of individuals and those around them.[1] As with physical health, mental health fluctuates throughout one's life course and requires attention and maintenance.[2] Promotion of mental health should begin in the early years and continue throughout all phases of life given that good mental health during childhood is critical for psychological development, social relationships, and resilience.[3,4] In this study, we focused on the period of adolescence. During adolescence, critical emotional and developmental milestones are often achieved. Research suggests that more than half of mental health conditions experienced during adulthood can be traced back to adolescent experiences.[5]

Globally, approximately 1 in 7 (14%) youths aged 10 to 19 years experience mental health conditions, depression being among the leading causes of illness and disability among this group.[4] The World Health Organization defines depression as a mental illness characterized by persistent sadness and loss of interest in activities that one normally enjoys accompanied by an inability to carry out daily activities for at least 2 weeks.[6] Findings from the 2021 Youth Risk Behavior Survey (YRBS) revealed that, nationally, 42% of high school students felt so sad or hopeless almost every day for at least 2 weeks that they stopped doing their usual activities, representing a 5%

increase from 2019.[7] Furthermore, the percentage of high school students who experienced persistent feelings of sadness or hopelessness increased from 2011 to 2021 by 8% among male students and 21% among female students.[7]

Research recognizes violence (especially sexual violence and bullying) as an experience with enduring detriments to one's mental health.[4] Unfortunately, in the United States experiencing violence has become a common occurrence among our youths. Nationally, in 2019, approximately one half of high school students experienced at least 1 type of violence, and 1 in 7 experienced 2 or more types.[8] Persistent feelings of sadness or hopelessness were also reported by 42.6% of students who had experienced 1 type of violence and rose to 78.4% among students who experienced 3 or more types of violence.[8] Similar to violence, being bullied or bullying others remains a global problem and negatively affects everyone involved, including witnesses.[9] Nationally, in 2021, female students experienced bullying at school and electronically at higher rates than male students (17% vs 15% and 20% vs 11%, respectively).[7] Exposure to violence and bullying has been linked to poor mental health, substance use, high-risk sexual behavior, sleep difficulties, academic difficulties, and suicidal thoughts or behaviors.[9,10]

Physical activity and elevated screen time have been identified as factors that affect mental health. Research has established regular physical activity as an effective method for controlling mild to moderate depression.[11] Physical activity has also been found to help ameliorate associated burdens and stressors of depressive symptomology by enhancing an individual's mood or sleep quality.[11]

Conversely, elevated screen time has been found to contribute to depression, mood problems, and poor self- and body-image issues and to be associated with cyberbullying, experiences with violence, and risk-taking behaviors.[12] Several longitudinal studies have examined the relationship between screen time and mental health. Using data from the Adolescent Brain Cognitive Development Study, Nagata et al.[13] found prospective associations between higher total screen time and depressive, attention-deficit/hyperactivity, somatic, and conduct symptoms among adolescents. Moreover, Mougharbel et al.[14] found that changes in screen time over a 2-year period, whether increases or decreases, were associated with corresponding changes in depressive and anxiety symptoms.

Such findings are alarming given that digital media and technology are integral parts of our daily lives and that much of adolescents' leisure time is spent using electronic devices.[15] On average, adolescents in the United States spend up to 9 hours a day watching or using screens, almost 5 times more than the American Academy of Pediatrics recommendation of 2 hours or less of daily sedentary screen time.[12,16]

The extant literature has depicted the association between persistent feelings of sadness or hopeless, bullying, and suicidal behaviors. However, little research has focused on the association between persistent feelings of sadness or hopelessness and violence-related experiences according to the screen time use frequency or sex-based differences. Addressing this gap, we explored the association between persistent feelings of sadness or hopelessness, violence-related experiences, in-school bullying, cyberbullying, and screen time. We hypothesized that persistent feelings of sadness or hopelessness would be positively associated with experiences of violence, in-school bullying, and cyberbullying and elevated rates of screen time and that these associations would vary by sex.

METHODS

We used data from the 2021 New York City (NYC) YRBS, a school-based anonymous, self-administered survey completed by public high school students in grades 9 through 12. The NYC YRBS is an ongoing collaboration involving the New York City Department of Health and Mental Hygiene, the New York City Department of Education, and the Centers for Disease Control and Prevention (CDC). The 99-item survey covered the topics of physical activity, mental health, dietary behaviors, bullying, violence, sexual behaviors, alcohol use, and substance use.[17]

The YRBS involves a stratified 2-stage cluster design. In the first stage, schools are randomly selected with probability proportional to school enrollment size from a list provided by the New York City Department of Education.[17] In the second stage, classrooms are placed in a sampling frame and randomly selected.[17] Once classes are selected, all students are eligible to participate; however, the survey is voluntary, and students can choose to opt out. Completed surveys are sent to the CDC, where the data are edited for missing data and inconsistencies.[17,18] A weighting factor is then applied to each student to adjust for nonresponses and varying selection probabilities, and final weights are scaled to match the

NYC public high school population.[17] The data presented here are the weighted population estimates.

In 2021, the survey was completed by 3944 students in 36 public, charter, and vocational high schools across the city.[19] There was a 72% school and student response rate and a 52% overall response rate.[19]

Measures

We examined persistent feelings of hopelessness and sadness and their association with violence-related experiences, in-school bullying, and cyberbullying. Persistent feelings of sadness or hopelessness were measured via the survey question "During the past 12 months, did you ever feel so sad or hopeless almost every day for two weeks or more in a row that you stopped doing some usual activities?" (yes or no). Five violence-related experiences and bullying victimization questions were assessed (Table A, available as a supplement to the online version of this article at https://ajph.org). Questions regarding screen time and physical activity were incorporated into bivariate and multivariable models as covariates (Table A); covariates included race/ethnicity, sex, sexual identity, and a question regarding transgender identity.

Statistical Analysis

Descriptive analyses were conducted to assess the distribution of demographic characteristics and study variables for the overall population and by persistent feelings of sadness of hopelessness. We used χ^2 tests to analyze bivariate associations between persistent feelings of sadness or hopelessness, violence-related experiences, in-school bullying, and cyberbullying overall and stratified by sex. Adjusted odds ratios (AORs) were generated via logistic regression models for the population overall and by sex. Models included demographic characteristics, physical activity, and elevated screen time as covariates. Logistic regression models with sex as an interaction term were also generated to examine whether sex interacted with the study variables.

All statistical tests were considered significant if significance levels were below .05, and estimates are reported with corresponding 95% confidence intervals (CIs). We performed all analyses with SAS-callable SUDAAN Statistical Software version 11.0.4 (Research Triangle Institute, Research Triangle Park, NC) using the provided primary sampling units, strata, and weights to account for the complex survey design and weighting.

RESULTS

Approximately half of the responding students were female (49.0%; Table 1). The race/ethnicity distribution among students included 39.7% Latino/a, 28.2% Black, 14.6% Asian, and 13.6% White; 4.0% of students identified as "other," including those who identified as American Indian/Alaska Native, Native Hawaiian/other Pacific Islander or as being of multiple races. Almost 3 in 4 students (72.5%) were heterosexual, 11.3% were bisexual, 5.3% questioned their sexual identity, 4.4% described their sexual identity some other way, 3.9% were gay or lesbian, and 2.6% were unsure what the sexual identity question was asking. Most students (92.8%) were not transgender; 3.0% (95% CI = 1.6%, 5.4%) were transgender, 2.2% were unsure whether they were transgender, and 2.1% were unsure what the question was asking. Overall, 32.3% of students reported being physically active, and most reported elevated screen time (77.3%).

A total of 38.2% of students (n = 1507) reported feelings of sadness or hopelessness almost every day for 2 consecutive weeks or more (Table 2). Among the racial/ethnic groups, Latino/a (41.9%) and Black (41.2%) students most frequently reported feelings of sadness or hopelessness. Among heterosexual students, 32.0% reported persistent feelings of sadness or hopelessness; among students who described their sexual identity some other way, 63.2% reported persistent feelings of sadness or hopelessness. Almost half of female students (48.4%) reported persistent feelings of sadness or hopelessness. Among transgender students, 71.1% (95% CI = 54.0%, 84.0%) reported persistent feelings of sadness and hopelessness.

The prevalence of persistent feelings of sadness or hopelessness was higher among female students than among male students (48.4% vs 28.2%; Table 3). Among students who reported persistent feelings of sadness or hopelessness, 58.6% did not go to school because of safety concerns, 66.1% (95% CI = 52.8%, 77.2%) were threatened or injured with a weapon on school property, 51.1% witnessed someone being physically hurt on purpose, 65.8% experienced in-school bullying, and 68.6% were cyberbullied.

There were associations between persistent feelings of sadness or hopelessness and violence-related experiences, in-school bullying, and cyberbullying, both overall and by sex. However, the prevalence was higher among female students than male students in the case of all violence-related

TABLE 1— Weighted Characteristics of New York City (NYC) High School Students: 2021

Characteristic	No. (Rounded)	% (95% CI)
Race/ethnicity		
White	36 000	13.6 (9.3, 19.5)
Black	75 000	28.2 (23.4, 33.5)
Latino/a	105 000	39.7 (34.2, 45.5)
Asian	39 000	14.6 (11.2, 18.7)
Other (American Indian/Alaska Native, Native Hawaiian/other Pacific Islander, multiple)	11 000	4.0 (3.1, 5.1)
What is your sex?		
Female	132 000	49.0 (43.9, 54.2)
Male	138 000	51.0 (45.8, 56.2)
Sexual identity		
Heterosexual (straight)	195 000	72.5 (68.6, 76.1)
Gay or lesbian	11 000	3.9 (2.8, 5.4)
Bisexual	30 000	11.3 (9.8, 13.0)
I describe my sexual identity some other way	12 000	4.4 (3.0, 6.3)
I am not sure about my sexual identity (questioning)	14 000	5.3 (4.0, 6.9)
I do not know what this question is asking	7 000	2.6 (2.0, 3.5)
Are you transgender?		
No, I am not transgender	253 000	92.8 (89.0, 95.3)
Yes, I am transgender	8 000	3.0[a] (1.6, 5.4)
I am not sure if I am transgender	6 000	2.2 (1.3, 3.7)
I do not know what this question is asking	6 000	2.1 (1.3, 3.2)
Physically active[b]		
Yes	71 000	32.3 (28.9, 36.0)
No	149 000	67.7 (64.0, 71.1)
Elevated screen time[c]		
Yes	171 000	77.3 (74.2, 80.1)
No	50 000	22.7 (19.9, 25.8)

Note. CI = confidence interval. Data were derived from the 2021 NYC Youth Risk Behavior Survey. Data are weighted to the NYC public high school population and are not age adjusted. For the purposes of this tabulation, Latino/a includes individuals of Hispanic, Latino, or Spanish origin, as identified via the survey question, "Are you Hispanic or Latino?" and regardless of race. The Black, White, Asian, and other race categories excluded those who identified as Latino/a. Weighted population estimates are rounded to the nearest 1000.

[a]Estimate should be interpreted with caution. The estimate's relative standard error (a measure of estimate precision) is greater than 30%, the 95% confidence interval half width is greater than 10, or the sample size is too small, making the estimate potentially unreliable.

[b]At least 60 minutes per day on 5 or more days, including any kind of physical activity that increased students' heart rate and made them breathe hard some of the time during the 7 days before the survey.

[c]Including time spent in front of a TV, computer, smartphone, or other electronic device watching shows or videos, playing games, accessing the Internet, or using social media (not including time spent doing schoolwork) on an average day.

experiences and both in-school bullying and cyberbullying. Persistent feelings of sadness or hopelessness were also associated with elevated screen time but only among female students. Among students who reported persistent feelings of sadness or hopelessness and elevated screen time, 50.7% were female, a higher portion than in the overall sample (40.2%). There was no association between persistent feelings of sadness or hopelessness and being physically active either overall or by sex.

Logistic regression models with sex as an interaction term (data not shown) showed that sex had a positive interaction with elevated screen time and negative interactions with in-school bullying and cyberbullying. Overall, female students were twice as likely to report persistent feelings of sadness or hopelessness than male students (Table 4). Similarly, Black and Latino/a students were twice as likely as White students to report persistent feelings of sadness and hopelessness.

Gay or lesbian students, bisexual students, and students who described their sexual identity in another way had higher odds of experiencing feelings of sadness or hopelessness than heterosexual students. In addition, transgender students were 3 times as likely to experience feelings of sadness and hopelessness as nontransgender students. Cyberbullying (AOR = 2.94; 95% CI = 2.12, 4.08), in-school bullying (AOR = 2.06; 95% CI = 1.21, 3.50), witnessing someone being physically hurt on purpose (AOR = 2.03; 95% CI = 1.70, 2.42), not going to school because of safety concerns (AOR = 1.72; 95% CI = 1.23, 2.41), and elevated screen time (AOR = 1.52; 95% CI = 1.08, 2.15) were associated with higher odds of experiencing persistent feelings of sadness or hopelessness.

As with the overall model, the stratified models showed that lesbian female students were 3 times as likely to report persistent feelings of sadness and hopelessness as heterosexual female students. Also, transgender female students were 4 times as likely

TABLE 2— Prevalence of Persistent Feelings of Sadness and Hopelessness Among New York City (NYC) High School Students by Selected Demographic Characteristics: 2021

Characteristic	No. (Rounded)	% (95% CI)
Overall	102 000	38.2 (35.1, 41.5)
Race/ethnicity		
White	11 000	29.9 (23.5, 37.2)
Black	30 000	41.2 (36.8, 45.8)
Latino/a	43 000	41.9 (35.8, 48.2)
Asian	13 000	33.4 (27.1, 40.4)
Other (American Indian/Alaska Native, Native Hawaiian/other Pacific Islander, multiple)	4 000	37.4 (29.2, 46.4)
What is your sex?		
Female	63 000	48.4 (44.7, 52.1)
Male	38 000	28.2 (24.8, 32.0)
Sexual identity		
Heterosexual (straight)	61 000	32.0 (29.0, 35.2)
Gay or lesbian	6 000	58.9[a] (47.6, 69.4)
Bisexual	18 000	62.5 (56.1, 68.4)
I describe my sexual identity some other way	7 000	63.2 (55.1, 70.7)
I am not sure about my sexual identity (questioning)	7 000	48.4[a] (36.4, 60.7)
I do not know what this question is asking	1 000	20.6[a] (11.2, 34.7)
Are you transgender?		
No, I am not transgender	91 000	36.7 (34.0, 39.5)
Yes, I am transgender	5 000	71.1[a] (54.0, 84.0)
I am not sure if I am transgender	4 000	75.4[a] (62.5, 85.0)
I do not know what this question is asking	1 000	24.5[a] (14.5, 38.4)

Note. CI = confidence interval. Data were derived from the 2021 NYC Youth Risk Behavior Survey. Data are weighted to the NYC public high school population and are not age adjusted. For the purposes of this tabulation, Latino/a includes individuals of Hispanic, Latino, or Spanish origin, as identified via the survey question, "Are you Hispanic or Latino?" and regardless of race. The Black, White, Asian, and other race categories excluded those who identified as Latino/a. Weighted population estimates are rounded to the nearest 1000.

[a]Estimate should be interpreted with caution. The estimate's relative standard error (a measure of estimate precision) is greater than 30%, the 95% confidence interval half width is greater than 10, or the sample size is too small, making the estimate potentially unreliable.

to report persistent feelings of sadness and hopelessness as nontransgender female students. Both female and male students who witnessed someone being physically hurt on purpose or did not go to school because of safety concerns were twice as likely to report persistent feelings of sadness and hopelessness. Higher odds of reporting persistent feelings of sadness or hopelessness were observed among male students (AOR = 3.51; 95% CI = 2.08, 5.91) than female students (AOR = 2.44; 95% CI = 1.56, 3.83) who were cyberbullied.

Interestingly, the association between persistent feelings of sadness or hopelessness and in-school bullying was seen only among male students. Male students who were bullied at school had twice the odds of reporting persistent feelings of sadness or hopelessness (AOR = 2.27; 95% CI = 1.03, 4.98). An association with elevated screen time was found only among female students. Female students reporting elevated screen time had twice the odds of experiencing persistent feelings of sadness as female students reporting less than 3 hours of screen time.

DISCUSSION

Persistent feelings of sadness or hopelessness are widespread among NYC students, as nearly 40% of public high school students reported such feelings in 2021. This is of concern because these feelings are a predictor of depression. Experiences with violence and bullying have been identified as determinants of depression, and depression has been determined to be a strong predictor of youth suicidal behavior.[8] Understanding potential factors that correlate with persistent feelings of sadness and hopelessness is crucial in reducing these rates. It is also necessary to investigate disparities by sex, sexual identity, and transgender identity because we found that the prevalence of these feelings is higher among female students, sexual minority students, and transgender students.

The results of this study support our hypothesis and previous research showing that persistent feelings of sadness or hopelessness are associated with violence-related experiences, in-school bullying, and cyberbullying among both female and male students; however, higher rates were observed among female students. The higher prevalence among female students echoes previous findings from the CDC indicating that female adolescents are more likely to experience 3 or more types of violence than male adolescents and more often report dating

TABLE 3— Bivariate Associations of Persistent Feelings of Sadness and Hopelessness With Violence-Related Experiences, Bullying Victimization, Physical Activity, and Elevated Screen Time, Overall and by Sex: New York City (NYC), 2021

	Overall			Female			Male		
	No. (Rounded)	% (95% CI)	P	No. (Rounded)	% (95% CI)	P	No. (Rounded)	% (95% CI)	P
Overall	102 000	38.2 (35.1, 41.5)		63 000	48.4 (44.7, 52.1)		38 000	28.2 (24.8, 32.0)	
Did not go to school because of feeling unsafe at school or on the way to or from school[a]			<.001			<.001			<.001
Yes	19 000	58.6 (53.0, 64.0)		11 000	74.1 (63.2, 82.6)		7 000	44.3 (37.8, 51.1)	
No	83 000	35.4 (31.7, 39.4)		51 000	44.9 (40.8, 49.0)		31 000	26.1 (22.0, 30.7)	
Threatened or injured with a weapon on school property[b]			<.001			.004			.001
Yes	9000	66.1[c] (52.8, 77.2)		4 000	80.5[c] (64.7, 90.3)		5 000	59.2[c] (43.5, 73.2)	
No	93 000	36.8 (33.6, 40.1)		59 000	47.2 (43.4, 51.0)		33 000	26.3 (22.7, 30.2)	
Witnessed someone being physically hurt on purpose[d]			<.001			<.001			<.001
Yes	51 000	51.1 (47.0, 55.1)		32 000	62.2 (57.2, 67.0)		19 000	38.9 (34.0, 44.1)	
No	49 000	30.3 (26.4, 34.5)		30 000	39.3 (34.9, 43.8)		19 000	22.4 (18.1, 27.4)	
Bullied on school property[e]			<.001			<.001			.001
Yes	18 000	65.8 (58.2, 72.7)		10 000	69.5 (61.0, 76.9)		8 000	61.4[c] (50.0, 71.7)	
No	83 000	34.9 (31.5, 38.4)		53 000	45.7 (41.7, 49.8)		29 000	24.3 (21.0, 28.0)	
Cyberbullied[f]			<.001			<.001			<.001
Yes	24 000	68.6 (61.6, 74.8)		14 000	72.4 (64.7, 79.0)		9 000	63.6 (53.4, 72.6)	
No	77 000	33.3 (29.7, 37.0)		48 000	43.7 (39.9, 47.7)		28 000	23.5 (20.2, 27.2)	
Physically active[g]			.8			.82			.44
Yes	26 000	37.7 (31.9, 44.0)		15 000	47.0 (38.2, 56.0)		12 000	30.2 (24.1, 37.1)	
No	56 000	38.4 (34.8, 42.4)		36 000	48.0 (43.6, 52.5)		19 000	27.4 (22.7, 32.8)	
Elevated screen time[h]			.002			<.001			.78
Yes	67 000	40.2 (35.9, 44.7)		44 000	50.7 (46.2, 55.1)		22 000	28.4 (23.5, 33.8)	
No	14 000	30.2 (25.2, 35.6)		6 000	33.9 (25.2, 43.9)		7 000	27.1 (20.8, 34.5)	

Note. CI = confidence interval. Data were derived from the 2021 NYC Youth Risk Behavior Survey. Data are weighted to the NYC public high school population and are not age adjusted. Weighted population estimates are rounded to the nearest 1000.

[a]On at least 1 day during the 30 days before the survey.

[b]Such as a gun, knife, or club 1 or more times during the 12 months before the survey.

[c]Estimate should be interpreted with caution. The estimate's relative standard error (a measure of estimate precision) is greater than 30%, the 95% confidence interval half width is greater than 10, or the sample size is too small, making the estimate potentially unreliable.

[d]Includes being hit, slammed into something, or injured with an object or weapon 1 or more times during the 12 months before the survey.

[e]During the past 12 months.

[f]Including being bullied through texting, Instagram, Facebook, or other social media during the 12 months before the survey.

[g]At least 60 minutes per day on 5 or more days, including any kind of physical activity that increased students' heart rate and made them breathe hard some of the time during the 7 days before the survey.

[h]Including in front of a TV, computer, smartphone, or other electronic device watching shows or videos, playing games, accessing the Internet, or using social media (not including time spent doing schoolwork) on an average day.

TABLE 4— Adjusted Logistic Association of Persistent Feelings of Sadness and Hopelessness With Violence-Related Experiences, Bullying Victimization, Physical Activity, and Elevated Screen Time, Overall and by Sex: New York City (NYC), 2021

Characteristic	Overall AOR (95% CI)	Female AOR (95% CI)	Male AOR (95% CI)
Race/ethnicity			
White (ref)	1	1	1
Black	1.82 (1.34, 2.48)	1.58 (0.95, 2.62)	1.89 (0.91, 3.91)
Latino/a	1.86 (1.20, 2.89)	1.53 (0.79, 2.97)	2.23 (1.13, 4.38)
Asian	1.47 (0.94, 2.29)	1.63 (1.01, 2.61)	1.18 (0.48, 2.90)
Other (American Indian/Alaska Native, Native Hawaiian/other Pacific Islander, multiple)	1.65 (0.95, 2.87)	1.49 (0.63, 3.54)	1.76 (0.74, 4.21)
What is your sex?			
Female	1.98 (1.64, 2.38)	...	...
Male (ref)	1	...	...
Sexual identity			
Heterosexual (straight) (ref)	1	1	1
Gay or lesbian	2.85 (1.26, 6.48)	3.13 (1.01, 9.68)	1.63 (0.54, 4.98)
Bisexual	1.85 (1.37, 2.50)	1.79 (1.34, 2.37)	2.42 (0.70, 8.38)
I describe my sexual identity some other way	3.33 (1.84, 6.05)	2.95 (1.32, 6.59)	4.59 (0.43, 49.14)
I am not sure about my sexual identity (questioning)	1.65 (0.92, 2.93)	1.37 (0.76, 2.48)	2.48 (1.47, 4.20)
I do not know what this question is asking	0.59 (0.23, 1.53)	0.34 (0.07, 1.63)	0.76 (0.28, 2.02)
Are you transgender?			
No, I am not transgender (ref)	1	1	1
Yes, I am transgender	3.36 (2.14, 5.25)	3.55 (1.66, 6.34)	3.01 (0.57, 15.78)
I am not sure if I am transgender	3.67 (1.27, 10.59)	2.06 (0.89, 4.47)	14.99 (1.30, 140.58)
I do not know what this question is asking	0.37 (0.21, 0.65)	0.74 (0.34, 1.62)	0.15 (0.04, 0.61)
Did not go to school due to safety concerns[a]			
No (ref)	1	1	1
Yes	1.72 (1.23, 2.41)	2.03 (1.01, 4.09)	1.65 (1.13, 2.41)
Threatened or injured with a weapon on school property[b]			
No (ref)	1	1	1
Yes	2.04 (0.90, 4.62)	2.84 (0.57, 14.09)	1.66 (0.81, 3.41)
Witnessed someone being physically hurt on purpose[c]			
No (ref)	1	1	1
Yes	2.03 (1.70, 2.42)	2.02 (1.51, 2.71)	2.08 (1.51, 2.87)
In-school bullying[d]			
No (ref)	1	1	1
Yes	2.06 (1.21, 3.50)	1.69 (0.81, 3.51)	2.27 (1.03, 4.98)
Cyberbullying[e]			
No (ref)	1	1	1
Yes	2.94 (2.12, 4.08)	2.44 (1.56, 3.83)	3.51 (2.08, 5.91)
Physically active[f]			
No (ref)	1	1	1
Yes	1.11 (0.83, 1.48)	0.96 (0.66, 1.40)	1.32 (0.87, 1.98)

Continued

TABLE 4— Continued

Characteristic	Overall AOR (95% CI)	Female AOR (95% CI)	Male AOR (95% CI)
Elevated screen time[g]			
No (ref)	1	1	1
Yes	1.52 (1.08, 2.15)	1.87 (1.20, 2.90)	1.24 (0.75, 2.03)

Note. AOR = adjusted odds ratio; CI = confidence interval. Data were derived from the 2021 NYC Youth Risk Behavior Survey. Data are weighted to the NYC public high school population and are not age adjusted. For the purposes of this tabulation, Latino/a includes individuals of Hispanic, Latino, or Spanish origin, as identified via the survey question, "Are you Hispanic or Latino?" and regardless of race. The Black, White, Asian, and other race categories excluded those who identified as Latino/a.
[a]On at least 1 day during the 30 days before the survey.
[b]Such as a gun, knife, or club 1 or more times during the 12 months before the survey.
[c]Includes being hit, slammed into something, or injured with an object or weapon 1 or more times during the 12 months before the survey.
[d]During the past 12 months.
[e]Including being bullied through texting, Instagram, Facebook, or other social media during the 12 months before the survey.
[f]At least 60 minutes per day on 5 or more days, including any kind of physical activity that increased students' heart rate and made them breathe hard some of the time during the 7 days before the survey.
[g]Including in front of a TV, computer, smartphone, or other electronic device watching shows or videos, playing games, accessing the Internet, or using social media (not including time spent doing schoolwork) on an average day.

violence, sexual violence, and bullying.[8,20] Our findings underscore the sex-based disparities in the association between persistent feelings of sadness or hopelessness, violence, and bullying and show that there is a demonstrable need for greater support among this population.

Furthermore, our results emphasize the need for continuous support for sexual minority and transgender adolescents. Our outcomes corroborate and extend existing research showing that sexual minority and transgender youths are at heightened risk for depression and peer victimization, including bullying and threatening behavior.[21,22]

We also found racial differences in reports of persistent feelings of sadness or hopelessness, with a higher prevalence among Black and Latino/a students. Our finding highlights previous literature indicating that minorities experience higher levels of depressive symptoms across early life than Whites.[23] In addition, Sen[24] found that Black, Asian, and Hispanic adolescents were more likely to suffer from depressed mood than White adolescents. Even with such findings, racial/ethnic minority adolescents are affected disproportionately by unmet treatment needs.[25] Although our results strengthen existing research, they show the further need to understand and diminish the disparities other racial groups experience regarding mental health.

Unexpectedly, physical activity was not shown to be helpful in preventing persistent feelings of sadness and hopelessness. Specifically, there was no difference between students who were and were not physically active regarding reported feelings of sadness and hopelessness. Given this finding, additional research is needed to better understand the role of physical activity in mental health. Interestingly, although there was a relationship between elevated screen time and persistent feelings of sadness or hopelessness, the relationship was observed only among female students, even after control for cyberbullying, in-school bullying, violence, and physical activity. A previous population-level study discussed this relationship and suggested that adolescent girls who engage in screen time for longer may do so because of social and emotional difficulties (e.g., social isolation), which can negatively affect their mental health.[26]

In addition, our results are consistent with a previous population-based study showing that youths reporting elevated screen time were twice as likely to be diagnosed with depression or anxiety or to need treatment for mental or behavioral health conditions as youths not reporting elevated screen time.[15] Furthermore, research has shown that media activities vary by sex, with adolescent girls spending more time on smartphones, social media, and computers in general and boys spending more time gaming and on electronic devices in general.[27] The fact that there was no association between screen time and persistent feelings of sadness or hopelessness among male students shows that the focus should be not only on screen time but on the types of media activities engaged in while on screens, especially given that screen time in this study encompassed time spent on a range of media sources including social media, computers, smartphones, television, and video games.

Limitations

This study involved several limitations. First, the NYC YRBS is administered only to NYC public high school students, so our results can be generalized to that population but not to others, including private school students and public high school students outside of NYC. Future studies would benefit from considering the full youth population in NYC to understand whether differences are present.

Second, the NYC YRBS is a cross-sectional study and, as a result of its design, causality cannot be established. However, because the survey questions are asked over multiple years, a repeated cross-sectional time trend analysis can be conducted to further understand the relationships between the variables included in our study.

Third, the NYC YRBS involves self-reported data, which have the potential of introducing bias. Students may not answer questions accurately for numerous reasons such as embarrassment, fear, or simply not remembering certain events. This can lead to overestimation or underestimation of the resulting data.

Finally, screen time included being in front of a TV, computer, smartphone, or other electronic device watching shows or videos, playing games, accessing the Internet, or using social media. Although there was an association between elevated screen time and experiencing persistent feelings of sadness or hopelessness among female students, a particular screen time type cannot be specified.

Social media has been a recent topic of interest with mixed findings regarding its impact on mental health. Adolescents with positive perceptions describe social media as a place that encourages self-expression and can contribute to well-being as a source of peer support and social engagement.[28] However, recent data show that in the United States, youths spend an average of 5 hours per day on social media, and research has established associations between social media use and increased levels of depression and anxiety, lower self-esteem, and poorer sleep quality.[29,30] Notably, a recent mental health survey administered to NYC youths revealed that those who used social media experienced anxiety and depression at higher rates than those who did not.[31]

If the types of activities occurring on devices with screens are separated, differences in associations with experiences of persistent sadness or hopelessness can be investigated. For example, is there a difference in experiencing persistent feelings of sadness or hopelessness between students who spend 3 or more hours per day watching TV and those who spend 3 or more hours per day playing video games?

Public Health Implications

Overall, our study strengthens existing research on persistent feelings of sadness or hopelessness and violence-related experiences, cyberbullying, and in-school bullying. Given widespread reporting of persistent feelings of sadness or hopelessness among NYC high school students, identifying factors that may contribute to their emergence is essential. In addition, our findings point to the need to address the sex, sexual identity, and transgender-based inequities we observed. The prevalence of violence-related experiences, cyberbullying, and in-school bullying was higher among female students than among male students. Also, gay or lesbian students, students who described their sexual identity in another way, students who questioned their sexual identity, transgender students, and students who were unsure whether they were transgender had higher odds of experiencing persistent feelings of sadness or hopelessness than heterosexual and nontransgender students.

Our study findings also highlight the need for programs, interventions, and resources for students who experience violence or bullying and the need for bullying and violence prevention programs. Importantly, elevated screen time was shown to be an independent factor only among female students after control for violence-related experiences, in-school bullying, cyberbullying, and physical activity. This result underscores the need for further research on the types of screen-based activities that contribute to poorer mental health among this population and the need for interventions and policies.

Our findings point to the need to create safe spaces for those who engage in screen time, especially given that 77% of students reported screen times of 3 or more hours per day. The New York City Public Schools Digital Citizenship Curriculum and the New York City Department of Health and Mental Hygiene's Social Media and Youth Mental Health: A Guide for Parents and Caregivers are examples of guidelines and resources. The Digital Citizenship Curriculum provides guidance for parents, students, and teachers to help students act in ways that lead to effective digital learning, remain safe online, and become good digital citizens.[32] The Social Media and Youth Mental Health Guide aims to achieve an open dialogue between parents and their children about social media use while also enabling parents to learn more about social media, youth mental health, and ways to reduce exposure to harmful content.[33] Through the use of such resources and programs, NYC is working toward creating a safer and more positive media space for young people. AJPH

ABOUT THE AUTHORS

Jaynisha Jackson, Meghan Hamwey, and Nicole Stratton are with the Bureau of Children, Youth, Families and Developmental Disabilities, New York City Department of Health and Mental Hygiene, Long Island City, NY. At the time of this study, Ashwin Vasan was with the Office of the Commissioner, New York City Department of Health and Mental Hygiene, New York, NY.

CORRESPONDENCE

Correspondence should be sent to Jaynisha Jackson, MS, New York City Department of Health and Mental Hygiene, 42-09 28th St, Long Island City, NY 11101 (e-mail: jjackson11@health.nyc.gov). Reprints can be ordered at https://www.ajph.org by clicking the "Reprints" link.

PUBLICATION INFORMATION

Full Citation: Jackson J, Hamwey M, Stratton N, Vasan A. Persistent sadness, violence, and bullying and associations with screen time among New York City public high school students, 2021. *Am J Public Health*. 2025;115(9):1397–1407.

Acceptance Date: January 31, 2025.

DOI: https://doi.org/10.2105/AJPH.2025.308051

ORCID iDs:

Jaynisha Jackson https://orcid.org/0009-0001-1121-9927

Meghan Hamwey https://orcid.org/0000-0002-8687-0749

Nicole Stratton https://orcid.org/0009-0006-4519-2933

CONTRIBUTORS

J. Jackson conceptualized and designed the study, performed the data analysis, and drafted the article. M. Hamwey, N. Stratton, and A. Vasan provided critical revisions. N. Stratton assisted with the data analysis and provided analytic support.

ACKNOWLEDGMENTS

We thank the Center for Population Health Data Science for its assistance with data analysis and interpretation. We also thank Jordan Fenlon for his assistance in the editing and revision process.

CONFLICTS OF INTEREST

The authors have no conflicts of interest to declare.

HUMAN PARTICIPANT PROTECTION

This study was approved by the institutional review board of the New York City Department of Health and Mental Hygiene. The study data are publicly available.

REFERENCES

1. US Department of Health and Human Services. US surgeon general's advisory: protecting youth mental health. Available at: https://www.hhs.gov/sites/default/files/surgeon-general-youth-mental-health-advisory.pdf. Accessed July 22, 2024.
2. Gautam S, Jain A, Chaudhary J, Gautam M, Gaur M, Grover S. Concept of mental health and mental well-being, it's determinants and coping strategies. *Indian J Psychiatry*. 2024;66(suppl 2):S231–S244. https://doi.org/10.4103/indianjpsychiatry.indianjpsychiatry_707_23
3. Cho SM, Shin YM. The promotion of mental health and the prevention of mental health problems in child and adolescent. *Korean J Pediatr*. 2013;56(11):459–464. https://doi.org/10.3345/kjp.2013.56.11.459
4. World Health Organization. Mental health of adolescents. Available at: https://www.who.int/news-room/fact-sheets/detail/adolescent-mental-health. Accessed July 16, 2024.
5. Kessler RC, Berglund P, Demler O, Jin R, Merikangas KR, Walters EE. Lifetime prevalence and age-of-onset distributions of DSM-IV disorders in the National Comorbidity Survey replication. *Arch Gen Psychiatry*. 2005;62(6):593–602. https://doi.org/10.1001/archpsyc.62.6.593
6. World Health Organization. Depression. Available at: https://www.who.int/india/health-topics/depression. Accessed August 30,2024.
7. Centers for Disease Control and Prevention. Youth Risk Behavior Survey data summary and trends report 2011–2021. Available at: https://www.cdc.gov/healthyyouth/data/yrbs/pdf/yrbs_data-summary-trends_report2023_508.pdf. Accessed June 27, 2024.
8. David-Ferdon C, Clayton HB, Dahlberg L, et al. Vital signs: prevalence of multiple forms of violence and increased health risk behaviors and conditions among youths—United States, 2019. *MMWR Morb Mortal Wkly Rep*. 2021;70(5):167–173. https://doi.org/10.15585/mmwr.mm7005a4
9. Centers for Disease Control and Prevention. About bullying. Available at: https://www.cdc.gov/youth-violence/about/about-bullying.html. Accessed June 27, 2024.
10. National Center for Injury Prevention and Control. CDC vital signs: violence impacts teens' lives. Available at: https://stacks.cdc.gov/view/cdc/136372. Accessed July 22, 2024.
11. Samsudin N, Bailey RP, Ries F, Hashim SNAB, Fernandez JA. Assessing the impact of physical activity on reducing depressive symptoms: a rapid review. *BMC Sports Sci Med Rehabil*. 2024;16(1):107. https://doi.org/10.1186/s13102-024-00895-5
12. American Academy of Child and Adolescent Psychiatry. Screen time and children. Available at: https://www.aacap.org/AACAP/Families_and_Youth/Facts_for_Families/FFF-Guide/Children-And-Watching-TV-054.aspx. Accessed June 28, 2024.
13. Nagata JM, Al-Shoaibi AAA, Leong AW, et al. Screen time and mental health: a prospective analysis of the Adolescent Brain Cognitive Development (ABCD) Study. *BMC Public Health*. 2024;24(1):2686. https://doi.org/10.1186/s12889-024-20102-x
14. Mougharbel F, Chaput JP, Sampasa-Kanyinga H, et al. Longitudinal associations between different types of screen use and depression and anxiety symptoms in adolescents. *Front Public Health*. 2023;11:1101594. https://doi.org/10.3389/fpubh.2023.1101594
15. Twenge JM, Campbell WK. Associations between screen time and lower psychological well-being among children and adolescents: evidence from a population-based study. *Prev Med Rep*. 2018;12:271–283. https://doi.org/10.1016/j.pmedr.2018.10.003
16. Santos RMS, Mendes CG, Sen Bressani GY, et al. The associations between screen time and mental health in adolescents: a systematic review. *BMC Psychol*. 2023;11(1):127. https://doi.org/10.1186/s40359-023-01166-7
17. New York City Department of Health and Mental Hygiene. Comprehensive YRBS High School Methods Report. Available at: https://www.nyc.gov/assets/doh/downloads/pdf/survey/yrbs-methods-report.pdf. Accessed July 2,2024.
18. Mpofu JJ, Underwood JM, Thornton JE, et al. Overview and methods for the Youth Risk Behavior Surveillance System—United States, 2021. *MMWR Suppl*. 2023;72(1):1–12. https://doi.org/10.15585/mmwr.su7201a1
19. New York City Department of Health and Mental Hygiene. New York City High School Survey—survey summary. Available at: https://www.nyc.gov/assets/doh/downloads/pdf/episrv/survey-summary-yrbs-2021.pdf. Accessed June 13, 2024.
20. Clayton HB, Kilmer G, DeGue S, et al. Dating violence, sexual violence, and bullying victimization among high school students—Youth Risk Behavior Survey, United States, 2021. *MMWR Suppl*. 2023;72(suppl 1):66–74. https://doi.org/10.15585/mmwr.su7201a8
21. Guz S, Kattari SK, Atteberry-Ash B, Klemmer CL, Call J, Kattari L. Depression and suicide risk at the cross-section of sexual orientation and gender identity for youth. *J Adolesc Health*. 2021;68(2):317–323. https://doi.org/10.1016/j.jadohealth.2020.06.008
22. Norris AL, Orchowski LM. Peer victimization of sexual minority and transgender youth: a cross-sectional study of high school students. *Psychol Violence*. 2020;10(2):201–211. https://doi.org/10.1037/vio0000260
23. Adkins DE, Wang V, Elder GH Jr. Structure and stress: trajectories of depressive symptoms across adolescence and young adulthood. *Soc Forces*. 2009;88(1):31–60. https://doi.org/10.1353/sof.0.0238

24. Sen B. Adolescent propensity for depressed mood and help seeking: race and gender differences. *J Ment Health Policy Econ.* 2004;7(3):133–145.
25. Chang AR, Slopen N. Racial and ethnic disparities for unmet needs by mental health condition: 2016 to 2021. *Pediatrics.* 2024;153(1):e2023062286. https://doi.org/10.1542/peds.2023-062286
26. Oberle E, Ji XR, Kerai S, Guhn M, Schonert-Reichl KA, Gadermann AM. Screen time and extracurricular activities as risk and protective factors for mental health in adolescence: a population-level study. *Prev Med.* 2020;141:106291. https://doi.org/10.1016/j.ypmed.2020.106291
27. Twenge JM, Martin GN. Gender differences in associations between digital media use and psychological well-being: evidence from three large datasets. *J Adolesc.* 2020;79(1):91–102. https://doi.org/10.1016/j.adolescence.2019.12.018
28. Popat A, Tarrant C. Exploring adolescents' perspectives on social media and mental health and well-being—a qualitative literature review. *Clin Child Psychol Psychiatry.* 2023;28(1):323–337. https://doi.org/10.1177/13591045221092884
29. Rosewell J. How parenting and self-control mediate the link between social media use and youth mental health. Available at: https://ifstudies.org/ifs-admin/resources/briefs/ifs-gallup-parenting socialmediascreentime-october2023-1.pdf. Accessed August 13, 2024.
30. Woods HC, Scott H. #Sleepyteens: social media use in adolescence is associated with poor sleep quality, anxiety, depression and low self-esteem. *J Adolesc.* 2016;51(1):41–49. https://doi.org/10.1016/j.adolescence.2016.05.008
31. Hamwey M, Gordon K, Stratton N, Jackson J, Abdelnabi J. Special report on social media and mental health. Available at: https://www.nyc.gov/assets/doh/downloads/pdf/mh/social-media-mental-health-report-2024.pdf?trk=public_post_comment-text. Accessed August 13, 2024.
32. New York City Public Schools. Digital citizenship. Available at: https://www.schools.nyc.gov/school-life/school-environment/digital-citizenship. Accessed August 13, 2024.
33. New York City Department of Health and Mental Hygiene. Social media and youth mental health: a guide for parents and caregivers. Available at: https://www.nyc.gov/assets/doh/downloads/pdf/mh/social-media-guide-parents.pdf. Accessed August 13, 2024.

Cost-Effectiveness of an Economic Empowerment and Family Intervention on Mental Health Among School-Going Adolescent Girls in Uganda, 2017–2022

Fred M. Ssewamala, PhD, Yesim Tozan, PhD, Rachel Brathwaite, PhD, Joshua Kiyingi, PhD, Phionah Namatovu, MPH, Ozge Sensoy Bahar, PhD, Proscovia Nabunya, PhD, Portia B. Nartey, MSW, and Torsten B. Neilands, PhD

See also Adolescent Mental Health, pp. 1377–1453.

Objectives. To assess the cost-effectiveness of an economic empowerment and family intervention on mental health outcomes among school-going adolescent girls in Uganda from 2017 to 2022.

Methods. We randomized adolescent girls aged 14 to 17 years into 3 arms: (1) health and sex education (usual care; n = 408), (2) youth development accounts (YDAs; n = 471), and (3) a combination intervention (YDA plus multiple family group [MFG]; n = 381). We fitted mixed-effects models and estimated intervention costs prospectively using the microcosting approach.

Results. The combination intervention had a statistically significant impact on mental health outcomes (depressive symptoms, hopelessness, self-concept) at 12 and 24 months, except self-esteem at 24 months, relative to usual care, with incremental cost–effectiveness ratios ranging from $51 to $100 per 0.2-SD change at 12 months, and $53 to $157 at 24 months per 0.2-SD change.

Conclusions. The combination intervention positively and significantly impacted a higher number of mental health outcomes among school-going adolescent girls compared with YDA alone. The benefits were sustained in the short and long term, with the incremental cost-per-unit effect remaining comparable. Findings support the integration of combination interventions in school settings to promote adolescent girls' positive mental health functioning.

Trial Registration. ClinicalTrials.gov registration no. NCT03307226. (*Am J Public Health*. 2025;115(9): 1408–1416. https://doi.org/10.2105/AJPH.2025.308135)

Despite the progress made in improving access to effective HIV prevention, treatment, and care programs over the past few decades,[1] HIV continues to be a significant public health burden in sub-Saharan Africa (SSA).[1–3] SSA was estimated to be home to 71% of people with HIV (PWH) and accounted for approximately 65% of new HIV infections worldwide in 2021.[1] Within SSA, adolescent girls and young women face multiple vulnerabilities to HIV, including biological, behavioral, and socio-structural risk factors.[4] A healthy adolescence is critical for a successful transition into adulthood.[5] Yet, poverty and limited access to health care, education, and social support can undermine this essential developmental stage. Adolescence is a period when various health risks and challenges often emerge, including exploratory sexual behaviors, substance use, and poor mental health.[6] Globally, adolescents are increasingly representing a substantial portion of people living with HIV.[7] UNICEF reports that around 360 000 adolescents and young people aged 15 to 24 years were newly infected with HIV in 2023, with 140 000

AJPH September 2025, Vol. 115, No. 9

of these new infections occurring among those aged 15 to 19 years.[8] Moreover, the most recent data indicate that only 29% of adolescent girls in East and Southern Africa are aware of their HIV status.[8] In SSA, new HIV infections among adolescent girls were nearly 6 times more frequent than among their male peers.[8]

Adolescents in SSA also face a substantial burden of mental health issues, with research showing that girls experience these challenges at a disproportionately higher rate compared with boys.[9–11] Furthermore, mental health problems, such as depression, low self-esteem, and anxiety, are known to be associated with increased HIV risk.[12] Against this background, a multilevel response has been called for to address the complex and multidimensional drivers of HIV risk among adolescent girls in SSA to reach the 95-95-95 Joint United Nations Program on HIV/AIDS goal by 2030.[4] These targets aim for 95% of PWH to know their status, 95% of those diagnosed to receive sustained antiretroviral therapy (ART), and 95% of those on ART to achieve viral suppression. This strategy is critical for reducing onward transmission, improving health outcomes among PWH, and advancing efforts to end the HIV/AIDS epidemic. Poverty significantly affects sexual risk behaviors and mental health outcomes of adolescents.[13] Existing theories and evidence suggest that social protection programs, such as savings-led economic empowerment interventions, can help mitigate the risks faced by children affected by HIV/AIDS. In particular, savings-led interventions may help reduce sexual risk-taking and improve mental health outcomes among adolescents.[14] In addition, family strengthening programs have significantly improved children's mental health functioning in SSA.[15,16]

In the Central Region of Uganda, which has a disproportionately high HIV prevalence of 10.6% compared with the national mean of 7.4%,[17] a randomized controlled trial titled "Suubi4Her" was implemented between 2017 and 2022.[18] Aimed at addressing the multidimensional drivers of HIV risk, the Suubi4Her intervention combined an asset-based financial inclusion and economic empowerment model with a family-strengthening approach to reduce HIV risk behaviors among adolescent girls. Evaluation of this combination intervention revealed that adolescent girls in the treatment arms showed a significant reduction in depressive symptoms and feelings of hopelessness, along with improvements in self-concept, at both 12 and 24 months after the intervention.[19,20]

Economic empowerment and mental health interventions can address the diverse needs of HIV-at-risk adolescents in resource-limited settings.[14–16] To justify public investment, it is essential to pair effectiveness evidence with cost data. Cost–effectiveness analyses identify interventions offering the greatest benefits relative to costs, aiding resource allocation amid competing priorities. However, evidence on cost–effectiveness for improving adolescent girls' health outcomes remains limited. In this study, we evaluated the economic value of a combined intervention in Uganda, featuring a savings-led economic empowerment program (using youth development accounts [YDAs]) and a family strengthening approach (multiple family group [MFG]). The study aims to reduce sexual risk-taking and improve mental health among disadvantaged adolescent girls.

Our earlier research showed that this combined intervention improved mental health in at-risk adolescent girls compared with usual care in the short term.[16,19,21] However, key questions remain about the duration of these benefits and their associated costs. Using 12- and 24-month follow-up data, we examined the intervention's sustained efficacy and cost–effectiveness over time. Specifically, we evaluated the intervention's impact on 4 mental health outcomes—depressive symptoms, hopelessness, self-concept, and self-esteem—over 2 years postintervention compared with usual care.

METHODS

The current analysis utilized baseline, 12-month, and 24-month follow-up data from the Suubi4Her trial. Suubi4Her was a 5-year (2017–2022) randomized controlled trial designed to evaluate the efficacy and cost-effectiveness of a combined intervention aimed at reducing sexual risk-taking behaviors and improving mental health among adolescent girls in low-resource settings in Uganda. The study recruited 1260 adolescents from 47 secondary schools across 5 districts in Southern Uganda (Figure A, available as a supplement to the online version of this article at http://www.ajph.org).

Participants were randomized at the school level into 3 study arms:

1. Usual care: This group (n = 408 girls; 16 schools) received educational materials about sexual and reproductive health, approved by the Ministry of Education of Uganda.
2. Incentivized YDAs: This group (n = 471 girls; 16 schools) received YDAs in the form of incentivized savings with a 1-to-1 match rate. The funds were deposited at a

national financial institution, with matched funds kept separately to safeguard these funds for education-related expenses. This prevented families from pressuring girls to withdraw the savings for other purposes. Participants could use up to 30% of their combined savings for income-generating activities, while the remaining 70% was strictly for their education and skills development.

3. Combination intervention (YDA+MFG): This group (n = 381 girls; 15 schools) received both YDA and MFG. MFG is a 16-session evidence-based family-strengthening intervention designed to enhance youth behavior by strengthening family relationships and addressing mental health challenges that commonly occur in adolescence. MFG fosters family support by creating a safe space where parents and children can connect with other families facing similar challenges. This peer-to-peer learning allows families to learn from each other's experiences. The 16-session MFG curriculum was facilitated by trained community health workers and parent peers, and focused on building essential skills for healthy family functioning. These included setting clear rules, establishing responsibilities, building strong relationships, fostering respectful communication, managing stress, and strengthening social support.

Adolescent girls were recruited on the basis of the following criteria: (1) enrolled in the first year of secondary school, (2) aged 14 to 17 years, and (3) living within a family setting (not in orphanages or foster homes). Written consent was obtained from participants' guardians, while the girls provided voluntary assent in a private setting.

Measures

Depressive symptoms were assessed with a 20-item Beck Depression Inventory scale (Cronbach $\alpha = 0.85$).[22] The scale measures characteristic attitudes and symptoms of depression, including suicidal ideation. All items in the scale were summed to create a continuous variable, with higher scores indicating higher levels of depressive symptoms. Hopelessness was measured with the 20-item Beck Hopelessness Scale (Cronbach $\alpha = 0.73$).[23] The Hopelessness Scale measures pessimistic attitudes toward the future, with 9 reverse-coded items summed into a continuous variable; higher scores indicate greater hopelessness. Self-concept[24,25] was assessed with the Tennessee Self-Concept Scale (Cronbach $\alpha = 0.85$), with 20 items (10 reverse-coded) summed into a continuous variable; higher scores reflect better self-concept. Self-esteem was measured with the Rosenberg Self-Esteem Scale (Cronbach $\alpha = 0.71$),[26] with 10 items summed into a continuous variable; higher scores indicate greater self-esteem.

Intervention Efficacy

We analyzed and presented baseline characteristics of participants using counts and percentages for categorical variables, while we summarized continuous variables using means and SDs. To evaluate the impact of the intervention on the 4 mental health outcomes, we fitted 3-level linear mixed-effects models. The 3-level models accounted for the nested structure of the data, with repeated measurements (level 1) nested within individuals (level 2), and individuals nested within schools (level 3). This hierarchical structure reflects the study design and ensures accurate estimation of fixed and random effects while appropriately modeling the variability at each level. Each model included fixed categorical effects for the study group, time, and the interaction between study group and time, as well as a random intercept at the school level. The group-by-time interaction term was included to test whether the intervention's impact on mental health outcomes differed across time points. We included a random intercept at the school level to account for between-school variability, as schools can influence mental health outcomes through shared environmental factors or intervention delivery. This random effect allows the model to partition variance attributable to differences between schools while improving precision in the fixed-effect estimates. We employed an unstructured residual-error covariance matrix to account for residuals from repeated assessments of the same participants, allowing for variability in residuals across groups. We computed variance–covariance matrices of parameter estimates using robust Huber–White standard errors. We assessed omnibus effects for the study group, time, and the group-by-time interaction. In addition, we computed within-group effects across time, regardless of the significance of the group-by-time interaction effect. We conducted all analyses with Stata version 17 (StataCorp LP, College Station, TX).

Intervention Costs

We calculated intervention costs for the usual care, YDA, and YDA+MFG arms from a health care provider perspective using a combination of activity-based and ingredients-based costing approaches. This involved identifying all activities within each study arm, then measuring and valuing the resources used for each activity, including program overheads and capital costs. Activities included identification of schools, recruitment of study participants, opening and contributions to YDAs, delivery of financial literacy training education workshops and MFG sessions, and stakeholder engagement. All costs were recorded alongside the implementation of the Suubi4Her trial, and the costing analysis has been published elsewhere.[27] We calculated per-participant costs for each cost category using the treatment-on-the-treated (TOT) sample and summed these costs to estimate the total per-participant cost for each arm over the intervention period. We adjusted all costs for inflation using the Ugandan Consumer Index, discounted at an annual rate of 3% to the start year of the trial, and presented in 2018 US dollars.

Cost–Effectiveness Analysis

The cost–effectiveness analysis was based on the cost data collected throughout the Suubi4her trial from project inception to closeout. We collected outcome data at baseline, 12 months, and 24 months. We calculated incremental cost-effectiveness ratios (ICERs) with the cost difference between each treatment arm (YDA and YDA+MFG) and the usual care arm as the numerator, and the difference in mean treatment effects between these arms as the denominator. This analysis aimed to determine the cost of achieving per unit of effect with YDA or YDA+MFG compared with usual care. We used the per-participant cost from each study arm based on TOT sample. We assessed the effects of the intervention on mental health outcomes using intention-to-treat (ITT) sample. We calculated standardized mean differences between each treatment arm and the usual care arm, referred to as effect sizes, with a 0.2-SD change considered as a small effect size according to Cohen's guidelines.[28] Finally, we calculated ICERs using the aforementioned formulation and determined the per-participant cost per 0.2-SD change for each study outcome. The analysis was reported in accordance with the Consolidated Health Economic Evaluation Reporting Standards.

Sensitivity Analysis

We performed a sensitivity analysis by using the 95% confidence intervals (CIs) of the effect sizes and adjusting the total per-participant costs of the intervention within a range of 80% and 120% of the original estimate. We calculated ICERs across these ranges to assess pessimistic (high cost/low effectiveness) and optimistic (low cost/high effectiveness) scenarios for YDA and YDA+MFG.

RESULTS

The study recruited 1260 adolescent girls, with 408 in usual care, 471 in YDA-only, and 381 in YDA+MFG. Participants' mean age was 15.4 years (±0.9 SD). Approximately 83% were nonorphans, 1.9% double orphans, and 15.2% single orphans. More than 76% lived with biological parents, and 11.1% with grandparents. About 23% of care givers were formally employed, and 25.3% had completed some secondary education. The mean household size was 7 (±2.7 SD). Further details are in Table 1.

Table 2 presents the effects of the intervention on the mental health outcomes as determined by 3-level linear regression analysis. At 12 months, adolescent girls in the YDA+MFG intervention had significantly fewer depressive symptoms (b = −2.13; 95% CI = −2.18, −0.36; P = .006) and feelings of hopelessness (b = −0.55; 95% CI = −0.94, −0.16; P = .005) than girls receiving usual care. Girls receiving the YDA+MFG intervention displayed higher levels of self-concept (b = 1.81; 95% CI = 0.02, 3.61; P = .047) and self-esteem (b = 1.63; 95% CI = 0.60, 2.66; P = .002) compared with those in the usual care arm. These findings suggest that the YDA+MFG intervention had a meaningful and significant impact on improving mental health, with better outcomes on key indicators of emotional distress. In addition, girls receiving YDA only displayed higher levels of self-concept (b = 1.85; 95% CI = 0.28, 3.43; P = .021) and self-esteem (b = 0.94; 95% CI = 0.01, 1.87; P = .047) compared with those in the usual care arm. These positive effects suggest that YDA alone can enhance the sense of self-worth and self-perception among adolescent girls. At 24 months, the YDA+MFG intervention continued to have a statistically significant impact on depressive symptoms (b = −2.04; 95% CI = −2.18, −0.36; P = .003) and hopelessness (b = −0.69; 95% CI = −1.16, −0.22; P = .047), as well as self-concept (b = 2.74; 95% CI = 0.57, 4.92; P = .013) among adolescent girls compared with those who received usual care. These sustained improvements indicate that the YDA+MFG intervention had a long lasting positive effect on mental health outcomes.

Table 3 outlines the total per-participant costs using the TOT sample for each of the 3 study arms. The cost

TABLE 1— Baseline Characteristics of the Study Population: Uganda, 2017–2022

Characteristics	Total (n = 1260), Mean ±SD or No. (%)	Usual Care (n = 408), Mean ±SD or No. (%)	YDA (n = 471), Mean ±SD or No. (%)	YDA+MFG (n = 381), Mean ±SD or No. (%)
Age, y	15.4 ±0.9	15.2 ±0.9	15.5 ±0.8	15.4 ±0.9
Orphanhood status				
Double orphan	24 (1.9)	7 (1.7)	8 (1.7)	9 (2.4)
Single orphan	191 (15.2)	59 (14.5)	72 (15.3)	60 (15.8)
Nonorphan	1045 (82.9)	342 (83.8)	391 (83.0)	312 (81.9)
Primary caregiver				
Biological parents	965 (76.6)	312 (76.5)	370 (78.6)	283 (74.3)
Grandparents	140 (11.1)	46 (11.3)	54 (11.5)	40 (10.5)
Other relatives or nonrelatives	155 (12.3)	50 (12.2)	47 (10.0)	58 (15.2)
Primary caregiver employment status				
Formally employed	292 (23.2)	102 (25.0)	104 (22.1)	86 (22.6)
Not formally employed	968 (76.8)	306 (75.0)	367 (77.9)	295 (77.4)
Primary caregiver education level				
Did not go to school or completed all or part of primary-level education	496 (39.4)	144 (35.3)	186 (39.5)	166 (43.6)
Completed all or part of secondary-level education	319 (25.3)	115 (28.2)	110 (23.3)	94 (24.7)
Completed technical diploma or university degree	137 (10.9)	40 (9.8)	59 (12.5)	38 (10.0)
Don't know	308 (24.4)	109 (26.7)	116 (24.6)	83 (21.8)
Household size	7.0 ±2.7	6.8 ±2.6	7.0 ±2.7	7.2 ±2.9

Note. MFG = multiple family group; YDA = youth development account.

per participant for the usual care arm was US $272, US $476 for the YDA-only arm, and US $812 for the YDA+MFG arm.

Table 4 presents the ICERs for mental health outcomes for which the effects of YDA and YDA+MFG were statistically significant compared with the usual care arm at 12 and 24 months. At 12 months, the ICER of YDA for self-concept was US $22 (95% CI = 12, 146) per 0.2 SD, and for self-esteem US $43

TABLE 2— Linear Mixed Effects Models Evaluating the Intervention Effects on Mental Health Outcomes: Uganda, 2017–2022

Model Components	Depressive Symptoms	Hopelessness	Self-Concept	Self-Esteem
Study group, $\chi2$ (*P*)	16.46 (<.001)	2.54 (.28)	6.75 (.034)	10.74 (.005)
YDA, b (95% CI)	−1.36 (−2.82, 0.10)	0.09 (−0.34, 0.52)	0.45 (−1.43, 2.33)	0.48 (−0.14, 1.11)
YDA+MFG, b (95% CI)	0.76 (−5.07, −3.54)	0.23 (−0.17, 0.64)	0.30 (−1.42, 2.02)	−0.11 (−0.83, 0.62)
Group#time, $\chi2(4)$ (*P*)	13.08 (.011)	11.77 (.019)	10.14 (.038)	13.68 (.008)
12 mo#YDA, b (95% CI)	−0.91 (−2.18, 0.36)	−0.41 (−0.90, −0.09)	1.85 (0.28, 3.43)	0.94 (0.01, 1.87)
12 mo#YDA+MFG, b (95% CI)	−2.13 (−2.18, −0.36)	−0.55 (−0.94, −0.16)	1.81 (0.02, 3.61)	1.63 (0.60, 2.66)
24 mo#YDA, b (95% CI)	−0.02 (−1.34, 1.31)	−0.39 (−0.86, 0.08)	1.51 (−0.34, 3.37)	−0.14 (−0.81, 0.52)
24 mo#YDA+MFG, b (95% CI)	−2.04 (−3.37, −0.72)	−0.69 (−1.16, −0.22)	2.74 (0.57, 4.92)	0.64 (−0.14, 1.43)
Constant, b (95% CI)	19.20 (18.16, 20.24)	4.87 (4.59, 5.14)	80.61 (79.19, 82.03)	32.85 (32.34, 33.36)
No. of participants	1260	1260	1260	1260
No. of observations	3644	3644	3409	3643

Note. # = interaction term; CI = confidence interval; MFG = multiple family group; YDA = youth development account. The control group is the reference group.

TABLE 3— Itemized Total Per-Participant Costs Using the Treatment-on-Treated: Uganda, 2017–2022

Costs	Usual Care	YDA	YDA+MFG
Personnel	752 852	1 319 618	2 245 824
Identification of schools and school visits	948	821	1 015
Screening and recruitment of study participants	16 097	16 084	17 935
Usual care	96 730	83 792	103 585
YDAs	...	77 490	86 578
Delivery of FLT sessions	...	18 854	25 795
Delivery of IGA sessions	...	4 874	5 084
Training of MFG facilitators	...	...	1 438
Delivery of MFG sessions	...	...	99 326
Donated resources	4 504	9 691	23 769
Program overheads	123 245	213 388	367 650
Stakeholder engagement and dissemination	12 266	16 662	26 157
Capital costs	7 259	12 724	21 654
Total costs	1 013 900	1 773 997	3 025 810
Total costs (in 2018 US $)	272	476	812

Note. FLT = financial literacy training; IGA = income generating activities; MFG = multiple family group; YDA = youth development account. All costs are in 2018 Ugandan shillings unless otherwise indicated.

(95% CI = 22, 4080) per 0.2 SD relative to the usual care arm. For YDA+MFG, the ICERs were higher, at US $60 (95% CI = 30, 5400) per 0.2 SD for self-concept and US $66 (95% CI = 41, 180) per 0.2 SD for self-esteem. The ICER of YDA+MFG for depressive symptoms was US $51 (95% CI = 50, 300) per 0.2 SD and for hopelessness US $100 (95% CI = 115, 675) per 0.2 SD relative to the usual care arm.

At 24 months, the ICERs for depressive symptoms, hopelessness, and self-concept for YDA+MFG relative to usual care were US $53 (95% CI = 32, 150), US $157 (95% CI = 93, 491), and US $39 (95% CI = 22, 189) per 0.2 SD, respectively. Overall, YDA+MFG had a statistically significant impact on all mental health outcomes at both 12 and 24 months, except for self-esteem at 24 months, relative to usual care, with ICERs ranging from $51 to $100 per 0.2-SD change at 12 months, and $53 to $157 at 24 months per 0.2-SD change. These findings indicate that the combination intervention yielded a significant and lasting impact on a greater number of mental health outcomes in adolescents compared with YDA alone, with comparable incremental costs per unit effect.

Table A (available as a supplement to the online version of this article at https://ajph.org) shows sensitivity analysis results and ICERs for significant mental health outcomes at 12 and 24 months under optimistic (high-cost/low-effectiveness) and pessimistic (low-cost/high-effectiveness) scenarios. The findings align with the primary analysis, showing that YDA+MFG's cost for a

TABLE 4— Incremental Cost-Effectiveness Ratios (ICERs) for Mental Health Outcomes of YDA and YDA+MFG at 12- and 24-Month Follow-Up: Uganda, 2017–2022

	12 Months		24 Months	
Mental Health Outcome	YDA, ICER (95% CI)	YDA+MFG, ICER (95% CI)	YDA, ICER (95% CI)	YDA+MFG, ICER (95% CI)
Depressive symptoms	45 (−0.2, 113)	51 (50, 300)	2040 (−81, 31)	53 (32, 150)
Hopelessness	100 (−45, 453)	100 (115, 675)	105 (−47, 510)	157 (93, 491)
Self-concept	22 (12, 146)	60 (30, 5400)	27 (−120, 12)	39 (22, 189)
Self-esteem	43 (22, 4080)	66 (41, 180)	291 (−50, 78)	169 (−771, 76)

Note. CI = confidence interval; MFG = multiple family group; YDA = youth development account.

0.2-SD improvement relative to usual care remained consistent. ICERs ranged from $24 to $6480, reflecting cost and effectiveness variations. This range underscores the sensitivity of cost–effectiveness estimates to key parameter changes, highlighting the need to consider potential fluctuations in costs and effectiveness when interpreting results.

DISCUSSION

In this study, we evaluated the efficacy and cost-effectiveness of a savings-led intervention targeting adolescent girls in Uganda, focusing on 4 mental health outcomes: depressive symptoms, hopelessness, self-concept, and self-esteem. At 12 months postintervention, adolescent girls receiving YDA+MFG reported lower levels of depressive symptoms and hopelessness compared with those in the YDA and usual care arms (Table 2). For self-concept and self-esteem, outcomes were similar across the YDA and YDA+MFG arms (Table 2). Specifically, adolescent girls in both treatment conditions had improvements compared with those in the usual care arm, but the YDA+MFG arm had higher ICERs compared with the YDA arm for the statistically significant mental health outcomes (Table 4). This indicates that YDA was more cost–effective, with lower ICERs for achieving a 0.2-SD change relative to usual care.

At 24 months, YDA+MFG showed significant effects on depressive symptoms, hopelessness, and self-concept compared with usual care, with ICERs ranging from US $39 to US $157 per 0.2-SD change (Table 4). ICERs for depressive symptoms and hopelessness increased, reflecting decreasing effectiveness, while ICERs for self-concept decreased as the intervention's impact improved. Overall, 24-month ICERs (US $50 to US $100 per 0.2-SD change; Table 4) were higher than at 12 months, indicating reduced intervention effects over time.

Per-participant costs were conservatively calculated using the TOT sample. Based on the intention-to-treat sample, costs would be lower: $264 for usual care, $534 for YDA, and $737 for YDA+MFG (Table B, available as a supplement to the online version of this article at https://ajph.org), leading to less conservative ICER estimates per 0.2-SD change. Given Suubi4Her's resource-intensive strategy, per-participant costs are expected to decrease when integrated into broader health care systems, with further reductions possible through scaled-up delivery.

The Suubi4Her study targeted multiple mental health outcomes for Ugandan adolescent girls, presenting ICERs for each outcome. At 24 months, YDA+MFG showed sustained improvements in depressive symptoms, hopelessness, and self-concept compared with usual care, with ICERs ranging from US $39 to US $157 per 0.2-SD change (Table 4). This indicates that adding MFG to YDA provided lasting mental health benefits, while YDA alone's effects diminished. YDA+MFG demonstrated more sustained impacts, suggesting that combination interventions hold promise in resource-limited settings. Higher matching rates have shown long-term mental health benefits for AIDS-affected adolescents in SSA. Future studies should explore higher matching rates and replicate findings to build an evidence base for policy development.

MFG and savings-led economic empowerment interventions have been proven to significantly improve health outcomes among vulnerable households in low-resource settings.[15,16,29] Several studies that have implemented family strengthening and savings-led economic empowerment interventions have attempted to report the associated costs. The SMART Africa study in Uganda, which implemented MFG interventions with children and adolescents, demonstrated improvements in self-concept and reductions in depressive symptoms over time.[16] This study estimated a per-participant cost of approximately $255 per child for the MFG intervention.[30] In South Africa, a similar family-strengthening intervention resulted in improved mental health outcomes among adolescents living with HIV,[15] though no costing or cost–effectiveness analysis was conducted. Another South African study estimated the cost of a parenting program aimed at preventing violence against adolescents to be US $504 per family, with a cost of US $1837 per incident of physical or emotional abuse averted.[31] In Malawi, a savings-led economic empowerment program led by the government successfully improved the mental health outcomes of children over time, yet no cost data were reported.[32] Another Ugandan study implemented a family-based savings-led economic empowerment intervention aimed at improving health and mental health outcomes of children and adolescents affected by HIV/AIDS. This study reported the cost of the intervention to range between US $418 and $426 per child, with ICERs between $224 and $298 per 0.2-SD change.[33] However, evidence suggests that economic empowerment interventions alone may not be sufficient to achieve significant improvements in mental health outcomes.[29]

Our study uniquely contributes to mental health intervention literature by combining incentivized microsavings-led economic empowerment with MFG, a novel approach lacking established cost–effectiveness benchmarks. This gap complicates the interpretation of our results. However, our rigorous analysis of efficacy and cost data for 2 treatment arms—YDA and YDA+MFG—at 12- and 24-month follow-ups offers valuable insights into their relative impacts and costs, advancing understanding of this innovative intervention model.

Overall, our findings suggest that the combination intervention had a positive impact on mental health outcomes among adolescent girls in low-resource settings, demonstrating benefits both in the short and long term. The significant and sustained improvements across various critical mental health outcomes in this high-risk population underscore the importance and value of investing in interventions that combine savings-led economic empowerment and family strengthening (i.e., MFG) components. This evidence supports the ongoing development and implementation of such interventions to effectively promote mental health among adolescent girls in resource-limited contexts.

This study had limitations. We used self-reported data to assess mental health and sexual risk-taking behaviors, reflecting participants' perceptions rather than clinical diagnoses. While self-reports are prone to social desirability bias, measures like anonymity, validated tools, and consistent protocols were employed to reduce its impact. However, some bias, particularly for mental health outcomes, may persist. The cost–effectiveness findings were derived solely from quantitative methods, though qualitative insights could enhance understanding of context and intervention mechanisms. A follow-up qualitative study highlighted the acceptability of the intervention among adolescent girls.[34] Future research should combine qualitative and quantitative methods to explore causal pathways and broader impacts, validate findings across contexts, and establish cost–effectiveness benchmarks. This will strengthen the evidence for savings-led economic empowerment and family-strengthening interventions in resource-limited settings. AJPH

ABOUT THE AUTHORS

Fred M. Ssewamala, Rachel Brathwaite, Ozge Sensoy Bahar, Proscovia Nabunya, and Portia B. Nartey are with Brown School, Washington University in St. Louis, MO. Yesim Tozan is with New York University School of Global Public Health, New York, NY. Joshua Kiyingi and Torsten B. Neilands are with the Division of Prevention Science, University of California, San Francisco. Phionah Namatovu is with the International Center for Child Health and Development, Masaka, Uganda.

CORRESPONDENCE

Correspondence should be sent to Fred M. Ssewamala, William E. Gordon Distinguished Professor, Brown School, Washington University in St. Louis, St. Louis, MO 63130 (e-mail: fms1@wustl.edu). Reprints can be ordered at https://www.ajph.org by clicking the "Reprints" link.

PUBLICATION INFORMATION

Full Citation: Ssewamala FM, Tozan Y, Brathwaite R, et al. Cost-effectiveness of an economic empowerment and family intervention on mental health among school-going adolescent girls in Uganda, 2017–2022. *Am J Public Health*. 2025;115(9): 1408–1416.

Acceptance Date: March 23, 2025.

DOI: https://doi.org/10.2105/AJPH.2025.308135

ORCID iDs:

Rachel Brathwaite https://orcid.org/0000-0002-9363-3581

Joshua Kiyingi https://orcid.org/0000-0001-7264-6976

Portia B. Nartey https://orcid.org/0000-0001-8929 6028

Torsten B. Neilands https://orcid.org/0000-0001-7936-9123

CONTRIBUTORS

F. M. Ssewamala conceptualized and designed the Suubi4Her Study on which this article is based, acquired funding for the Suubi4Her study, supervised the work, and reviewed and edited the article. J. Kiyingi and Y. Tozan performed the data analysis and wrote the initial draft of the article. R. Brathwaite, O. Sensoy Bahar, P. Nabunya, P. Namatovu, P. B. Nartey, and T. B. Neilands reviewed and edited the article. All authors provided critical inputs and edits to the article and its revisions and approved the final article for submission.

ACKNOWLEDGMENTS

This study was supported by the National Institute of Mental Health (NIMH) under award 1R01MH113486-01 (Principal Investigator: Fred M. Ssewamala, PhD).

We extend our gratitude to the staff at the International Center for Child Health and Development field office in Uganda for their invaluable contributions to the study's design and implementation, as well as to our implementation partners, including Reach the Youth Uganda, Rakai Health Sciences Program, and the partnering financial institutions that managed the savings accounts for study participants. Special thanks to the Ugandan Ministry of Education and the 47 secondary schools that participated in the Suubi4Her study.

Note. The content in this article is solely the responsibility of the authors and does not necessarily represent the official views of NIMH or the National Institutes of Health.

CONFLICTS OF INTEREST

The authors declare no conflicts of interest.

HUMAN PARTICIPANT PROTECTION

The Suubi4Her study was conducted in accordance with the Declaration of Helsinki and approved by the Washington University in St. Louis institutional review board (IRB no. 201703102), the Uganda Virus Research Institute (GC/127/17/07/619), and the Uganda National Council of Science and Technology (SS4406). The study is also registered in the ClinicalTrials.gov database (identifier: NCT03307226).

REFERENCES

1. World Health Organization. HIV and AIDS. July 22, 2024. Available at: https://www.who.int/news-room/fact-sheets/detail/hiv-aids. Accessed August 2, 2024
2. Ramjee G, Daniels B. Women and HIV in Sub-Saharan Africa. *AIDS Res Ther*. 2013;10(1):30. https://doi.org/10.1186/1742-6405-10-30
3. Moyo E, Moyo P, Murewanhema G, et al. Key populations and Sub-Saharan Africa's HIV response. *Front Public Health*. 2023;11:1079990. https://doi.org/10.3389/fpubh.2023.1079990
4. *Global Health Sector Strategy on HIV, Viral Hepatitis, and Sexually Transmitted Infections for the Period 2022–2030*. Geneva, Switzerland: World Health Organization; 2022.

5. Ahmed Zaky E. Adolescence; a crucial transitional stage in human life. *J Child Adolesc Behav.* 2016;4(6). https://doi.org/10.4172/2375-4494.1000e115
6. Janighorban M, Boroumandfar Z, Pourkazemi R, Mostafavi F. Barriers to vulnerable adolescent girls' access to sexual and reproductive health. *BMC Public Health.* 2022;22(1):2212–2216. https://doi.org/10.1186/s12889-022-14687-4
7. Calabrese S, Perkins M, Lee S, et al. Adolescent and young adult research across the HIV prevention and care continua: an international programme analysis and targeted review. *J Int AIDS Soc.* 2023;26(3):e26065. https://doi.org/10.1002/jia2.26065
8. UNICEF Data. Adolescent HIV prevention. Available at: https://data.unicef.org/topic/hivaids/adolescents-young-people. Accessed August 2, 2024
9. Abbo C, Kinyanda E, Kizza RB, et al. Prevalence, comorbidity and predictors of anxiety disorders in children and adolescents in rural north-eastern Uganda. *Child Adolesc Psychiatry Ment Health.* 2013;7(1):21. https://doi.org/10.1186/1753-2000-7-21
10. Campbell OLK, Bann D, Patalay P. The gender gap in adolescent mental health: a cross-national investigation of 566,829 adolescents across 73 countries. *SSM Popul Health.* 2021;13:100742. https://doi.org/10.1016/j.ssmph.2021.100742
11. Cortina MA, Sodha A, Fazel M, Ramchandani PG. Prevalence of child mental health problems in sub-Saharan Africa: a systematic review. *Arch Pediatr Adolesc Med.* 2012;166(3):276–281. https://doi.org/10.1001/archpediatrics.2011.592
12. Goin DE, Pearson RM, Craske MG, et al. Depression and incident HIV in adolescent girls and young women in HIV Prevention Trials Network 068: targets for prevention and mediating factors. *Am J Epidemiol.* 2020;189(5):422–432. https://doi.org/10.1093/aje/kwz238
13. Mabrouk A, Mbithi G, Chongwo E, et al. Mental health interventions for adolescents in sub-Saharan Africa: a scoping review. *Front Psychiatry.* 2022;13:937723. https://doi.org/10.3389/fpsyt.2022.937723
14. Cluver L, Boyes M, Orkin M, et al. Child-focused state cash transfers and adolescent risk of HIV infection in South Africa: a propensity-score-matched case–control study. *Lancet Glob Health.* 2013;1(6):e362–e370. https://doi.org/10.1016/S2214-109X(13)70115-3
15. Bhana A, Mellins CA, Petersen I, et al. The VUKA family program: piloting a family-based psychosocial intervention to promote health and mental health among HIV infected early adolescents in South Africa. *AIDS Care.* 2014;26(1):1–11. https://doi.org/10.1080/09540121.2013.806770.
16. Ssewamala FM, Brathwaite R, Sensoy Bahar O, et al. The post-intervention impact of Amaka Amasanyufu on behavioral and mental health functioning of children and adolescents in low-resource communities in Uganda: analysis of a cluster-randomized trial from the SMART Africa-Uganda Study (2016–2022). *J Adolesc Health.* 2023;72(5S):S3–S10. https://doi.org/10.1016/j.jadohealth.2022.09.035
17. Government of Uganda. Uganda HIV/AIDS country progress report July 2017–June 2018. 2018. Available at: https://uac.go.ug/images/2024/jar-2024/jar-report-2018.pdf. Accessed July 22, 2024.
18. Ssewamala FM, Bermudez LG, Neilands TB, et al. Suubi4Her: a study protocol to examine the impact and cost associated with a combination intervention to prevent HIV risk behavior and improve mental health functioning among adolescent girls in Uganda. *BMC Public Health.* 2018;18(1):693. https://doi.org/10.1186/s12889-018-5604-5
19. Byansi W, Ssewamala FM, Neilands TB, et al. The short-term impact of a combination intervention on depressive symptoms among school-going adolescent girls in Southwestern Uganda: the Suubi4Her Cluster Randomized Trial. *J Adolesc Health.* 2022;71(3):301–307. https://doi.org/10.1016/j.jadohealth.2022.04.008
20. Ssewamala FM, Brathwaite R, Neilands TB. Economic empowerment, HIV risk behavior, and mental health among school-going adolescent girls in Uganda: longitudinal cluster-randomized controlled trial, 2017–2022. *Am J Public Health.* 2023;113(3):306–315. https://doi.org/10.2105/AJPH.2022.307169
21. Filiatreau LM, Tutlam N, Brathwaite R, et al. Effects of a combination economic empowerment and family strengthening intervention on psychosocial well-being among Ugandan adolescent girls and young women: analysis of a cluster randomized controlled trial (Suubi4Her). *J Adolesc Health.* 2023;72(5 suppl):S33–S40. https://doi.org/10.1016/j.jadohealth.2022.11.250
22. Beck AT, Ward CH, Mendelson M, Mock J, Erbaugh J. An inventory for measuring depression. *Arch Gen Psychiatry.* 1961;4:561–571. https://doi.org/10.1001/archpsyc.1961.01710120031004
23. Beck AT, Weissman A, Lester D, Trexler L. The measurement of pessimism: the hopelessness scale. *J Consult Clin Psychol.* 1974;42(6):861–865. https://doi.org/10.1037/h0037562
24. TCS Education System Libraries. Tennessee Self-Concept Scale: TSCS-2. Available at: https://search.tcsedsystem.edu/permalink/01TCSEDSYSTEM_INST/dcoso6/alma991000097949706756. Accessed July 6, 2024.
25. Outcome Measure Tennessee Self-Concept Scale-2 (TSCS-2). Available at: https://movingahead.psy.unsw.edu.au/documents/research/outcome%20measures/adult/Measures%20of%20Self/Website%20TSCS-2.pdf. Accessed July 6, 2024. doi:10.1080/02699050400005218
26. Rosenberg M. *Society and the Adolescent Self-Image.* Princeton, NJ: Princeton University Press; 1965. https://doi.org/10.1515/9781400876136
27. Tozan Y, Kiyingi J, Kim S, Namuwonge F, et al. Costing of a combination intervention (Suubi4Her) to prevent HIV risk behaviors and improve mental health functioning among school-going adolescent girls in southwestern Uganda. *PLOS Ment Health.* 2024; 1(7):e0000201. https://doi.org/10.4269/ajtmh.23-0485
28. Sullivan GM, Feinn R. Using effect size—or why the *P* value is not enough. *J Grad Med Educ.* 2012;4(3):279–282. https://doi.org/10.4300/JGME-D-12-00156.1
29. Maara J, Cirillo C, Angeles G, Malawi SCT Evaluation Team., et al. Impacts of cash transfer and "cash plus" programs on self-perceived stress in Africa: evidence from Ghana, Malawi, and Tanzania. *SSM Popul Health.* 2023;22:101403. https://doi.org/10.1016/j.ssmph.2023.101403
30. Tozan Y, Capasso A, Namatovu P, et al. Costing of a multiple family group strengthening intervention (SMART Africa) to improve child and adolescent behavioral health in Uganda. *Am J Trop Med Hyg.* 2022;106(4):1078–1085. https://doi.org/10.4269/ajtmh.21-0895
31. Redfern A, Cluver LD, Casale M, Steinert JI. Cost and cost-effectiveness of a parenting programme to prevent violence against adolescents in South Africa. *BMJ Glob Health.* 2019;4(3):e001147. https://doi.org/10.1136/bmjgh-2018-001147
32. Kilburn K, Handa S, Angeles G, Mvula P, Tsoka M. Short-term impacts of an unconditional cash transfer program on child schooling: experimental evidence from Malawi. *Econ Educ Rev.* 2017;59:63–80. https://doi.org/10.1016/j.econedurev.2017.06.002
33. Tozan Y, Sun S, Capasso A, et al. Evaluation of a savings-led family-based economic empowerment intervention for AIDS-affected adolescents in Uganda: a four-year follow-up on efficacy and cost-effectiveness. *PLoS One.* 2019;14(12):e0226809. https://doi.org/10.1371/journal.pone.0226809
34. Sensoy Bahar O, Nabunya P, Namuwonge F, et al. "It gives you a road map of what to do to solve your problems": acceptability of a combination HIV prevention intervention among adolescent girls in Uganda. *BMC Public Health.* 2023;23(1):249. https://doi.org/10.1186/s12889-023-15083-2

Authenticity, Racial Discrimination, Depression, and Suicidal Ideation Among Young Black Men, United States, 2024

Donte T. Boyd, PhD, MSW, Myles I. Durkee, PhD, Deon W. Brown, PhD, and Andrea S. Constant, MA

Objectives. To examine how perceived authenticity may buffer the impact of racial discrimination on depressive symptoms and suicidal ideation among young Black/African American men.

Methods. In 2024, we collected data online in the United States using Qualtrics. Participants were 350 Black men aged 18 to 24 years (mean = 21.49; SD = 1.96), most of whom identified as heterosexual or straight and had completed a high school diploma or general equivalency diploma. We measured suicidal ideation, depressive symptoms, racial discrimination, and perceived authenticity through self-report questionnaires.

Results. Authenticity reduced suicidal ideation ($b = -0.24$; $P < .001$) and depressive symptoms ($b = -0.22$; $P < .001$). An interaction effect emerged for suicidal ideation ($b = -0.09$; $P = .045$) but not depressive symptoms ($b = 0.02$; $P = .58$).

Conclusions. Perceived authenticity served as a protective factor for young Black men.

Public Health Implications. Practitioners may consider incorporating strategies to enhance perceived authenticity as part of interventions aimed at improving men's mental health. (*Am J Public Health*. 2025;115(9):1417–1425. https://doi.org/10.2105/AJPH.2025.308148)

AJPH September 2025, Vol. 115, No. 9

The high prevalence of depression and the increasing suicide rates among Black youths in the United States are significant public health concerns. Depression is among the most prevalent, costly, and debilitating psychiatric disorders in the country.[1] Although major depressive disorder is less common among Black individuals than White individuals, its chronicity and burden are often greater for Black individuals.[2] Over the past 2 decades, rates of depression among youths have increased significantly, and both Black youths and Black adults report a higher prevalence of persistent depressive disorder.[2–4] Recent research indicates that 34% of Black men aged 18 to 24 years attending college have experienced depression, anxiety, an eating disorder, nonsuicidal self-injury, or suicidal thoughts over the past year.[5]

Suicide is now the third leading cause of death among Black male adolescents and young adults.[6–7] Recent data indicate that Black boys and men account for the vast majority (81%) of completed suicides among Black Americans.[7] In 2021, the death rate from suicide for Black men was more than 4 times higher than the rate for Black women.[8] Furthermore, during this same period, the suicide rates among Black men increased by 25.3%, highlighting a public health crisis affecting this demographic.[9] A recent study in the Midwest United States found that Black men aged 18 to 24 years were more likely to experience suicidal ideation than were Black women and girls.[10] However, there is a pressing need for more research on suicide risk and protective mechanisms among Black young adult men, as they are often underrepresented in empirical studies.[11]

Racial discrimination is the behavioral aspect of racism; it is characterized by the marginalization, oppression, and exclusion of subordinate racial groups to benefit the power, influence, and wealth of dominant racial groups.[12]

Research indicates that experiences of racial discrimination are linked to a range of negative mental health outcomes.[13] Among Black youths, exposure to racial discrimination heightens the risk of mental health issues, including psychological distress,[14] suicidal ideation,[15] and psychiatric disorders such as anxiety[12] and depression.[16,17] Previous research has indicated that Black men may be more susceptible to the mental health impacts of discrimination than are Black women.[9] In a longitudinal study focusing on Black youths, findings revealed that an increase in racial discrimination was linked to heightened symptoms of anxiety and depression among men but not among women.[18] The increasing prevalence of depression and suicidal behaviors among Black men has become a significant public health concern. Therefore, it is crucial to conduct research on protective factors that can help alleviate these mental health challenges.

Authenticity can be defined as the perception that one's behavior is self-authored, internally motivated, and aligned with how individuals view themselves.[19–20] People who perceive themselves as more authentic are less prone to feelings of self-alienation, less susceptible to external influences, and more likely to act consistently with their true character across different contexts.[21] For instance, Black men in the US context, navigating societal expectations and cultural identities while striving for authenticity, may experience unique mental health implications.[21] The pressure to conform to external stereotypes or societal norms can lead to stress, anxiety, and identity conflict.[22] Conversely, embracing authentic self-expression may promote resilience and emotional well-being.[20]

Previous research has advanced our understanding of how perceived authenticity is linked to mental health outcomes.[19–20,23] Research has indicated that individuals who view themselves as more authentic tend to report lower levels of depression and greater life satisfaction.[23–25] Additionally, research has established a connection between higher levels of dispositional authenticity—the unimpeded expression of one's core or true self in daily life—and multiple positive outcomes, including increased self-esteem and increased well-being overall.[19,25–26] These findings hold across college undergraduates from the United States and the United Kingdom as well as racially diverse community groups. However, limited research has specifically examined the protective psychological benefits of perceived authenticity among Black men. Investigating the role of authenticity as a protective factor that could potentially mitigate the harmful effects of racial discrimination on depressive symptoms and suicidal ideation will provide valuable insights for researchers and practitioners seeking to promote protective mechanisms for at-risk populations.

CURRENT STUDY

The phenomenological variant of ecological systems theory is the guiding theoretical framework that helps us to understand how the interplay between individual social identities, stressors, and ecological factors (e.g., family, culture, and society) influence authenticity, suicidal ideation, and depressive symptoms.[27–29] Authenticity, or the ability to express oneself honestly, can influence emotional well-being by reducing stress and fostering positive identity development. Suicidal ideation may emerge as a maladaptive response when individuals face overwhelming stressors influenced by cultural, familial, or socioeconomic pressures.

Similarly, depressive symptoms might develop as a chronic response to such stressors, affecting one's ability to adapt. The phenomenological variant of ecological systems theory provides a conceptual framework to explore and address these issues in broader ecological and cultural contexts. It promotes interventions that strengthen identity resources and modify stressor-laden environments to foster resilience. This comprehensive approach helps to address significant gaps in the existing literature, particularly the lack of research focusing on risk and protective factors related to depressive symptoms and suicidal ideation among Black men.

To our knowledge, our study is the first quantitative empirical investigation to examine whether perceived authenticity functions as a buffer against depressive symptoms and suicidal ideation. Specifically, we explored the following research questions: Is racial discrimination associated with increased depressive symptoms and suicidal ideation? Is perceived authenticity associated with fewer depressive symptoms and less suicidal ideation? Does perceived authenticity function as a protective factor that moderates the association between racial discrimination and mental health outcomes, such as depressive symptoms and suicidal ideation?

METHODS

We designed our study to examine the factors that contribute to the overall health and well-being of Black/African American men aged 18 to 24 years. We recruited a sample of Black emerging adult men from across the United States using Qualtrics Panels (Qualtrics, Seattle, WA/Provo, UT), a professional online recruitment service that helped us identify eligible participants in the target population. To qualify for the study, participants had to reside in the United States, self-identify as Black/African American, be between 18 and 24 years, and be fluent in English. We sent eligible participants an e-mail invitation to participate, and they were required to provide consent before proceeding with the online survey. The survey collected self-reported data from participants and took approximately 20 minutes to complete. Participants were compensated with a $30 gift card for their participation.

Participants

The study involved 350 Black men aged 18 to 24 years (mean = 21.49; SD = 1.96) living in the United States; 94% of the sample identified as Black/African American, 4% identified as Caribbean, and 1% as Continental African or Afro-Latinx. Regarding sexual orientation, the majority identified as heterosexual or straight (88%), with smaller percentages identifying as homosexual or gay (5%), bisexual (4%), pansexual (1%), bicurious (0.3%), queer (0.3%), or another orientation (2%). Most participants had a high school diploma or general equivalency diploma (63%), with 14% holding an associate's degree and 11% possessing a bachelor's degree or higher. Whereas 37% of the sample was enrolled in college at the time of participation, 63% was not. Concerning the highest education level attained by their mothers, 56% had completed high school or obtained a general equivalency diploma, and 23% had earned a bachelor's degree or higher. Most participants were raised in a single-parent family (47%) or a 2-parent family (38%). In terms of household income, 42% of participants came from households earning less than $30 000 per year, 29% from households earning between $30 000 and $60 000 per year, and 28% from households earning more than $60 000 per year.

Measures

We assessed suicidal ideation using the Suicidal Ideation Attributes Scale (SIDAS).[30] The SIDAS was designed to detect and assess the severity of suicidal thoughts. It consists of 5 items intended to capture the following attributes of suicidal ideation: frequency, controllability, closeness to an attempt, level of distress, and impact on daily functioning. Sample items include "In the past month, how often have you had thoughts about suicide?" and "In the past month, how close have you come to making a suicide attempt?" Participants responded on a scale from 0 (never) to 10 (always), and we reverse-coded 1 item before summing all items to create a total score ranging from 0 to 50, with higher scores indicating greater severity of suicidal thoughts. The scale demonstrated strong reliability in this study ($\alpha = 0.84$).

We evaluated depressive symptoms using a brief version of the Center for Epidemiologic Studies Depression Scale,[30] which screens for depressive symptoms experienced in the past week. The scale comprises 10 items, including statements such as "I felt depressed" and "I felt hopeless about the future." We rated responses on a scale from 0 (rarely/none of the time) to 3 (all of the time). We reverse-coded 2 items before summing all items to create a total score ranging from 0 to 30, with higher scores indicating more severe depressive symptoms. The scale demonstrated acceptable reliability in this study ($\alpha = 0.77$).

We measured racial discrimination using the 18-item Daily Life Experiences subscale from the Racism and Life Experiences Scales.[31] This subscale measures racial microaggressions—subtle racial slights and insults—that people of color may experience in their daily lives. Example items include "being ignored, overlooked, or not given service" and "others reacting to you as if they were afraid or intimidated." The response scale ranged from 1 (never) to 6 (once a week or more). The items were averaged to create a mean composite score, with higher scores indicating more frequent experiences of racial discrimination. The scale demonstrated excellent reliability in this study ($\alpha = 0.96$).

We assessed authenticity using the authenticity scale.[19] This 12-item measure is grounded in the person-centered model of authenticity and evaluates the degree to which a person leads an authentic lifestyle, conforms to the expectations of others, and experiences alienation from their true self. Sample items include "I always stand by what I believe in" and "I do not know how I really feel inside." The response scale ranged from 1 (does not describe me at all) to 6 (describes me very well). One item ("I live in accordance with my values and beliefs") was unintentionally omitted from the online survey, resulting in a final scale comprising 11 items. We reverse-coded 8 items before we averaged all items to create a mean composite score, with higher scores indicating a greater sense of perceived authenticity. The scale demonstrated acceptable reliability in this study ($\alpha = 0.77$).

We also collected demographic variables, including the participant's age, college enrollment status, and total household income. These variables served as demographic covariates in the analyses.

Statistical Analysis

We conducted linear regression analyses using SPSS version 29 (IBM, Somers, NY) to examine the direct associations of racial discrimination and authenticity on suicidal ideation and depressive symptoms (model 1). Additionally, we examined 2-way interactions between racial discrimination and authenticity on suicidal ideation and depressive symptoms (model 2) using the PROCESS 4.0 macro[26] in SPSS. We mean-centered independent variables before constructing interaction terms, probed statistically significant 2-way interactions, and graphed them at 1 SD above and below the mean for each independent variable to assess the significance of simple slopes.[32] We adjusted each model for the following covariates: participant's age, college enrollment, and household income.

RESULTS

Means, SDs, and bivariate correlations for all variables are depicted in Table 1. The average level of depressive symptoms was 12.55 (SD = 5.77). Research guidelines indicate that a cutoff score of 10 or greater is used to identify individuals at risk for depression,[23] and 71% of our sample met this threshold. The average level of suicidal ideation in our sample was 15.60 (SD = 13.28). Guidelines indicate that a cutoff score of 21 or greater is used to identify individuals at high risk for suicidal behaviors,[22] and 39% of the sample met this threshold.

TABLE 1— Means ±SD and Pearson Correlations Among Study Variables: United States, 2024

Variable	Mean ±SD	Suicidal Ideation, r^a	Depressive Symptoms, r	Racial Discrimination, r	Perceived Authenticity, r	Age, r	Household Income, r	College Enrollment, r
Suicidal ideation	15.60 ±13.28	...	...	...	...	...	...	...
Depressive symptoms	12.55 ±5.77	0.42***	...	...	...	...	...	...
Racial discrimination	2.93 ±1.21	0.47***	0.55***	...	...	...	...	...
Perceived authenticity	3.77 ±0.84	−0.36***	−0.36***	−0.28***	...	...	...	...
Age	21.49 ±1.96	0.07	0.06	0.01	0.01	...	...	...
Household income	4.81 ±3.17	−0.10	−0.13*	−0.02	0.07	0.02	...	...
College enrollment[b]	1.37 ±0.49	−0.01	−0.14**	−0.06	−0.01	−0.07	0.15**	...

Note. The sample size was n = 353.
[a]Values are Pearson correlation coefficients.
[b]College enrollment: 1 = not enrolled, 2 = enrolled.
*$P < .05$; **$P < .01$; ***$P < .001$.

TABLE 2— Linear Regression Models Predicting Suicidal Ideation and Depressive Symptoms: United States, 2024

	Suicidal Ideation		Depressive Symptoms	
Variable	**Model 1, b (SE); *P***	**Model 2, b (SE); *P***	**Model 1, b (SE); *P***	**Model 2, b (SE); *P***
Racial discrimination	4.44 (0.52); <.001	4.33 (0.52); <.001	2.26 (0.21); <.001	2.27 (0.21); <.001
Perceived authenticity	−3.78 (0.75); <.001	−4.02 (0.76); <.001	−1.54 (0.31); <.001	−1.51 (0.31); <.001
Age	0.47 (0.31); .128	0.39 (0.31); .209	0.14 (0.13); .279	0.15 (0.13); .253
Household income	−0.31 (0.19); .106	−0.30 (0.19); .119	−0.15 (0.08); .061	−0.15 (0.08); .059
College enrollment	0.88 (1.27); .488	0.92 (1.26); .464	−1.22 (0.52); .019	−1.22 (0.52); .019
Discrimination × authenticity	...	−1.13 (0.56); .045	...	0.13 (0.23); .585

Note. P values refer to models predicting scores on the Suicidal Ideation Attributes Scale (SIDAS), ranging from 0 to 50 and the Center for Epidemiologic Studies Depression Scale (CES-D-10), ranging from 0 to 30.

Suicidal Ideation

Direct associations. Model 1 in the linear regression analyses revealed that experiencing higher levels of racial discrimination was significantly associated with increased suicidal ideation (b = 4.44; SE = 0.52; *P* < .001). Conversely, perceived authenticity was significantly associated with reduced suicidal ideation (b = −3.78; SE = 0.75; *P* < .001; Table 2).

Interactions. Model 2 indicated that perceived authenticity moderated the relationship between racial discrimination and suicidal ideation (b = −1.13; SE = 0.56; *P* = .045). When perceived authenticity was 1 SD below the mean (−1 SD), racial discrimination had the largest association with greater suicidal ideation (b = 5.28; 95% confidence interval [CI] = 3.97, 6.59; *P* < .001). At the mean level of perceived authenticity, racial discrimination remained significantly associated with heightened suicidal ideation (b = 4.33; 95% CI = 3.30, 5.35; *P* < .001), although the association was less pronounced. When perceived authenticity was 1 SD above the mean (+1 SD), the protective buffering effect increased and racial discrimination continued to have a significant association with greater suicidal ideation (b = 3.38; 95% CI = 1.93, 4.83; *P* < .001), but the association was even less pronounced (Figure 1).

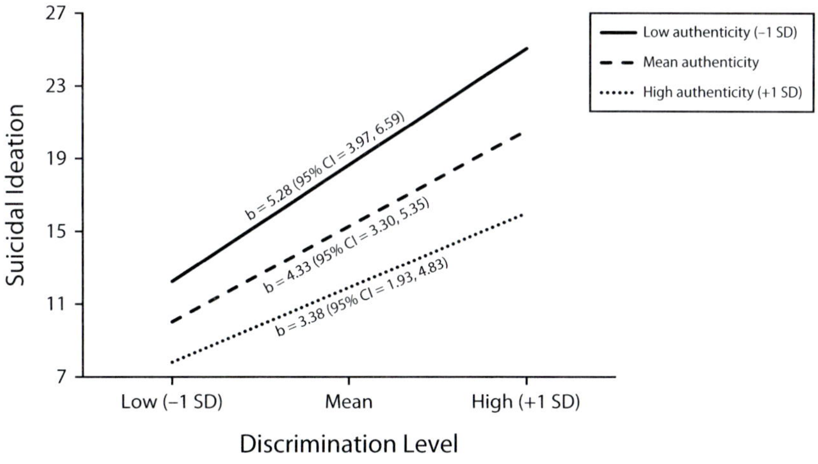

FIGURE 1— Interaction Between Racial Discrimination and Perceived Authenticity on Suicidal Ideation: United States, 2024

Note. CI = confidence interval. The model adjusted for the following covariates: participant's age, household income, and college enrollment status. We assessed suicidal ideation using the Suicidal Ideation Attributes Scale, which includes 5 items measuring frequency, controllability, proximity to an attempt, distress level, and impact on daily functioning. Participants rated their experiences on a scale from 0 (never) to 10 (always), and we calculated a total score from 0 to 50, with higher scores indicating greater severity of suicidal thoughts.

Depressive Symptoms

Direct associations. Model 1 revealed that higher levels of racial discrimination were significantly associated with greater depressive symptoms ($b = 2.26$; $SE = 0.21$; $P < .001$). Conversely, perceived authenticity was significantly associated with fewer depressive symptoms ($b = -1.54$; $SE = 0.31$; $P < .001$; Table 2).

Interactions. Model 2 indicated that perceived authenticity did not moderate the relationship between racial discrimination and depressive symptoms ($b = 0.13$; $SE = 0.23$; $P = .585$). Consequently, we did not examine simple slopes because of the absence of a statistically significant interaction.

DISCUSSION

In our study, guided by the phenomenological variant of ecological systems theory framework, we examined the relationships between racial discrimination, authenticity, depressive symptoms, and suicidal ideation among young Black men. Approximately 71% of the sample met the criteria for being at risk for depression, and 39% met the criteria for risk of suicide. Rates of depressive symptoms were notably higher in this sample than in large samples such as that in the Healthy Minds Study, which found that 34% of Black male college undergraduates faced major mental health challenges, including depression, anxiety, suicidal ideation, or self-injury.[33] Therefore, our sample of Black male emerging adults, aged 18 to 24 years, showed higher depressive symptoms and suicidal ideation than similar populations in other studies. We are not aware of any other studies investigating the protective role of perceived authenticity in buffering racial discrimination's effects on depression and suicidal ideation.

Suicidal Ideation

Our results indicate that racial discrimination is associated with suicidal ideation. The findings also suggest that perceived authenticity is linked to lower suicidal ideation. Notably, Black men who reported higher levels of perceived authenticity experienced a smaller increase in suicidal ideation as the rates of racial discrimination increased. Conversely, when racial discrimination was experienced more frequently, the detrimental link with suicidal ideation was more severe for Black men who reported lower levels of authenticity. Our results support previous research indicating that racial discrimination has profound negative impacts on mental health,[10,14–15] leading to an increase in suicidal ideation among Black men. Moreover, our study makes a significant contribution to the public health literature by demonstrating that perceived authenticity protects against suicidal ideation. This is important because other empirical research indicates that authenticity positively correlates with stronger social bonds, greater relationship satisfaction, and positive mental health.[34] Therefore, a logical explanation for our findings regarding perceived authenticity is that Black male emerging adults who report higher levels of authenticity may also possess more robust social connections, providing them with additional outlets to cope with racial discrimination and reducing the likelihood of experiencing negative emotions[30] or suicidal ideation.[10]

This explanation suggests that Black men can use their social support systems to foster their authenticity by increasing perceived closeness in their networks, potentially enhancing perceived authenticity. Black men with a strong sense of authenticity may feel more agency and control, which can empower them to navigate societal challenges, such as racial discrimination, with resilience. This may reduce vulnerability to negative mental health effects, including suicidal ideation. Thus, promoting authenticity is critical for Black men frequently facing racial discrimination, as it promotes healthy relationships and provides essential coping mechanisms.

Depressive Symptoms

Our study highlights the significant impact of racial discrimination on depressive symptoms among Black men aged 18 to 24 years.[28] Notably, our findings demonstrate a strong association between racial discrimination and increased depressive symptoms, emphasizing the considerable ecological stressors and systemic inequalities this population faces. The prevalence of depressive indicators, with 71% of participants meeting the threshold for being at risk for depression, underscores the critical need to address racial discrimination as a central factor influencing mental health. Interestingly, although perceived authenticity was associated with fewer depressive symptoms, it did not buffer the effect of racial discrimination on these symptoms in our sample. Authenticity, or being true to oneself, is generally recognized as enhancing mental well-being,[24–25] but it appeared to be less effective for this highly depressed group. This discrepancy suggests that perceived authenticity alone may not counteract the intense impact of racial discrimination. It is also possible that intersecting stressors, such as systemic racism and economic hardship, mitigate the protective role of authenticity. For instance, 42% of our participants reported a household income of less than $30 000 per year, potentially compounding the negative effects of racial discrimination.

For Black men confronting racially biased environments and negative stereotypes, fostering authenticity may involve identifying positive role models who exemplify behaviors that support the development of their true selves.[35] However, the complex interplay of race-related stress and economic challenges may undermine the benefits of authenticity for mental health. To effectively mitigate depressive symptoms and enhance resilience, public health strategies must address both the protective role of authenticity and the broader systemic issues that Black men face. This requires comprehensive approaches combining culturally competent interventions with efforts to alleviate economic and racial stressors.

Authenticity Across Contexts

Our study highlights that perceived authenticity acts as a protective mechanism against depressive symptoms and suicidal ideation among Black male emerging adults. However, we must consider the significant impact of ecological factors. Although we aim to encourage Black men to embrace authenticity in all settings, many mainstream US environments remain racially oppressive and emotionally restrictive. These environments often force Black men to suppress their emotional experiences, diminishing their sense of authenticity and compromising their mental health. Given the value placed on authenticity in Black communities, alongside the aspiration for Black men to express their emotions without fear of repercussions, our findings underscore the importance for mental health practitioners to emphasize strategies that nurture authenticity. By fostering environments that allow genuine self-expression, these approaches may serve as a crucial mechanism for reducing suicidal ideation during this critical stage of development.

Limitations

Although our study enhances understanding of perceived authenticity and racial discrimination in relation to major mental health outcomes among Black emerging men, it is important to acknowledge its limitations. First, the data were cross-sectional, which limited our ability to draw causal inferences or determine the temporal ordering between independent and dependent variables. Second, a single item from the authenticity scale was unintentionally omitted from the survey, thus limiting the overall validity of this measurement. Nonetheless, the authenticity scale demonstrated acceptable internal reliability ($\alpha = 0.77$). Third, the findings from this study can be generalized only to Black emerging men in the United States, especially those at greater risk for depression. Therefore, future research should seek to replicate these findings with other demographic groups and developmental stages. Additionally, future studies should include perceived authenticity, social relationship dynamics, and emotional control measures to determine how these important mechanisms interact to promote positive mental health outcomes.

Public Health Implications

Understanding perceived authenticity as a protective mechanism against the negative impacts of racial discrimination on mental health has significant public health implications for Black men. Recognizing the role of authenticity can guide the development of interventions aimed at reducing suicidal ideation and depressive symptoms for Black men. By fostering authenticity, early intervention programs can encourage discussions about identity in schools, workplaces, and community settings, helping mitigate suicidal ideation risks. Mental health professionals can potentially integrate authenticity into therapeutic practices to offer culturally competent care aligned with Black men's experiences and identities. This approach can strengthen support systems and promote self-expressive behaviors, enhancing mental health outcomes. Moreover, reducing mental health stigma in communities of color, emphasizing authenticity and self-acceptance, can encourage help-seeking behaviors.

Our findings indicate that racial discrimination correlates with increased suicidal ideation and depressive symptoms, whereas perceived authenticity correlates with lower levels of these adverse outcomes. Emphasizing authenticity as a protective factor amid pervasive racism highlights the need for targeted public health interventions. Practitioners must focus on culturally competent, community-centered strategies that champion authenticity and bolster resilience. By addressing systemic inequities, fostering supportive environments, and promoting self-acceptance, these efforts can improve overall mental health and well-being among Black men facing racial discrimination. AJPH

ABOUT THE AUTHORS

Donte T. Boyd is with the College of Social Work, The Ohio State University, Columbus. Myles I. Durkee is with the Department of Psychology, University of Michigan, Ann Arbor. Deon W. Brown is with the

Program in the Human Development and Family and Sciences, Department of Psychological, Health and Learning Sciences, College of Education, University of Houston, Houston, TX. Andrea S. Constant is with the Department of Sociology, The Ohio State University, Columbus.

CORRESPONDENCE

Correspondence should be sent to Donte T. Boyd, 1047 College Rd, #325K, Columbus, OH 43215 (e-mail: Boyd.465@osu.edu). Reprints can be ordered at https://www.ajph.org by clicking the "Reprints" link.

PUBLICATION INFORMATION

Full Citation: Boyd DT, Durkee MI, Brown DW, Constant AS. Authenticity, racial discrimination, depression, and suicidal ideation among young Black men, United States, 2024. *Am J Public Health*. 2025;115(9):1417–1425.

Acceptance Date: April 1, 2025.

DOI: https://doi.org/10.2105/AJPH.2025.308148

ORCID iDs:

Donte T. Boyd https://orcid.org/0000-0001-9952-3116

Myles I. Durkee https://orcid.org/0000-0003-2617-7384

Andrea S. Constant https://orcid.org/0009-0009-0084-3917

CONTRIBUTORS

D. T. Boyd and M. I. Durkee conceptualized and designed the study. M. I. Durkee analyzed and interpreted the results. All authors wrote and edited the main article, reviewed the results, and approved the final version of the article.

CONFLICTS OF INTEREST

The authors declare no competing interests.

HUMAN PARTICIPANT PROTECTION

All procedures performed in the study were in accordance with the Declaration of Helsinki. The Ohio State University institutional board approved the protocol for this study, which was conducted in compliance with the standards for ethical research with human participants. All study participants provided digital informed consent.

REFERENCES

1. Hudson DL, Eaton J, Banks A, Sewell W, Neighbors H. "Down in the sewers": perceptions of depression and depression care among African American men. *Am J Mens Health*. 2018;12(1):126–1425. https://doi.org/10.1177/1557988316654864
2. Lindsey MA, Banks A, Cota CF, Scott ML, Joe S. A review of treatments for young Black males experiencing depression. *Res Soc Work Pract*. 2018;28(3):320–329. https://doi.org/10.1177/1049731517703747
3. Lindsey MA, Mufson L, Vélez-Grau C, et al. Engaging Black youth in depression and suicide prevention treatment within urban schools: study protocol for a randomized controlled pilot. *Trials*. 2024;25(1):112. https://doi.org/10.1186/s13063-024-07947-8. [Correction in: *Trials*. 2024;25(1):253. https://doi.org/10.1186/s13063-024-08084-y]
4. Bernard DL, López CM, Banks DE, Hahn AM, Danielson CK. Developmental differences in the impact of racial discrimination on depression and anxiety among Black youth: examining rumination as a mechanism. *Am J Orthopsychiatry*. 2023;93(4):293–303. https://doi.org/10.1037/ort0000679
5. Watkins DC, Brown BR, Abelson JM, Ellis J. First-generation Black college men in the United States and the value of cohort-based programs: addressing inequities through the YBMen project. In Smith JA, Watkins DC, Griffith DM, eds. *Health Promotion With Adolescent Boys and Young Men of Colour: Global Strategies for Advancing Research, Policy, and Practice in Context*. Cham, Switzerland: Springer; 2023:53–71.
6. Centers for Disease Control and Prevention. Web-based Injury Statistics Query and Reporting System (WISQARS). 2005. Available at: https://www.cdc.gov/injury/wisqars. Accessed September 13, 2024.
7. Adams LB, Thorpe RJ Jr. Achieving mental health equity in Black male suicide prevention. *Front Public Health*. 2023;11:1113222. https://doi.org/10.3389/fpubh.2023.1113222
8. Centers for Disease Control and Prevention. Deaths: final data for 2021. *Natl Vital Stat Rep*. 2024;(8):CS351103. https://doi.org/10.15620/cdc/158787
9. Meza JI, Patel K, Bath E. Black youth suicide crisis: prevalence rates, review of risk and protective factors, and current evidence-based practices. *Focus (Am Psychiatr Publ)*. 2022;20(2):197–203. https://doi.org/10.1176/appi.focus.20210034
10. Boyd DT, Quinn CR, Durkee MI, et al. Perceived discrimination, mental health help-seeking attitudes, and suicide ideation, planning, and attempts among Black young adults. *BMC Public Health*. 2024;24(1):2019. https://doi.org/10.1186/s12889-024-19519-1
11. Goodwill JR. Reasons for suicide in Black young adults: a latent class analysis. *J Racial Ethn Health Disparities*. 2024;11(1):425–440. https://doi.org/10.1007/s40615-023-01530-8
12. Seaton EK, Iida M. Racial discrimination and racial identity: daily moderation among Black youth. *Am Psychol*. 2019;74(1):117–127. https://doi.org/10.1037/amp0000367
13. Neblett EW Jr. Racial, ethnic, and cultural resilience factors in African American youth mental health. *Annu Rev Clin Psychol*. 2023;19:361–379. https://doi.org/10.1146/annurev-clinpsy-072720-015146
14. Assari S, Moazen-Zadeh E, Caldwell CH, Zimmerman MA. Racial discrimination during adolescence predicts mental health deterioration in adulthood: gender differences among Blacks. *Front Public Health*. 2017;5:104. https://doi.org/10.3389/fpubh.2017.00104
15. Boyd DT, Gale A, Quinn CR, et al. Do we belong? Examining the associations between adolescents' perceptions of school belonging, teacher discrimination, peer prejudice and suicide. *J Racial Ethn Health Disparities*. 2024;11(3):1454–1464. https://doi.org/10.1007/s40615-023-01622-5
16. Levine DS, Himle JA, Abelson JM, Matusko N, Dhawan N, Taylor RJ. Discrimination and social anxiety disorder among African-Americans, Caribbean Blacks, and non-Hispanic Whites. *J Nerv Ment Dis*. 2014;202(3):224–230. https://doi.org/10.1097/NMD.0000000000000099
17. Assari S, Watkins DC, Caldwell CH. Race attribution modifies the association between daily discrimination and major depressive disorder among Blacks: the role of gender and ethnicity. *J Racial Ethn Health Disparities*. 2015;2(2):200–210. https://doi.org/10.1007/s40615-014-0064-9
18. Assari S. Unequal gain of equal resources across racial groups. *Int J Health Policy Manag*. 2018;7(1):1–9. https://doi.org/10.15171/ijhpm.2017.90
19. Wood AM, Linley PA, Maltby J, Baliousis M, Joseph S. The authentic personality: a theoretical and empirical conceptualization and the development of the Authenticity Scale. *J Couns Psychol*. 2008;55(3):385–399. https://doi.org/10.1037/0022-0167.55.3.385
20. Bunker CJ, Balcerowska JM, Precht LM, Margraf J, Brailovskaia J. Perceiving the self as authentic on social media precedes fewer mental health symptoms: a longitudinal approach. *Comput Hum Behav*. 2024;152:108056. https://doi.org/10.1016/j.chb.2023.108056
21. Perkins T, Smith RE II, Durkee MI. Understanding authenticity through social identity processes. In: Vess M, Schlegel RJ, Hicks JA, eds. *Oxford Handbook of Authenticity*. New York, NY: Oxford University Press. In Press.
22. Nguyen J, Anthony AK. Black authenticity: defining the ideals and expectations in the construction of "real" Blackness. *Sociol Compass*. 2014;8(6):770–779. https://doi.org/10.1111/soc4.12171
23. Wenzel AJ, Lucas-Thompson RG. Authenticity in college-aged males and females, how close others are perceived, and mental health outcomes. *Sex Roles*. 2012;67(5–6):334–350. https://doi.org/10.1007/s11199-012-0182-y
24. Mun IB, Kim H. Influence of false self-presentation on mental health and deleting behavior on Instagram: the mediating role of perceived popularity. *Front Psychol*. 2021;12.660484. https://doi.org/10.3389/fpsyg.2021.660484
25. Goldman BM, Kernis MH. The role of authenticity in healthy psychological functioning and subjective well-being. *Ann Am Psychother Assoc*. 2002;5(6):18–20.
26. Kernis MH, Goldman BM. A multicomponent conceptualization of authenticity: theory and research. *Adv Exp Soc Psychol*. 2006;38:283–357. https://doi.org/10.1016/S0065-2601(06)38006-9
27. Velez G, Spencer MB. Phenomenology and intersectionality: using PVEST as a frame for adolescent identity formation amid intersecting ecological systems of inequality. *New Dir Child Adolesc Dev*. 2018;2018(161):75–90. https://doi.org/10.1002/cad.20247
28. Hill RM, Rooney EE, Mooney MA, Kaplow JB. Links between social support, thwarted belongingness, and suicide ideation among lesbian, gay, and bisexual college students. *J Fam Strengths*. 2017;17(2):6. https://doi.org/10.58464/2168-670X.1350
29. Boyd DT, Sterrett-Hong E, Scott ED, Allen JL, Smith B, Quinn CR. Family as a pathway to suicidal behaviors through depression symptoms and

internalized homophobia. *J Racial Ethn Health Disparities.* 2025;12(2):1228–1239. https://doi.org/10.1007/s40615-024-01956-8

30. Andresen EM, Malmgren JA, Carter WB, Patrick DL. Screening for depression in well older adults: evaluation of a short form of the CES-D (Center for Epidemiologic Studies Depression Scale). *Am J Prev Med.* 1994;10(2):77–84.
31. Harrell SP, Merchant MA, Young SA. Psychometric properties of the racism and life experiences scales (RaLES). Paper presented at: the 105th Annual Meeting of the American Psychological Association. Chicago, IL; August 15–19, 1997.
32. Aiken LS, West SG. *Multiple Regression: Testing and Interpreting Interactions.* Thousand Oaks, CA: Sage; 1991.
33. Lipson SK, Kern A, Eisenberg D, Breland-Noble AM. Mental health disparities among college students of color. *J Adolesc Health.* 2018;63(3):348–356. https://doi.org/10.1016/j.jadohealth.2018.04.014
34. Lopez FG, Rice KG. Preliminary development and validation of a measure of relationship authenticity. *Journal of Counseling Psychology.* 2006;53(3):362–371. https://doi.org/10.1037/0022-0167.53.3.362
35. Goodwill JR, Anyiwo N, Williams E-DG, Johnson NC, Mattis JS, Watkins DC. Media representations of popular culture figures and the construction of Black masculinities. *Psychol Men Masculinity.* 2019;20(3):288–298. https://doi.org/10.1037/men0000164

Mental Health of Emerging Adults in New York City in 2023

Rachel Suss, MPH, Jo-Anne Caton, MPH, Melanie Close, PhD, Dewi Sihaloho, MPH, Ellenie Tuazon, MPH, and Christina Norman, PhD

See also Adolescent Mental Health, pp. 1377–1453.

Objectives. To investigate the prevalence of serious psychological distress (SPD), mental health treatment, unmet need for mental health treatment, social isolation, and barriers to treatment access among emerging adults, aged 18 to 24 years, and compared with older adults.

Methods. We use data from the New York City (NYC) Neighborhood Wellness Survey (2023), a representative survey of adults in NYC (n = 43 606), to calculate weighted prevalence estimates and fit logistic regression models controlling for sociodemographic characteristics.

Results. Emerging adults had higher odds of SPD and social isolation than adults aged 35 to 44 years, 45 to 64 years, and 65 years or older, and lower odds of past-year mental health treatment among those with SPD compared with all other age groups. Emerging adults reported different reasons for unmet need for mental health treatment than other age groups. Among emerging adults, individuals who identified as noncisgender, bisexual, or unsure of their sexual orientation, or who experienced financial strain, violence, or discrimination, had poorer mental health outcomes.

Conclusions. These findings demonstrate the need for expanded efforts to increase mental health treatment access focused on those aged 18 to 24 years, as their needs may differ from those of other age groups. (*Am J Public Health*. 2025;115(9):1426–1435. https://doi.org/10.2105/AJPH.2025.308163)

AJPH September 2025, Vol. 115, No. 9

Age has been established as a robust predictor of mental health outcomes; recent data show concerning trends in mental health outcomes for younger people.[1,2] On top of stressors including rising income inequality, racism, gun violence, and climate change, today's youths faced widespread disruption to schooling, employment, and socialization during the COVID-19 pandemic.[3] Ubiquitous use of social media also has the potential to directly and indirectly harm youth mental health.[4,5]

While the domain of youth mental health is often thought of as ending at age 18 years, another closely related group of concern is individuals aged 18 to 24 years who are transitioning from adolescence to adulthood. By using 18 years as the age to separate adolescence from adulthood, researchers risk overlooking the unique experiences and challenges of this transitionary age group. Service provision and policy often do not align with the cut-off at 18 years, as many health services for youths are offered until age 21 or 24 years (e.g., New York City [NYC] Family and Youth Peer Support Program[6]). In addition, becoming an adult is a longer social process than in previous generations, as more young people pursue further schooling and start families later.[7,8] The period between 18 and 24 years is a unique, nonhomogeneous, transitionary period that can be considered "late adolescence" or "emerging adulthood."[9]

There are several reasons to investigate the mental health of emerging adults. Previous literature has established poorer mental health outcomes among emerging adults compared with older age groups.[1,2] Emerging adulthood is a critical period in the development of psychiatric disorders, with 62.5% of people experiencing a mental disorder having an onset when aged younger than 25 years.[10] While many serious mental health problems emerge in late adolescence, this period is simultaneously associated with a large drop in service utilization, because of factors such as decreased parental oversight, difficulty navigating the transition between child and adult services, and changes to insurance.[11] Stressors unique to this transitionary period include major life transitions such as living independently for the first time or adjusting to a new job or school. Contemporary 18- to 24-year-old adults are among the first of Gen Z (born between 1997 and 2012) to transition to adulthood, and they are the first generation who had smartphones and social media throughout their youth.[12] They experienced high susceptibility to food insecurity and employment loss during the COVID-19 pandemic, which has been associated with anxiety and depression.[13,14] Young adults may also be especially vulnerable to social isolation, which is highly correlated with psychological distress.[15,16]

Furthermore, among emerging adults, there may be inequities in mental health outcomes. Individuals who identify as lesbian, gay, bisexual, transgender, queer, or other identities (LGBTQ+) face stigma and discrimination that can harm their mental health.[17,18] Social drivers of health shape an individual's ability to lead a healthy life and their physical and mental health status; experiencing adverse social drivers of health, such as financial strain, intimate partner violence (IPV), neighborhood violence, or racial or ethnic discrimination, may further harm the mental health of this vulnerable population.[19]

Our aims were to (1) investigate mental health outcomes and differences in outcomes by sociodemographic characteristics and social drivers of health among individuals aged 18 to 24 years (emerging adults), (2) compare mental health outcomes among emerging adults to older age groups, and (3) compare reported barriers to mental health treatment among those aged 18 to 24 years with other age groups.

METHODS

We used data from the NYC Neighborhood Wellness Survey (NWS), a sample of noninstitutionalized adults aged 18 years and older in NYC. The NYC NWS was conducted from May 2023 to September 2023 through a collaboration between the NYC Health Department and the City University of New York (CUNY) Graduate School of Policy and Public Health. The NWS used a probability-based approach using address-based sampling methods to mail surveys to randomly selected households in NYC. The adult aged 18 years or older with the "next birthday" was eligible for the survey. Most surveys were completed by mail, with some online completion. The paper survey was available in English and Spanish and online in English, Spanish, Traditional Chinese, Simplified Chinese, French Creole, and Russian. The response rate using the 2023 American Association for Public Opinion Research calculator was 21.3%.[20]

We weighted survey data to adjust for design, nonresponse, and population representation. The design weight adjusted for probability of selection. Respondent values used for weighting included age, sex assigned at birth, education, race, Hispanic or Latino/a ethnicity, household income, and homeownership. We imputed missing values for sex at birth using first name and cell-based imputation and imputed missing values for the other weighting variables using random hot-deck imputation. We matched and weighted respondent and population demographic characteristics at the borough and city level. We applied multivariate adjustments, or "raking," to the weights using demographic characteristic distributions from the 2021 American Community Survey to ensure these distributions aligned.

We checked the variables not imputed for weighting for levels of missingness. Most covariate and outcome variables were 1% or less missing, except SPD, insurance status, and sexual orientation, which were less than 5% missing. We conducted sensitivity analyses to test the impact of the missing data; the direction and significance of the findings did not change.

Outcome Variables

The main outcomes of interest for this study were (1) SPD, (2) mental health treatment among those with SPD, (3) unmet need for mental health treatment among those with SPD, and (4) social isolation. We defined SPD as having a score greater than or equal to 13 on the Kessler 6 (K6) scale, a validated six-item scale developed to identify people highly likely to have a diagnosable mental illness and associated functional limitations. K6 scores range from 0 to 24 and are calculated by scoring the frequency of 6 symptoms of psychological distress (e.g., feeling nervous, hopeless) in the past 30 days.[21] We defined mental health treatment as answering yes to 1 or both of the following questions about the past 12 months: "Did you take any prescription medication for your emotions, nerves, or mental health?" and "Did you receive any therapy or counseling for your emotions, nerves, or mental health?" We defined unmet need as reporting that there was a time in the past 12 months when the individual needed treatment for their emotions, nerves, or mental health, but did not get it. We adapted treatment and unmet need items from the NYC Community Health Survey.[22] We defined social isolation, adapted from the Brief Grief Questionnaire,[23] as answering "somewhat" or "a lot" to the question: "In the past 30 days, how much have you been feeling cut off or distant from other people?"

Additional outcomes of interest included reported barriers to mental health treatment, adapted from the National Survey on Drug Use and Health.[24] Individuals who reported an unmet need for mental health treatment selected from 8 multiple-choice reasons for their unmet need (e.g., could not afford the cost). Participants could select multiple reasons and could also select "other" and write in a response. Three independent coders (R. S., J. C., M. C.) coded "other" responses to identify additional barriers to treatment.

Sociodemographics and Social Drivers

Sociodemographic characteristics and social drivers of health included in the descriptive analyses were collected by multiple choice survey items and defined in Table 1: race and ethnicity, gender identity, sexual orientation, LGBTQ+ identity, financial strain, place of birth, employment status, insurance status, experienced racial or ethnic discrimination, experienced IPV, and witnessed neighborhood violence. Adjusted regression models included the covariates of race and ethnicity, gender identity, sexual orientation, and financial strain. We hypothesized these covariates based on literature to be associated with both the exposure (age) and outcome variables.

Statistical Analysis

We calculated the weighted prevalence of the main outcome variables by sociodemographic and social drivers of health variables among those aged 18 to 24 years. Using SAS version 9.4 (SAS Institute Inc, Cary, NC) with callable SUDAAN 11.0.1 (Research Triangle Institute, Research Triangle Park, NC) to analyze the data, we evaluated the differences in prevalence estimates using the 2-sided t test with a level of significance of $P < .05$. When comparing 2 groups, the SUDAAN PROC DESCRIPT's CONTRAST statement performs the independent 2-sample t test to test the difference between the means or percentages of the 2 groups. SUDAAN applies logistic regression to categorical variables to obtain a common variance to calculate a t test statistic. We used unadjusted and adjusted logistic regression models to calculate odds ratios (ORs) and 95% confidence intervals (CIs) for the outcomes of interest with age group (18–24, 25–34, 35–44, 45–64, and ≥ 65 years) as the predictor variable and 18 to 24 years as the reference group.

RESULTS

The final analytic sample contained 43 606 adult New Yorkers. Characteristics of the analytic sample are found in Table 1.

Serious Psychological Distress

The prevalence of SPD among those aged 18 to 24 years was 13.0%. Those with another gender identity had a higher prevalence of SPD (30.6%) compared with cisgender men (11.0%) and cisgender women (13.0%). Bisexual emerging adults (23.3%) and emerging adults not sure of their sexual orientation (17.6%) had a higher prevalence of SPD compared with heterosexual emerging adults (10.4%). Select social drivers of health, including financial strain, experiencing IPV, and witnessing neighborhood violence, were also associated with SPD among emerging adults. SPD increased as the frequency of experiencing discrimination based on race and ethnicity increased (10.5% never or rarely, 15.3% sometimes, 21.7% often or always; Table 2). Unemployed emerging adults also had a higher prevalence of SPD than employed adults (23.8% vs 12.3%; Table A, available as a supplement to the online version of this article at https://ajph.org). Additional results for all outcomes are in Table A.

Mental Health Treatment

Among emerging adults with SPD (unweighted n = 253), 38.5% had received mental health treatment in the past year. Groups with a higher prevalence of past-year mental health treatment included those with another gender identity (68.2%) compared with cisgender men (32.0%) and cisgender women (37.7%), bisexual adults compared with heterosexual adults (51.9% vs 31.2%), and those who experienced IPV compared with those who did not (55.7% vs 34.4%; Table 2).

More than half (54.8%) of emerging adults with SPD reported an unmet need for mental health treatment in the past year. Among emerging adults with SPD, bisexual adults reported a higher prevalence of unmet need than heterosexual adults (78.8% vs 48.0%). Emerging adults with SPD who witnessed violence in their neighborhood

TABLE 1— Sociodemographic Characteristics of New York City Neighborhood Wellness Survey Sample: 2023

	Unweighted No. (Weighted %)				
	Aged 18–24 Years	Aged 25–34 Years	Aged 35–44 Years	Aged 45–64 Years	Aged ≥ 65 Years
Overall	2028 (100)	6775 (100)	6824 (100)	14438 (100)	13541 (100)
Race and ethnicity[a]					
Asian/Pacific Islander	518 (22.2)	1386 (17.3)	1320 (17.8)	2065 (13.3)	1611 (11.4)
Black	223 (15.7)	659 (14.8)	974 (19.4)	3251 (26.5)	2878 (25.3)
Latino	643 (35.1)	1624 (27.3)	1735 (28.6)	3757 (27.4)	2820 (20.4)
White[b]	557 (24.9)	2804 (38.3)	2492 (31.9)	4733 (30.8)	5792 (41.5)
Another race[c]	87 (2.1)	302 (2.2)	303 (2.3)	632 (2.1)	440 (1.4)
Gender identity					
Cisgender man	783 (46.8)	2385 (45.1)	2510 (47.0)	5466 (45.9)	5421 (41.0)
Cisgender woman	1163 (49.1)	4179 (52.1)	4224 (51.8)	8861 (53.4)	8025 (58.4)
Another gender identity[d]	82 (4.1)	211 (2.8)	90 (1.2)	111 (0.7)	95 (0.6)
Sexual orientation					
Gay or lesbian	120 (5.6)	585 (8.4)	429 (5.7)	706 (4.1)	342 (2.8)
Heterosexual	1453 (75.1)	5126 (78.8)	5751 (87.2)	12497 (91.3)	11578 (92.5)
Bisexual	207 (9.0)	635 (8.0)	251 (3.3)	279 (1.7)	154 (1.0)
Something else	32 (1.9)	89 (1.3)	56 (0.8)	68 (0.5)	90 (0.9)
Not sure	171 (8.5)	226 (3.6)	184 (3.1)	324 (2.4)	333 (2.7)
LGBTQ+ identity					
Cisgender and heterosexual	1445 (74.6)	5098 (78.3)	5736 (86.8)	12446 (90.9)	11531 (92.1)
LGBTQ+	539 (25.4)	1564 (21.7)	940 (13.2)	1426 (9.1)	971 (7.9)
Place of birth					
Born outside the United States and US territories	465 (24.1)	1921 (29.9)	2817 (45.9)	6218 (47.3)	5601 (43.6)
US born, including US territories	1555 (75.9)	4837 (70.1)	3987 (54.1)	8118 (52.7)	7804 (56.4)
Employment					
Employed	1128 (49.9)	5550 (79.7)	5474 (79.3)	9731 (67.9)	2529 (18.8)
Unemployed	319 (16.8)	754 (12.7)	752 (11.5)	1454 (10.2)	528 (4.0)
Not in labor force[e]	576 (33.3)	439 (7.6)	561 (9.2)	3091 (21.9)	10280 (77.1)
Insurance status					
Insured	1891 (95.8)	6321 (94.1)	6386 (93.9)	13616 (96.2)	13082 (99.1)
Not insured	80 (4.1)	339 (5.9)	319 (6.0)	467 (3.7)	97 (0.8)
Financial strain[f]					
No financial strain	1008 (50.2)	3844 (52.6)	3688 (50.3)	7377 (48.7)	8474 (61.2)
Some financial strain	750 (37.6)	2143 (34.5)	2234 (35.5)	5167 (38.2)	3947 (30.8)
High financial strain	250 (12.3)	755 (12.9)	864 (14.2)	1786 (13.1)	995 (8.0)
Experienced intimate partner violence					
No	1788 (90.5)	5428 (81.9)	5311 (81.0)	11590 (83.3)	11931 (90.3)
Yes	235 (9.5)	1324 (18.1)	1479 (19.0)	2726 (16.7)	1429 (9.7)
Experienced discrimination on basis of race and ethnicity					
Never or rarely	1176 (59.6)	4127 (60.2)	3935 (57.0)	7836 (54.7)	8478 (64.0)
Sometimes	635 (30.3)	1952 (29.2)	2159 (32.2)	4844 (33.7)	3799 (28.0)
Often or always	214 (10.1)	658 (10.6)	702 (10.8)	1680 (11.6)	1155 (8.0)

Continued

TABLE 1— Continued

	Unweighted No. (Weighted %)				
	Aged 18-24 Years	Aged 25-34 Years	Aged 35-44 Years	Aged 45-64 Years	Aged ≥65 Years
Witnessed violence in neighborhood					
No	1 455 (72.5)	4 862 (71.6)	4 797 (71.2)	10 721 (75.7)	11 445 (86.2)
Yes	557 (27.5)	1 858 (28.4)	1 941 (28.8)	3 524 (24.3)	1 858 (13.8)

Note. LGBTQ+ = lesbian, gay, bisexual, transgender, queer, or other identities.
[a]Latino includes people of Hispanic or Latino origin, as identified by the survey question "Are you Hispanic or Latino?" and regardless of reported race. All other race categories exclude Latino ethnicity.
[b]White race includes Middle Eastern or North African.
[c]Another race includes respondents who are multiple races, American Indian/Alaska Native, or selected "other race."
[d]Another gender identity includes respondents who identified as transgender, nonbinary or genderqueer, or "other gender identity."
[e]Not in labor force includes student, homemaker, retired, and unable to work.
[f]Financial strain was measured using the question, "In the PAST 12 MONTHS, how hard was it for you to pay for basic needs, like food, housing, utilities, and medical care?" Response options were "not hard" (no financial strain), "somewhat hard" (some financial strain), and "very hard" (high financial strain).

were more likely to report an unmet need for mental health treatment (65.1% vs 48.8%; Table 2).

Social Isolation

Among emerging adults, 50.1% felt socially isolated. Groups more likely to feel socially isolated included cisgender women (52.3%) and those with another gender identity (63.1%) compared with cisgender men (46.6%), and gay or lesbian (64.0%) and bisexual adults (68.5%) compared with heterosexual adults (47.3%). Social isolation was also higher among emerging adults experiencing financial strain, experiencing IPV, witnessing neighborhood violence, or experiencing discrimination on the basis of race and ethnicity (Table 2).

Associations Between Study Outcomes and Age Group

Emerging adults had a higher prevalence of SPD (13.0%) compared with all other age groups (Table B, available as a supplement to the online version of this article at https://ajph.org). In adjusted models, odds of SPD were significantly higher among those aged 18 to 24 years versus those aged 35 to 44 years (OR = 0.65; 95% CI = 0.53, 0.80), 45 to 64 years (OR = 0.55; 95% CI = 0.45, 0.67), and 65 years or older (OR = 0.43; 95% CI = 0.35, 0.53), but not those aged 25 to 34 years.

Among individuals with SPD, all older age groups had more than double the adjusted odds of past-year mental health treatment compared with those aged 18 to 24 years. Among individuals with SPD, the adjusted odds of reporting a past-year unmet need for mental health treatment did not differ significantly between those aged 18 to 24 years and 25 to 34 years or 35 to 44 years but was higher among emerging adults compared with those aged 45 to 64 years and 65 years or older (Table 3).

The adjusted odds of reporting social isolation most or all of the time was also higher among emerging adults compared with all older age groups except those aged 25 to 34 years (Table 3).

Barriers to Mental Health Treatment

Among emerging adults reporting an unmet need for mental health treatment in the past year (unweighted n = 439), 58.0% reported that their reason for unmet need was that they thought they could handle their mental health without treatment. The next most cited reasons were that they did not know who to contact or where to go (50.5%) and they could not afford the cost (46.0%; Table C, available as a supplement to the online version of this article at https://ajph.org). The most cited barrier in the "other" category was insurance (e.g., respondent did not have insurance, could not find a provider that accepted their insurance, or had difficulty navigating their insurance; unweighted n = 224). All remaining barrier categories were cited by fewer than 150 respondents and are not presented here. Among all adults with past-year unmet need (unweighted n = 5728), emerging adults had higher adjusted odds than all other age groups of reporting that their reason for unmet need was that they thought they could

TABLE 2— Prevalence of Mental Health Outcomes Among 18- to 24-Year-Old Adults: New York City, 2023

	Serious Psychological Distress (SPD)		Past-Year Mental Health Treatment Among Those With SPD[a]		Past-Year Unmet Need for Mental Health Treatment Among Those With SPD[a]		Social Isolation	
	Weighted % (95% CI)	P^b	Weighted % (95% CI)	P^b	Weighted % (95% CI)	P^b	Weighted % (95% CI)	P^b
Emerging adults (ages 18–24 y)	13.0 (11.4, 14.9)		38.5 (31.7, 45.7)		54.8 (47.5, 61.9)		50.1 (47.5, 52.7)	
Gender identity								
Cisgender man (Ref)	11.0 (8.8, 13.8)		32.0 (21.8, 44.2)		48.5 (36.6, 60.5)		46.6 (42.6, 50.6)	
Cisgender woman	13.5 (11.2, 16.1)	.18	37.7 (28.8, 47.6)	.45	60.7 (50.7, 69.8)	.13	52.3 (48.9, 55.8)	.032
Another gender identity[c]	30.6 (20.4, 43.1)	.001	68.2 (43.8, 85.5)	.004	49.8 (28.8, 70.9)	.92	63.1 (50.2, 74.3)	.012
Sexual orientation								
Gay or lesbian	19.2 (11.7, 30.0)	.06	49.4 (24.9, 74.3)	.21	52.3 (26.9, 76.5)	.77	64.0 (53.5, 73.3)	.002
Heterosexual (Ref)	10.4 (8.6, 12.4)		31.2 (23.3, 40.5)		48.0 (38.7, 57.5)		47.3 (44.3, 50.3)	
Bisexual	23.3 (16.9, 31.1)	.001	51.9 (34.8, 68.6)	.039	78.8 (64.3, 88.5)	<.001	68.5 (60.6, 75.4)	<.001
Something else	26.1 (12.7, 46.2)	.07	69.7 (29.0, 92.8)	.045	35.3 (9.9, 73.1)	.51	56.8 (37.2, 74.5)	.35
Not sure	17.6 (11.8, 25.4)	.044	34.6 (17.8, 56.3)	.76	60.4 (39.4, 78.1)	.28	48.0 (39.4, 56.8)	.87
Financial strain[d]								
No financial strain (Ref)	7.3 (5.6, 9.5)		36.8 (24.6, 50.8)		49.0 (35.5, 62.6)		42.2 (38.6, 45.8)	
Some financial strain	16.1 (13.1, 19.5)	<.001	31.0 (22.1, 41.6)	.5	53.1 (42.2, 63.7)	.65	55.6 (51.4, 59.8)	<.001
High financial strain	29.0 (22.8, 36.1)	<.001	53.2 (39.8, 66.2)	.09	63.9 (50.4, 75.5)	.12	65.2 (57.8, 71.9)	<.001
Experienced discrimination on basis of race and ethnicity								
Never or rarely (Ref)	10.5 (8.6, 12.8)		36.9 (27.5, 47.5)		54.7 (44.0, 64.9)		43.6 (40.3, 47.0)	
Sometimes	15.3 (12.2, 19.0)	.019	35.9 (25.5, 47.9)	.9	55.4 (43.4, 66.8)	.93	59.0 (54.4, 63.5)	<.001
Often or always	21.7 (15.7, 29.2)	.002	48.0 (31.2, 65.2)	.29	53.9 (36.5, 70.4)	.94	61.3 (53.4, 68.7)	<.001
Experienced intimate partner violence								
No (Ref)	11.4 (9.7, 13.3)		34.4 (27.0, 42.5)		51.7 (43.5, 59.9)		47.2 (44.5, 50.0)	
Yes	27.5 (21.0, 35.1)	<.001	55.7 (40.3, 70.1)	.015	65.5 (49.8, 78.5)	.11	76.6 (69.5, 82.4)	<.001
Witnessed violence in neighborhood								
No (Ref)	11.4 (9.6, 13.6)		42.6 (33.8, 52.0)		48.8 (39.7, 58.1)		46.4 (43.4, 49.5)	
Yes	17.8 (14.3, 21.9)	.003	31.5 (22.0, 42.8)	.12	65.1 (53.5, 75.1)	.027	59.5 (54.7, 64.2)	<.001

[a]Unweighted n = 253.
[b]*T* test *P* value.
[c]Another gender identity includes respondents who identified as transgender, nonbinary or genderqueer, or "other gender identity."
[d]Financial strain was measured using the question, "In the PAST 12 MONTHS, how hard was it for you to pay for basic needs, like food, housing, utilities, and medical care?" Response options included "not hard" (no financial strain), "somewhat hard" (some financial strain), and "very hard" (high financial strain).

TABLE 3— Estimated Adjusted Odds Ratios for Associations Between Mental Health Outcomes and Age Group: New York City, 2023

	Serious Psychological Distress (SPD), AOR[a] (95% CI)	Past-Year Mental Health Treatment Among Those With SPD,[b] AOR[a] (95% CI)	Past-Year Unmet Need for Mental Health Treatment Among Those With SPD,[b] AOR[a] (95% CI)	Social Isolation, AOR[a] (95% CI)
Age group, y				
18–24 (Ref)	1	1	1	1
25–34	0.83 (0.68, 1.02)	2.14 (1.46, 3.14)	0.82 (0.57, 1.19)	0.97 (0.85, 1.10)
35–44	0.65 (0.53, 0.80)	2.31 (1.53, 3.49)	0.72 (0.49, 1.06)	0.72 (0.64, 0.82)
45–64	0.55 (0.45, 0.67)	2.31 (1.57, 3.38)	0.62 (0.43, 0.89)	0.55 (0.48, 0.62)
≥65	0.43 (0.35, 0.53)	2.43 (1.62, 3.66)	0.42 (0.28, 0.63)	0.44 (0.39, 0.50)

Note. AOR = adjusted odds ratio; CI = confidence interval.
[a]Adjusted regression models included the covariates of race and ethnicity, gender identity, sexual orientation, and financial strain.
[b]Unweighted n = 3 049.

handle their mental health without treatment, that they did not know who to contact or where to go, or that they were worried that people would think badly of them (Table 4).

DISCUSSION

There are some groups of emerging adults for whom focused research and policy efforts to improve mental health outcomes are needed. An increasing number of Gen Z individuals identify as lesbian, gay, or bisexual compared with millennials at the same age, and they may face stigma and discrimination that can harm their well-being.[25] In our study, bisexual emerging adults showed particularly concerning trends across all mental health outcomes. Emerging adults unsure of their sexual orientation also showed higher rates of SPD than heterosexual individuals. This is consistent with previous research that found that bisexual youths and those questioning their sexuality have a higher risk of poor mental health outcomes compared with those with other sexual identities.[17]

The population of transgender and gender-diverse individuals is also

TABLE 4— Associations Between Mental Health Outcomes and Age Group (Among Those Reporting an Unmet Need): New York City, 2023

	Age Group (Ref = 18–24 Years), AOR[a] (95% CI)			
	25–34 Years	35–44 Years	45–64 Years	≥65 Years
Thought I could handle my mental health without treatment	0.69 (0.53, 0.91)	0.63 (0.47, 0.84)	0.58 (0.44, 0.77)	0.45 (0.33, 0.61)
Didn't know who to contact or where to go	0.64 (0.49, 0.83)	0.47 (0.36, 0.63)	0.44 (0.34, 0.59)	0.43 (0.31, 0.59)
Could not afford cost	1.35 (1.02, 1.77)	0.80 (0.60, 1.07)	0.60 (0.45, 0.80)	0.43 (0.31, 0.59)
Hours or locations were not convenient	1.10 (0.81, 1.48)	0.89 (0.64, 1.24)	0.79 (0.57, 1.09)	0.59 (0.40, 0.87)
Worried people would think badly of me	0.64 (0.44, 0.92)	0.57 (0.38, 0.85)	0.61 (0.42, 0.88)	0.61 (0.39, 0.95)
Worried it could affect my job	0.99 (0.63, 1.56)	0.99 (0.60, 1.63)	1.07 (0.68, 1.70)	0.28 (0.13, 0.59)
Could not find a provider who spoke my language or understood my culture	1.10 (0.65, 1.86)	1.13 (0.65, 1.99)	1.43 (0.84, 2.43)	1.33 (0.75, 2.36)
Problems using telehealth services	1.60 (0.98, 2.62)	1.10 (0.63, 1.93)	1.40 (0.83, 2.35)	2.97 (1.75, 5.02)
Insurance issues[b]	2.30 (1.11, 4.77)	2.82 (1.34, 5.95)	1.67 (0.76, 3.65)	0.80 (0.32, 2.01)

Note. AOR = adjusted odds ratio; CI = confidence interval. The unweighted number of those reporting an unmet need was 5728.
[a]Adjusted regression models included the covariates of race and ethnicity, gender identity, sexual orientation, and financial strain.
[b]Insurance issues was not included as an original multiple-choice answer option. Category derived from open-ended responses of "other, please specify."

growing, especially among youths. This group is currently facing stigma, violence, and attacks on their rights in the United States, which increases vulnerability to psychological distress.[18] Our findings show that emerging adults who identify with a gender identity besides cisgender reported high levels of SPD and social isolation. As Gen Z transitions from adolescence to adulthood, additional mental health resources should be allocated toward meeting the mental health needs of the LGBTQ+ population, along with efforts to address the discrimination and stigma that contribute to these health disparities.[8] It is notable that these inequalities persist in NYC despite the New York metropolitan area having the largest LGBTQ+ population in the country[26] and a relatively supportive political environment. While current antidiscrimination policies are a necessary first step, more action is needed at the city, state, and federal levels.

Another subpopulation on which to focus policy efforts is emerging adults experiencing adverse social drivers of health. Financial strain can influence mental health through multiple pathways, including increasing stress[27] and serving as a barrier to treatment. In our data, financial strain was associated with a higher prevalence of SPD and social isolation among emerging adults; emerging adults experiencing high financial strain had a prevalence of SPD 4 times higher than those not experiencing financial strain. Financial strain was not significantly associated with mental health treatment, suggesting that differential access to treatment is not driving the poor mental health outcomes. Financial strain is a particularly salient risk factor for mental illness among emerging adults, who are more susceptible to employment loss[13] and earn lower wages. Unemployment was also significantly associated with SPD among emerging adults in our study. In recent decades in the United States, poverty among those aged 18 to 24 years has spiked, with poverty rates for those aged 18 to 24 years among the highest across the entire age distribution, yet young adults are less likely to be eligible for public benefits compared with older adults.[28] To mitigate financial strain among emerging adults that can lead to poor mental health outcomes, it is necessary to expand the social safety net and eligibility for government antipoverty programs for this age group, as well as to implement broader redistributive policies to reduce economic inequality and poverty, such as raising the minimum wage and increasing the availability of public and affordable housing.[19,29]

Emerging adults experiencing IPV or neighborhood violence also had a higher prevalence of SPD and social isolation. Violence is a significant source of mental health problems among adolescents and emerging adults. Addressing this risk factor requires interventions at both the individual level (such as education about healthy relationships) and structural level (such as school policies to address sexual harassment[8] and blight remediation of buildings and land[30]). SPD also increased on a gradient as the frequency of discrimination based on race and ethnicity increased. Social media may contribute to increased exposure, both directly and vicariously, to bullying, racism, and hate speech among youths of color.[31]

Emerging adults reported a higher prevalence of SPD than all other age groups, supporting previous reports of increased burden of mental illness among this age group.[1,2] After controlling for sociodemographic variables, those aged 18 to 24 years had higher odds of both SPD and social isolation compared with those aged 35 to 44, 45 to 64, and 65 years or older, although they did not differ significantly from those aged 25 to 34 years. While those aged 18 to 24 years may share some unique characteristics, no strict age cut-off completely captures the experiences of an age group; future work should explore mental health among those aged 25 to 34 years.

A key finding from this study was that among individuals with SPD, emerging adults had lower odds of past-year mental health treatment compared with all other age groups. One potential explanation for this disparity is differences in perceived need for treatment. Emerging adults with SPD did not report higher levels of unmet need than those aged 25 to 34 or 35 to 44 years, despite lower treatment levels. Emerging adults who did report an unmet need were more likely than older adults to report that they thought they could handle their mental health on their own, with more than half reporting this barrier. Both findings suggest that those aged 18 to 24 years may have more difficulty identifying symptoms of psychological distress and when they may need professional help. Interventions such as Mental Health First Aid training, an evidence-based intervention that seeks to teach skills needed to identify and respond to signs of mental health challenges and crises, could help address this gap in awareness.[32]

In addition, stigma may play a role in emerging adults not seeking or receiving treatment. Emerging adults had higher odds than all other age groups of concern that others would think badly of them if they received mental health treatment. Campaigns targeted at this population, such as social media campaigns, could help reduce stigma and educate emerging adults about mental health.

Lower treatment rates among emerging adults may also reflect their uncertainty about how or where to access care. Emerging adults had higher odds than all other age groups of attributing their unmet need to not knowing who to contact or where to go for treatment. In addition to education campaigns, efforts to connect emerging adults to care in places they already frequent, such as community centers, athletic clubs, libraries, and schools, may help bridge the treatment gap. App-based mental health interventions have also shown promise for addressing some symptoms of mental illness in this age group.[33] Finally, young adults may have trouble navigating the transition from child to adult care systems. Efforts to enhance referral streams and shared planning between these 2 systems could help facilitate continuity of care and increase treatment rates.[11,34]

Interestingly, emerging adults were less likely to report that insurance or cost was the reason for their unmet need than those aged 25 to 34 years, perhaps because of access to treatment through their parent's insurance or school health services. However, cost was still 1 of the top reasons for unmet need, with nearly half of emerging adults (46%) reporting an unmet need identifying this barrier to treatment. There is a need to increase affordable and insurance-covered mental health treatment options for adults across all ages, which could be accomplished by a universal, publicly funded health care system.

The study's focus on NYC serves as both a strength and a limitation. The size and diversity of NYC allow for examination of different identities, such as noncisgender adults, which may face sample size constraints in other geographical areas. Furthermore, because NYC has made mental health a public priority,[35] an understanding of inequalities that persist can inform where additional efforts should be directed. While results may not be directly generalizable to populations outside NYC, many of the upstream determinants of mental health operate at the national and societal levels.

Major strengths of this study include that it is a large, representative sample. Limitations include that the NWS is cross-sectional and self-reported, so causality cannot be inferred, and there may have been respondent recall bias when reporting mental health symptoms. Small sample sizes of some populations occasionally resulted in unstable prevalence estimates. Sample size constraints also limited further analysis incorporating the intersection of gender identity and sexual orientation. Furthermore, because the survey sampling is address-based, homeless and institutionalized individuals are not represented by the data; efforts to reach these individuals should be made in future studies.

Public Health Implications

Overall, these findings demonstrate the need to expand efforts to address poor mental health and treatment needs among emerging adult populations. Additional resources should be allocated toward meeting the mental health needs of the growing Gen Z LGBTQ+ population, especially adults who identify as noncisgender or bisexual, or who are unsure of their sexual orientation. Campaigns to increase education about mental health stigma and help emerging adults navigate the transition from youth to adult care systems are needed. Finally, strategies to improve mental health outcomes should prioritize programs and policies that address upstream, systems-level drivers of mental health, such as poverty and discrimination. AJPH

ABOUT THE AUTHORS

Rachel Suss, Jo-Anne Caton, Melanie Close, Ellenie Tuazon, and Christina Norman are with the New York City (NYC) Health Department. Dewi Sihaloho was with the NYC Health Department at the time of this study.

CORRESPONDENCE

Correspondence should be sent to Rachel Suss, NYC Health Department, 42-09 28th St, Long Island City, NY 11101 (e-mail: rsuss2@health.nyc.gov). Reprints can be ordered at https://www.ajph.org by clicking the "Reprints" link.

PUBLICATION INFORMATION

Full Citation: Suss R, Caton J-A, Close M, Sihaloho D, Tuazon E, Norman C. Mental health of emerging adults in New York City in 2023. *Am J Public Health*. 2025;115(9):1426–1435.

Acceptance Date: April 12, 2025.

DOI: https://doi.org/10.2105/AJPH.2025.308163

ORCID iDs:

Rachel Suss https://orcid.org/0000-0002-0537-6694

Melanie Close https://orcid.org/0000-0002-8566-8389

Dewi Sihaloho https://orcid.org/0009-0008-8181-6904

Christina Norman https://orcid.org/0000-0003-1746-8622

CONTRIBUTORS

R. Suss, J. Caton, M. Close, and C. Norman contributed substantially to the conceptualization of the work, analysis and interpretation of data, and the drafting and revision of the work. D. Sihaloho contributed substantially to the analysis of the data and revision of the work. E. Tuazon contributed substantially to the drafting of the work and revision for important intellectual content. All authors gave final approval for the version to be published.

ACKNOWLEDGMENTS

The NYC Neighborhood Wellness Survey was funded by the NYC Health Department.

The authors would like to thank our many colleagues who contributed to the NYC Neighborhood Wellness Survey, including Sasha Fleary and Monique Millington at the City University of New

York (CUNY) Graduate School of Public Health and Health Policy. The authors would also like to thank Meghan Hamwey, Benjamin McCarthy, and Thinh Vu at the NYC Health Department for their writing support.

CONFLICTS OF INTEREST

All authors declare that they have no potential or actual conflicts of interest.

HUMAN PARTICIPANT PROTECTION

This study has been approved by the CUNY institutional review board.

REFERENCES

1. Czeisler MÉ, Lane RI, Petrosky E, et al. Mental health, substance use, and suicidal ideation during the COVID-19 pandemic—United States, June 24–30, 2020. *MMWR Morb Mortal Wkly Rep.* 2020;69(32):1049–1057. https://doi.org/10.15585/mmwr.mm6932a1
2. Goodwin RD, Weinberger AH, Kim JH, Wu M, Galea S. Trends in anxiety among adults in the United States, 2008–2018: rapid increases among young adults. *J Psychiatr Res.* 2020;130:441–446. https://doi.org/10.1016/j.jpsychires.2020.08.014
3. Office of the Surgeon General. *Protecting Youth Mental Health: The US Surgeon General's Advisory*. 2021. Available at: https://www.hhs.gov/sites/default/files/surgeon-general-youth-mental-health-advisory.pdf. Accessed September 4, 2024.
4. Shannon H, Bush K, Villeneuve PJ, Hellemans KG, Guimond S. Problematic social media use in adolescents and young adults: systematic review and meta-analysis. *JMIR Ment Health.* 2022;9(4):e33450. https://doi.org/10.2196/33450
5. Rasmussen EE, Punyanunt-Carter N, LaFreniere JR, Norman MS, Kimball TG. The serially mediated relationship between emerging adults' social media use and mental well-being. *Comput Hum Behav.* 2020;102:206–213. https://doi.org/10.1016/j.chb.2019.08.019
6. New York City Health Department. Youth services: community supports and services. Available at: https://www.nyc.gov/site/doh/health/health-topics/child-and-adolescent-mental-health-community-services.page. Accessed September 4, 2024.
7. Smith C, Crosnoe R, Chao SY. Family background and contemporary changes in young adults' school-work transitions and family formation in the United States. *Res Soc Stratif Mobil.* 2016;46(A):3–10. https://doi.org/10.1016/j.rssm.2016.01.006
8. Cattan M, Tifford S. *Mental Health Promotion.* Maidenhead, UK: McGraw-Hill Education; 2006.
9. Arnett JJ. Emerging adulthood. A theory of development from the late teens through the twenties. *Am Psychol.* 2000;55(5):469–480.
10. Solmi M, Radua J, Olivola M, et al. Age at onset of mental disorders worldwide: large-scale meta-analysis of 192 epidemiological studies. *Mol Psychiatry.* 2022;27(1):281–295. https://doi.org/10.1038/s41380-021-01161-7
11. Pottick KJ, Bilder S, Vander Stoep A, Warner LA, Alvarez MF. US patterns of mental health service utilization for transition-age youth and young adults. *J Behav Health Serv Res.* 2008;35(4):373–389. https://doi.org/10.1007/s11414-007-9080-4
12. Parker K, Igielnik R. On the cusp of adulthood and facing an uncertain future: what we know about Gen Z so far. Pew Research Center. May 14, 2020. Available at: https://www.pewresearch.org/social-trends/2020/05/14/on-the-cusp-of-adulthood-and-facing-an-uncertain-future-what-we-know-about-gen-z-so-far-2. Accessed July 3, 2024.
13. Ganson KT, Tsai AC, Weiser SD, Benabou SE, Nagata JM. Job insecurity and symptoms of anxiety and depression among US young adults during COVID-19. *J Adolesc Health.* 2021;68(1):53–56. https://doi.org/10.1016/j.jadohealth.2020.10.008
14. Carey N, Coley RL, Hawkins SS, Baum CF. Emerging adult mental health during COVID: exploring relationships between discrete and cumulative individual and contextual stressors and well-being. *J Adolesc Health.* 2024;75(1):26–34. https://doi.org/10.1016/j.jadohealth.2024.01.031
15. Hamwey M, Norman C, Suss R, et al. *The State of Mental Health of New Yorkers.* New York City Department of Health and Mental Hygiene. 2024. Available at: https://www.nyc.gov/assets/doh/downloads/pdf/mh/state-of-mental-health-new-yorkers.pdf. Accessed September 4, 2024.
16. Bruss KV, Seth P, Zhao G. Loneliness, lack of social and emotional support, and mental health issues—United States, 2022. *MMWR Morb Mortal Wkly Rep.* 2024;73(24):539–545. https://doi.org/10.15585/mmwr.mm7324a1
17. Russell ST, Fish JN. Mental health in lesbian, gay, bisexual, and transgender (LGBT) youth. *Annu Rev Clin Psychol.* 2016;12:465–487. https://doi.org/10.1146/annurev-clinpsy-021815-093153
18. Wittlin NM, Kuper LE, Olson KR. Mental health of transgender and gender diverse youth. *Annu Rev Clin Psychol.* 2023;19(1):207–232. https://doi.org/10.1146/annurev-clinpsy-072220-020326
19. World Health Organization. *Social Determinants of Mental Health.* 2014. Available at: https://www.who.int/publications/i/item/9789241506809. Accessed September 4, 2024.
20. The American Association for Public Opinion Research. Standard definitions: final dispositions of case codes and outcome rates for surveys. 2023. Available at: https://aapor.org/standards-and-ethics/standard-definitions. Accessed January 30, 2025.
21. Kessler RC, Andrews G, Colpe LJ, et al. Short screening scales to monitor population prevalences and trends in non-specific psychological distress. *Psychol Med.* 2002;32(6):959–976. https://doi.org/10.1017/s0033291702006074
22. New York City Health Department. Community Health Survey public use data. Available at: https://www.nyc.gov/site/doh/data/data-sets/community-health-survey-public-use-data.page. Accessed January 30, 2025.
23. Ito M, Nakajima S, Fujisawa D, et al. Brief measure for screening complicated grief: reliability and discriminant validity. *PLoS One.* 2012;7(2):e31209. https://doi.org/10.1371/journal.pone.0031209
24. Substance Abuse and Mental Health Services Administration. NSDUH 2023 Questionnaire. Available at: https://www.samhsa.gov/data/report/nsduh-2023-questionnaire. Accessed January 30, 2025.
25. Twenge JM, Wells BE, Le J. Increases in LGB identification among US adults, 2014–2021. *Sex Res Soc Policy.* 2024;21:863–878. https://doi.org/10.1007/s13178-023-00874-4
26. Conron K, Luhur W, Goldberg S. LGBT adults in large US metropolitan areas. UCLA School of Law Williams Institute. March 2021. Available at: https://williamsinstitute.law.ucla.edu/publications/lgbt-us-msa. Accessed January 30, 2025.
27. Steptoe A, Emch S, Hamer M. Associations between financial strain and emotional well-being with physiological responses to acute mental stress. *Psychosom Med.* 2020;82(9):830–837. https://doi.org/10.1097/PSY.0000000000000867
28. Hawkins J. The rise of young adult poverty in the US. Goldman School of Public Policy, University of California, Berkeley. June 2019. Available at: https://gspp.berkeley.edu/assets/uploads/page/poverty_FINAL_formatted.pdf. Accessed January 30, 2025.
29. Link BG, Phelan J. Social conditions as fundamental causes of disease. *J Health Soc Behav.* 1995; spec no.:80–94.
30. Kondo MC, Andreyeva E, South EC, MacDonald JM, Branas CC. Neighborhood interventions to reduce violence. *Annu Rev Public Health.* 2018;39:253–271. https://doi.org/10.1146/annurev-publhealth-040617-014600
31. Naslund JA, Bondre A, Torous J, Aschbrenner KA. Social media and mental health: benefits, risks, and opportunities for research and practice. *J Technol Behav Sci.* 2020;5(3):245–257. https://doi.org/10.1007/s41347-020-00134-x
32. Banh MK, Chaikind J, Robertson HA, et al. Evaluation of Mental Health First Aid USA using the Mental Health Beliefs and Literacy Scale. *Am J Health Promot.* 2019;33(2):237–247. https://doi.org/10.1177/0890117118784234
33. Leech T, Dorstyn D, Taylor A, Li W. Mental health apps for adolescents and young adults: a systematic review of randomised controlled trials. *Child Youth Serv Rev.* 2021;127:106073. https://doi.org/10.1016/j.childyouth.2021.106073
34. Davis M, Sondheimer DL. State child mental health efforts to support youth in transition to adulthood. *J Behav Health Serv Res.* 2005;32(1):27–42. https://doi.org/10.1007/BF02287326
35. New York City Health Department. Care, Community, Action: A Mental Health Plan for NYC. 2023. Available at: https://www.nyc.gov/assets/doh/care-community-action-mental-health-plan/index.html. Accessed January 30, 2025.

Social Vulnerability and Racial Disparities in Depression Screening of US Adolescents, 2016 to 2021

Kathleen Galper, MPH, Jillian M. Rung, PhD, Amber Shergill, MPH, Tyson S. Barrett, PhD, Demetrios Marousis, MA, and Emily Brignone, PhD

See also Adolescent Mental Health, pp. 1377–1453.

Objectives. To identify whether sociodemographic disparities exist by evaluating the association between rates of adolescent depression screening, social risk, and race.

Methods. We used a US nationwide sample of Highmark Health privately insured adolescents between 2016 and 2021 to estimate the odds of well-visit depression screening receipt as a function of social factors (Social Vulnerability Index [SVI], predicted race).

Results. Higher SVI was negatively associated with odds of screening and depended on predicted Black race (*P* for interaction < .01). Provider type was a strong predictor of screening, with pediatricians more likely to screen than other generalist specialties (odds ratio = 9.64; 95% confidence interval = 9.11, 10.2). Inclusion of variation at the practice location level attenuated the relationship with SVI and accounted for a large proportion of variability in screening (intraclass correlation coefficient = 0.76), although SVI remained significant (*P* < .01).

Conclusions. Adolescents are more likely to receive a depression screen if they reside in lower social-risk locations or, if likely to identify as Black, higher social-risk locations. Ultimately, screening has strong ties to where an adolescent lives and the type of provider they access. (*Am J Public Health*. 2025;115(9): 1436–1444. https://doi.org/10.2105/AJPH.2025.308149)

Adolescent depression is a significant and widespread public health concern, with a profound impact on various aspects of health, development, and natural life outcomes. Approximately 20% of adolescents experience a depressive episode before reaching adulthood,[1] which can impair academic performance, strain relationships, increase morbidity, and heighten risk of substance use disorders and suicidal behaviors.[2,3] Adolescent-onset depression is a strong predictor of recurrent depressive episodes and chronic mental health issues into adulthood, which pose further significant economic burdens from disability and loss of productivity.[4,5] The long-term impacts of adolescent depression underscore the need for early identification and intervention to mitigate extensive personal and societal costs.[6]

The connections between adolescent depression and socioeconomic status (SES) are complex and mediated by multiple factors. Adolescents from lower-SES backgrounds face higher rates of depression, which is attributable to a combination of chronic stressors, including financial and familial instability, limited access to mental health and educational resources, and higher exposure to violence.[1,2] Socioeconomic hardships can trigger some of these stressors, which then adversely affect adolescent mental health.[2] Taken together, low-SES adolescents routinely face barriers accessing quality and sufficient health care, which exacerbates the risk and severity of untreated or undertreated mental health disorders.[3]

The US Preventive Services Task Force (USPTF) recommends screening for major depressive disorder in adolescents aged 12 to 18 years,[4,5] ideally with support from systems that ensure accurate diagnosis, effective treatment, and proper follow-up. Health care professionals agree that adhering to screening guidelines is essential for effective identification, intervention, and management.[6] Despite that, screening rates remain low, even among privately insured adolescents, highlighting gaps in health care delivery and suggesting that systemic barriers continue to hinder screening implementation.[7–9] Given the external barriers and risk of double burden among a lower-SES population, lagging screening rates may pose outsize harm through delayed identification and treatment to those at highest risk. This conflict underscores the need for more robust screening practices and systems to ensure that all adolescents are appropriately assessed for mental health issues.

However, data are lacking on how the intersection of social risk, race/ethnicity, and care team characteristics may influence screening. Furthermore, there is limited understanding of current screening rates more broadly, as recent literature typically relies on data from single locations.[6,10] Information regarding the relationship between screening rates and social vulnerability can inform policy for the provision of education and resources that will empower providers to uniformly screen and treat adolescents at risk. As such, we extracted information on adolescent members and depression screening from a large health plan claims database and linked these data to the Social Vulnerability Index (SVI) from the Centers for Disease Control and Prevention (CDC) to investigate the relationship between SVI and adolescent depression screening.[11]

METHODS

The analytic cohort included adolescents aged 12 to 18 years across the United States who were enrolled in medical insurance through Highmark Health. To be eligible, adolescents had to be enrolled at some point between January 1, 2016 and April 30, 2021, with at least 1 well visit preceded by 6 months of enrollment. We identified well visits via outpatient claims with Current Procedural Terminology (CPT; American Medical Association, https://www.ama-assn.org/practice-management/cpt) codes (99381, 99382, 99383, 99384, 99385, 99391, 99392, 99393, 99394, 99395, 99461) or *International Classification of Diseases, 10th Revision* (*ICD-10*; Geneva, Switzerland: World Health Organization, 1992) codes (Z00121, Z00129, Z0000, Z0001). To avoid bias by member age or visit year, we selected a single random well visit as the index visit for each member. We identified depression screening from claims on the day of the index visit with the CPT/Healthcare Common Procedure Coding System (G0444, G8510, G8431, G8511, G8940, 96127) or *ICD-10* code (Z1331) in any position. We excluded individuals based on discontinuous medical coverage, missing covariate data, baseline depression diagnosis, antidepressant prescription, psychotherapy treatment, or (because of the requirements of the analytic method) residing in a zip code with fewer than 3 other individuals. Most exclusions resulted from prior diagnosis or treatment of depression, or lack of sufficient continuous medical coverage. Few members were excluded because of missing covariate data (< 0.1%; for flow diagram, see Figure B, available as a supplement to the online version of this article at http://www.ajph.org). The final sample meeting these criteria was 178 972.

Measures

We extracted the SVI from the CDC's 2018 estimates and appended it using geographic joining keys based on member residential address at index visit. The SVI is defined by 4 domains (Socioeconomic Status, Household Composition & Disability, Minority Status & Language, and Housing Type & Transportation) derived from 5-year averages of census tract data (2013–2018), and reported as an unweighted sum.[11] Although created to identify areas vulnerable to natural disaster, the SVI has frequently been implemented to demonstrate the importance of vulnerability in morbidity and mortality risk from chronic and noncommunicable disease.[12,13] We used the raw SVI in 2 ways: first as a categorical term with SVI broken into tertiles of low (SVI = 1.38–5.63), moderate (SVI = 5.64–7.21), and high (SVI = 7.22–13.1) social risk, and second as a standardized continuous term such that 1 unit represents 1 standard deviation. An additional version of SVI was used in select models, described where relevant in Methods.

Member characteristics were based on information from, or within, the 6-month look-back prior to the index well visit. This included sociodemographic factors, personal medical history, health care utilization (inpatient, emergency, and preventive encounters), and attributed provider specialty. Member age and gender were sourced from enrollment information, and medical history was quantified with the Agency for Healthcare Research and Quality's Pediatric Medical Complexity Algorithm (PMCA)[14] using all claims from the pre–well visit period. We calculated health care utilization based on unique service or admission dates. Well visit provider type was captured from the performing provider field on the index claim and categorized as "pediatric," "family medicine," or "other primary care" (e.g., multispecialty group, internal medicine) per specialty codes. We used identifiers for practice location of the performing provider to classify place of visit for sensitivity analysis.

Sociodemographic factors included predicted race and rurality of members' residence. Because the claims database does not contain member racial or ethnic identification, we computed a proxy term for race using RAND's Bayesian Improved Surname Geocoding (BISG) methodology. The BISG yields predicted probabilities for each of 5 race and ethnicity categories (White, Black, Hispanic, Asian, or Other) based on last name, age, gender, and census tract. We generated the BISG estimates for the cohort using the wru package.[15] Prior work has validated the BISG method within national health plans and found that the estimates are highly correlated with self-identified race (average concordance = 0.93).[15] For descriptive purposes only, predicted race was directly imputed based on the race or ethnicity category with the greatest predicted probability. However, all modeling incorporated the continuous predicted race probabilities, which better accounts for confidence and accuracy than direct categorical imputation. Because the BISG method includes Hispanic as its own category, predicted probabilities of race do not account for Hispanic ethnicity. Rurality designations were based on the US Department of Agriculture's Food Access Research Atlas categorization.[16] Residential zip code was additionally appended based on member address, per administrative claims, at time of index visit.

Statistical Analysis

We compared baseline characteristics by SVI tertile using Pearson's χ^2 test for categorical terms and Kruskal–Wallis rank sum test for continuous terms. We set statistical significance at $P < .05$ for all analyses.

To assess the relationship between SVI and likelihood of receiving a depression screen at a well visit, we used a hierarchical model building approach focusing first on fixed effects and then incorporating random effects. Unlike a stepwise approach, the order of variable inclusion is driven by theory rather than the magnitude of association with the outcome. The starting model contained SVI and a quadratic term to capture the nonlinear association between SVI and depression screening (evidenced by visual inspection of raw data; see Figure 1). Then, theoretically important variables (e.g., provider type, rurality) and relevant member characteristics were added to the model one at a time. To be retained

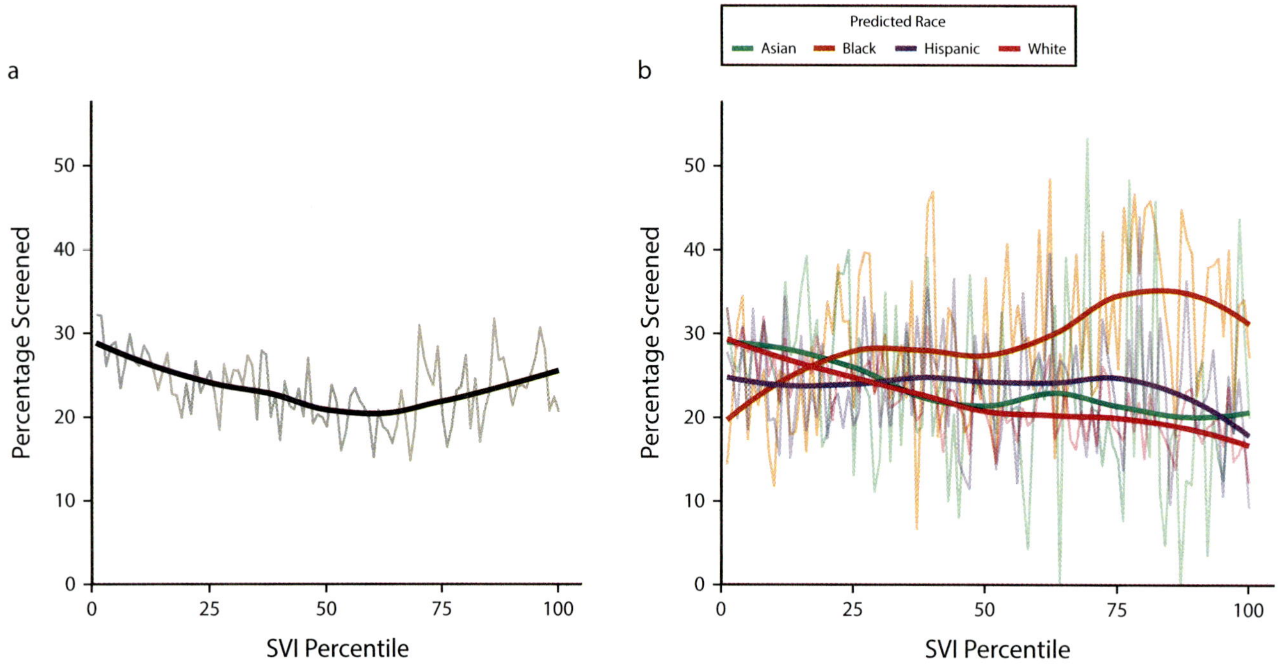

FIGURE 1— Percentage of Members Being Screened for Depression as a Function of Their Percentile-Transformed Social Vulnerability Index (SVI) for (a) the Full Sample and (b) as a Function of Those Who Met Threshold for Likely Identifying as Asian, Black, Hispanic, or White: United States, 2016–2021

Note. Raw data are represented by thinner, more transparent lines, with LOESS (locally estimated scatterplot smoothing) smoothed estimates overlaid in bold lines.

in the model, variable coefficients were required to be statistically significant and yield a significant improvement in the overall model based on a likelihood ratio test. Additionally, Akaike information criterion values were compared to ensure that significant improvements were also substantive, because negligible effects may be statistically significant given the large sample.

Included in the variable selection process was an interaction between SVI and predicted race, based on visual inspection of these variables and proportion screened (Figure 1b). We incorporated predicted race into models as the BISG predicted probability estimate of Black race. We used this single probability estimate based on its distinct trajectory (all others had similar, negative slopes) and nonsignificance of other race categories in the variable selection process. For all models fitted with predicted race, we removed the minority status and language domain from composite SVI to avoid overfitting as they rely on the same underlying census data.

Finally, variability in screening across years and community level clustering was accounted for with random intercepts for screening year and residential zip code, respectively. Their inclusion was subject to the same variable retainment criteria described in this subsection. We calculated the intraclass correlation coefficient to quantify the variance in screening attributable to year and zip code as the proportion of variance in the data explained by the random effects, without regard to the fixed effects (i.e., the adjusted intraclass correlation coefficient) using the distribution-specific variance.

Additional analyses explored potential contributors to gaps in screening and differences in the effect of SVI across categorical predictors. First, we conducted a sensitivity analysis to quantify variability explained by practice location clustering; for this, we created a subset of the cohort, which was limited to members attending a practice that performed well visits for at least 3 members in the sample. The final model was refitted with this smaller subset of the cohort and an additional random intercept for practice location. Of the 23 545 distinct practice locations attended by the initial 178 972-member sample, 13 552 practice locations met the sensitivity sample requirement with 167 235 members. Next, differences in the effect of SVI were identified through subgroup analyses refitting the final model with data split into subsets based on different levels of categorical predictors. We included member age in subgroup analyses based on younger (< 15 years) versus older members (≥ 15 years). Finally, we ran a supplemental Poisson regression at the practice location level to identify any variation in the rate of change in screening over time across practice locations (i.e., if different practices adopted guidelines at different rates).

We conducted all analyses using RStudio Workbench (version 1.4.1717-3) running R version 4.0.0. Package reference details are included in the methods citation section of the online Appendix.

RESULTS

Cohort characteristics stratified by SVI tertile are presented in Table 1. Figure 1 shows the proportion of members screened as a function of SVI and key sources of variability in screening rates that were subsequently explored in modeling analyses. Of 178 972 total members, 23% had a depression screen at their well visit; screening rates were not uniform by SVI (Figure 1a), with a rate of 25% in low SVI areas, 21% in moderate, and 23% in high. Graphical inspection by predicted race category further illustrated that those likely to identify as Black accounted for the increased screening rates in the highest SVI areas (Figure 1b). As shown in Table 1, most of the cohort had visits occurring between 2017 and 2020, and in that time frame the rate of screening increased from less than 15% to almost 40%. This trend in increasing rates of screening over time was evident across all SVI tertiles.

The initial unadjusted model (i.e., a linear and quadratic term for SVI and no random effects) had a very poor fit with R^2 0.002 and an area under the curve of 53%, although SVI was statistically significant ($P < .01$) and suggested a nonlinear relationship such that the odds of a screen initially decrease with increasing SVI up to the mean (SVI odds ratio [OR] = 0.94; 95% confidence interval [CI] = 0.93, 0.95), then increase again (quadratic SVI [OR] = 1.07; 95% [CI] = 1.06, 1.08). The iterative addition of other independent variables thought to be significant per baseline analysis (Table 1) included age, gender, predicted race, provider type, PMCA category, and rurality. All terms were statistically significant except for gender, but because of its theoretical importance, it was left in the model. Interaction terms were tested and, ultimately, a term for predicted Black probability × SVI was kept for its statistical significance, magnitude of association, and improvement in overall model fit. Finally, following the inclusion of all other covariates and random effects, the quadratic term for SVI no longer met criteria for inclusion and was ultimately removed from the model.

The significance and magnitude of the association between SVI and depression screening was maintained in the fully adjusted model despite the

TABLE 1— Baseline Characteristics of Cohort Across Social Vulnerability Index Tertiles: United States, 2016–April 2021

	Social Vulnerability Tertile, Mean ±SD or No. (%)				
Variable	Low (n = 58 937)	Moderate (n = 57 987)	High (n = 62 048)	P[a]	Effect Size[b]
Female	28 327 (48.1)	27 949 (48.2)	30 839 (49.7)	< .01	0.0
Age at well visit	15.0 ±2.0	15.0 ±2.0	14.9 ±2.0	< .01	0.0
BISG[c] race (direct imputation)				< .01	0.2
Asian	2 048 (3.5)	1 293 (2.2)	954 (1.5)		
Black	1 263 (2.1)	2 688 (4.6)	10 804 (17.4)		
Hispanic	2 700 (4.6)	3 863 (6.7)	10 733 (17.3)		
Other	33 (0.1)	40 (0.1)	382 (0.6)		
White	52 893 (89.7)	50 103 (86.4)	39 175 (63.1)		
Probability Black	0.1 ±0.1	0.1 ±0.2	0.2 ±0.3	< .01	0.0
Probability White	0.8 ±0.3	0.8 ±0.3	0.6 ±0.4	< .01	0.1
Probability Asian	0.0 ±0.2	0.0 ±0.1	0.0 ±0.1	< .01	0.0
Probability Hispanic	0.1 ±0.2	0.1 ±0.2	0.2 ±0.3	< .01	0.0
Probability other	0.0 ±0.0	0.0 ±0.0	0.0 ±0.1	< .01	0.0
Urban	42 793 ±72.6	34 077 ±58.8	43 630 ±70.3	< .01	0.1
Year of index visit				< .01	0.0
2016	6 700 (11.4)	6 668 (11.5)	5 814 (9.4)		
2017	10 828 (18.4)	11 133 (19.2)	10 316 (16.6)		
2018	11 466 (19.5)	11 851 (20.4)	13 838 (22.3)		
2019	12 087 (20.5)	11 926 (20.6)	14 053 (22.6)		
2020	13 577 (23.0)	12 481 (21.5)	13 284 (21.4)		
2021[d]	4 279 (7.3)	3 928 (6.8)	4 743 (7.6)		
Census region				<.01	0.1
Midwest	9 702 (16.5)	6 777 (11.7)	6 863 (11.1)		
Northeast	30 470 (51.7)	31 064 (53.6)	21 752 (35.1)		
South	15 961 (27.1)	17 698 (30.5)	29 601 (47.7)		
US territories/other	0 (0.0)	4 (0.0)	0 (0.0)		
West	2 804 (4.8)	2 444 (4.2)	3 832 (6.2)		
Emergency department	0.1 (0.3)	0.1 (0.3)	0.1 (0.4)	< .01	0.0
Inpatient stays[e]	3.6 (70.8)	3.9 (68.8)	5.2 (90.3)	< .01	0.0
Preventive care	0.2 (0.5)	0.2 (0.7)	0.2 (0.6)	0.5	0.0
Depression screen at visit	14 996 (25.4)	12 233 (21.1)	14 549 (23.4)	< .01	0.0
Medical complexity				< .01	0.0
Complex chronic	1 986 (3.4)	2 065 (3.6)	2 506 (4.0)		
Nonchronic	46 771 (79.4)	45 798 (79.0)	47 793 (77.0)		
Noncomplex chronic	10 180 (17.3)	10 124 (17.5)	11 749 (18.9)		
Provider type				< .01	0.1
Family medicine	6 325 (10.7)	9 846 (17.0)	8 976 (14.5)		
Other primary care	32 773 (55.6)	28 600 (49.3)	33 538 (54.1)		
Pediatric	19 839 (33.7)	19 541 (33.7)	19 534 (31.5)		

Note. The study cohort includes a sample of members of a national private payor. The total sample size was n = 178 972.
[a]Pearson's χ^2 test; Kruskal–Wallis rank sum test; Fisher's Exact Test for count data with simulated *P* value (based on 2000 replicates).
[b]Eta squared for Kruskal–Wallis, Cramer's V for χ^2.
[c]BISG = Bayesian Improved Surname Geocoding, a method for imputing race/ethnicity based on first/last name, date of birth, and census tract.
[d]Partial year, only runs through April 2021.
[e]Represented as rate per 1000 members.

significance of most individual and environmental predictors incorporated, as well as the random intercepts for year of screening and zip code. The interaction between race and SVI indicated that the relationship between SVI and depression screening depended on the likelihood of predicted Black race, where those likely to identify as Black in high SVI areas had higher predicted odds of screening than those unlikely to identify as Black in high SVI areas ($P < .01$; see Figure 2 for a depiction of the moderated association).

Subgroup analyses overall revealed little variation in the magnitude of the association between SVI and screening by individual member characteristics such as gender, age, medical complexity, or rurality (Figure B, available as a supplement to the online version of this article at http://www.ajph.org). However, models suggested differences by provider type such that SVI was not significantly associated with screening within family medicine providers, and was more strongly associated with reductions in screening within less specific provider specialties. Ultimately, the sensitivity model revealed that a large proportion of the variability in screening likelihood could be explained by clustering at the practice level: the addition of the random intercept representing practice location increased the intraclass correlation coefficient from 0.38 to 0.78 (see online Table A for full comparison of random effects variances across models). This addition attenuated both SVI and predicted Black race, although they remained statistically significant (Table 2). Ancillary Poisson analyses further demonstrated significant variability in the yearly trend (likelihood ratio test to reduced model $P < .01$) across practice locations (random slope, 0.18; full model output in online Table C).

DISCUSSION

The goal of this study was to describe patterns of adolescent depression screening at annual well visits by measures of social vulnerability. Our findings show that screening remains relatively low (approximately 23% of members), and that there is a nuanced relationship between the odds of screening and SVI. Although SVI is negatively associated with screening, the relationship depends on Black race, such that those most likely to identify

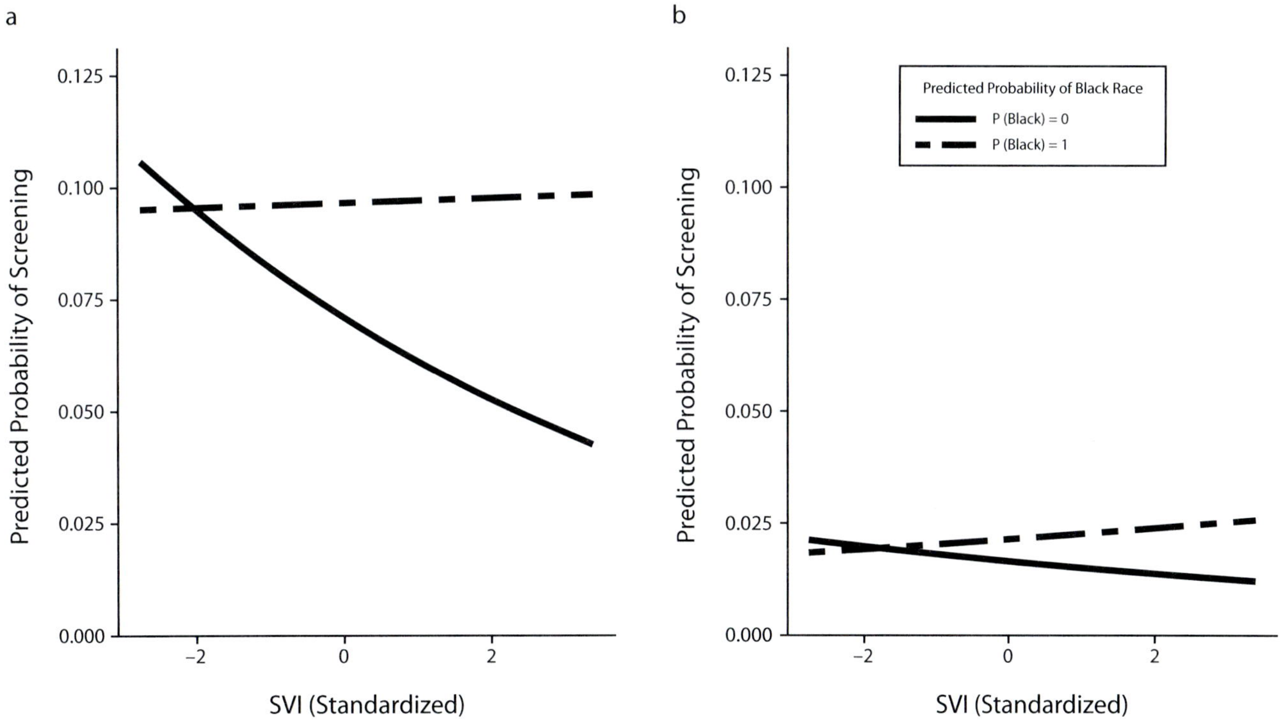

FIGURE 2— Predicted Probability of Being Screened for Depression as a Function of a High (P[Black] = 1) or Low (P[Black] = 0) Predicted Probability of Black Race From Generalized Linear Mixed Effects Models (a) Without (Fully Adjusted) and (b) With (Sensitivity) Terms to Control for Variability by Practice Location: United States, 2016–2021

Note. SVI = Social Vulnerability Index. Predictions are based on the midpoint of the study period for both models (year = 2019); for the sensitivity model, a random provider location whose percentage of members with depression screenings was at the average for that year (mean = 20%) was chosen.

TABLE 2— Odds of Depression Screening Receipt in the Context of a Well Visit as a Function of SVI and Other Predictors: United States, 2016–April 2021

	OR (95% CI)	
Characteristic	**Fully Adjusted**	**Sensitivity**
SVI	0.85 (0.84, 0.87)	0.91 (0.89, 0.94)
Provider type		
Family medicine (Ref)	1	1
Other primary care	2.17 (2.04, 2.31)	3.39 (2.92, 3.93)
Pediatric	9.64 (9.11, 10.2)	5.42 (4.59, 6.40)
Age	0.96 (0.95, 0.96)	1.00 (0.99, 1.01)
Rurality (Ref = urban)	1.16 (1.11, 1.20)	1.07 (1.02, 1.13)
BISG probability Black	1.40 (1.29, 1.52)	1.30 (1.16, 1.47)
Medical complexity		
Nonchronic (Ref)	1	1
Noncomplex chronic	1.05 (1.01, 1.08)	1.01 (0.96, 1.06)
Complex chronic	1.01 (0.94, 1.08)	0.80 (0.72, 0.88)
Gender (Ref = female)	0.98 (0.95, 1.00)	1.01 (0.97, 1.05)
SVI × BISG Probability Black	1.18 (1.10, 1.26)	1.16 (1.06, 1.27)

Note. BISG = Bayesian Improved Surname Geocoding (a method for imputing race/ethnicity based on first/last name, date of birth, and census tract); CI = confidence interval; OR = odds ratio; SVI = Social Vulnerability Index. The fully adjusted model includes the full sample cohort (n = 178 972); the sensitivity model includes a restricted sample of those attending a practice with at least 3 cohort members (n = 167 235). Study cohort includes a sample of members of a national private payor.

as Black residing in areas with the highest social risk had some of the greatest odds of screening across the SVI distribution. Of note, pediatricians far outpaced other provider types in screening. Ultimately, the sensitivity model clarified that much of the variability in depression screening across race and social risk can be explained by differences in group behaviors at the practice level.

The finding that provider type and degree of adherence to guidelines varied with geographic measures of social risk suggests that depression screening receipt is, in part, an issue of access and provider ability. Furthermore, the increased screening rates within higher SVI areas seen in the unadjusted data ultimately depended on a higher likelihood of identifying as Black. Members who were likely Black and resided in urban areas were seen by pediatricians at rates higher than any other race category (online Table B). It is possible that the density of urban areas allows for both greater proximity and greater availability of pediatric providers, and thus higher screening rates. The same providers may also be more empowered to screen, diagnose, and treat, as some pediatricians serving a primarily urban, high social risk case mix report higher rates of comanagement with pediatric mental health providers.[17]

Although increased screening rates among those likely to identify as Black is a positive sign, it is important to note that minority groups may also be disproportionately disadvantaged by living in less connected areas relative to their White peers. A study of pediatric access, availability, race, and mental health screening found that although Black, lower-SES children benefited from urban access, relatively short increases in drive time to a pediatrician had the strongest negative influence on screening rates among Black and Hispanic children.[18] Furthermore, in our sample, most of those unlikely to identify as Black in higher SVI areas had far lower model predicted odds of screening receipt, indicating persistent disparities by geography.

Evaluation of screening rates by broader indicators of social risk is uncommon, although there is existing evidence that general geographic factors like pediatrician access and availability are associated with screening.[18] Others have shown that screening completion can vary by individual factors such as native language, child demographics, insurance status, parental beliefs, or provider consistency, although reports are mixed on the direction and magnitude of association.[7,8,19] Our results showed that the bulk of variability in screening rates is primarily determined by practice-level tendencies, which may be more modifiable. Although education and training likely play a large role in these tendencies, published research suggests that resources may also be key, as providers cite time constraints, disagreement on the role of general pediatric providers in mental health management, and concern with a lack of available follow-up.[20–22] In the context of these findings, solutions that reduce direct time burdens on providers to perform screening, and ensure that providers have viable mental health care referral sources, could help improve screening guideline compliance. However, these solutions are speculative and would require direct study.

Although screening remains lower than ideal across studies, it appears that the USPTF guidelines have had a positive impact. A report on rates in the mid- to late 2010s found minimal screening overall, with just 1.8% of adolescents with a documented screen across a 5-year follow-up.[8] More recent analyses, as well as rates reported in this study (Table 1), show evidence of marked increases over time, although most existing estimates are often limited in scope.[6,10] Our supplemental analysis to identify variation in the rate of change in screening over time across providers revealed significant variation in adopting screening guidance, with some quick to change and others trailing behind. Although this study was not designed to identify specific provider tendencies that may influence screening, this finding and our primary results demonstrate the importance of the provider in closing screening gaps and the need for more research on the interface of provider behavior, geography, and individual determinants. Empowering physicians to better manage adolescents with depression and improving competency in pediatric mental health will be necessary to meet the needs of adolescents and avoid significant burden over the life course.

Limitations

This work presents a robust examination of the nuanced relationship between social risk, race, provider, and depression screening. Still, there are limitations. Although the BISG algorithm presents an opportunity to consider race where otherwise impossible, it is subject to misclassification. We attempted to account for the uncertainty in members' predicted race by incorporating continuous predicted probabilities as model terms rather than a direct imputation, although this can make interpretation more complex. Because members' index well visits occurred anywhere between 2016 and 2021, and all SVI data were from 2018 five-year estimates (spanning 2013–2018), there is a possibility that the SVI estimates may not reflect true area-level vulnerability across the study span. However, given that changes in geographic social risk are slow, it seems unlikely that using the 2018 estimates would yield substantive differences.

It is also important to note that claims-based measures of health status and utilization are subject to billing requirements, accuracy of data entry, and practitioners' time to comprehensively chart all elements of visits. As such, the estimates herein may reflect underestimates of actual use and experience. However, we used measures of health status validated for use with administrative data where possible. Although we cannot account for screens that occurred and were never recorded, we investigated whether excluding depression screenings at other visit types may have affected our findings by including any screen within 18 months of a member's randomly chosen well visit. The overall rate of screening increased only marginally (from 23% to 25%), and the pattern of results remained the same.

Despite these limitations, the opportunity to leverage administrative claims data from a large national payor allowed for the inclusion of adolescents and providers across a large geographic area and more accurate accounting of screening rates than single health system analyses or provider self-report.

Public Health Implications

Early identification of adolescent depression is needed to mitigate the burdens of and risks to adolescents' current health and longer-term impacts into adulthood; this is particularly important among those at higher risk because of social determinants or systemic inequalities. The USPTF recommends routine screening for depression in annual well visits to address this need, although our data show that uptake is still relatively low. Geographic-based social vulnerability is associated with a lower likelihood of screening, even after accounting for patient, geographic, and provider-level factors, although the nature of the association is complex and moderated by race. Ultimately, practice-level tendencies explain much of the variability in screening rates. Further study is needed to understand provider barriers and facilitators of screening across locations of varied social risk, which may lead to equitable solutions for improving identification and intervention. AJPH

ABOUT THE AUTHORS

Kathleen Galper, Jillian M. Rung, Amber Shergill, Tyson S. Barrett, and Emily Brignone are with Advanced Analytics at Highmark Health, and Highmark Health Research Institute, Pittsburgh, PA. Demetrios Marousis is with the Enterprise Behavioral Health Clinical Programs and Innovation Department at Highmark Inc, Pittsburgh, PA.

CORRESPONDENCE

Correspondence should be sent to Kathleen Galper, Highmark Health, Fifth Avenue Place, 120 Fifth Ave, Pittsburgh, PA 15222-3099 (e-mail: Kathleen.Galper@highmarkhealth.org). Reprints can be ordered at https://www.ajph.org by clicking the "Reprints" link.

PUBLICATION INFORMATION

Full Citation: Galper K, Rung JM, Shergill A, Barrett TS, Marousis D, Brignone E. Social vulnerability and racial disparities in depression screening of US adolescents, 2016 to 2021. *Am J Public Health*. 2025;115(9):1436–1444.

Acceptance Date: April 1, 2025.

DOI: https://doi.org/10.2105/AJPH.2025.308149

ORCID iDs:

Kathleen Galper https://orcid.org/0009-0009-6154-2106

Jillian M. Rung https://orcid.org/0000-0002-5945-6454

Amber Shergill https://orcid.org/0000-0002-5043-3002

Tyson S. Barrett https://orcid.org/0000-0002-2137-1391

Demetrios Marousis https://orcid.org/0009-0000-0999-9971

Emily Brignone https://orcid.org/0000-0001-7138-4775

CONTRIBUTORS

K. Galper made substantial contributions to the design, analysis, interpretation, drafting, revision, and final approval of the work. J. M. Rung made substantial contributions to the design, interpretation, revision, and final approval of the work. A. Shergill made substantial contributions to the drafting, revision, and final approval of the work. T. S. Barrett made substantial contributions to the design, revision, and final approval of the work. E. Brignone made substantial contributions to the design, interpretation, revision, and final approval of the work. D. Marousis made substantial contributions to the interpretation, revision, and final approval of the work.

ACKNOWLEDGMENTS

We thank Kira Riehm MsC, PhD, for her foundational work in developing this line of research.

CONFLICTS OF INTEREST

The authors have no conflicts of interest to disclose.

HUMAN PARTICIPANT PROTECTION

The study was approved by the institutional review board (IRB) of Allegheny Health Network Research Institute (acting IRB for Highmark Health). Informed consent was waived.

REFERENCES

1. Reiss F. Socioeconomic inequalities and mental health problems in children and adolescents: a systematic review. *Soc Sci Med.* 2013;90:24–31. https://doi.org/10.1016/j.socscimed.2013.04.026
2. Sampson RJ, Morenoff JD, Gannon-Rowley T. Assessing “neighborhood effects”: social processes and new directions in research. *Annu Rev Sociol.* 2002;28(1):443–478. https://doi.org/10.1146/annurev.soc.28.110601.141114
3. Tracy M, Zimmerman FJ, Galea S, McCauley E, Stoep AV. What explains the relation between family poverty and childhood depressive symptoms? *J Psychiatr Res.* 2008;42(14):1163–1175. https://doi.org/10.1016/j.jpsychires.2008.01.011
4. Mangione CM, Barry MJ, Nicholson WK, US Preventive Services Task Force, et al. Screening for depression and suicide risk in children and adolescents: US Preventive Services Task Force recommendation statement. *JAMA.* 2022;328(15):1534–1542. https://doi.org/10.1001/jama.2022.16946
5. US Preventive Services Task Force. Screening for depression in children and adolescents: recommendation statement. *American Family Physician.* 2016;93(6):506–508.
6. Beck KE, Snyder D, Toth C, et al. Improving primary care adolescent depression screening and initial management: a quality improvement study. *Pediatr Qual Saf.* 2022;7(2):e549. https://doi.org/10.1097/pq9.0000000000000549
7. Wissow LS, Brown J, Fothergill KE, et al. Universal mental health screening in pediatric primary care: a systematic review. *J Am Acad Child Adolesc Psychiatry.* 2013;52(11):1134–1147.e23. https://doi.org/10.1016/j.jaac.2013.08.013
8. Sekhar DL, Ba DM, Liu G, Kraschnewski JL. Major depressive disorder screening remains low even among privately insured adolescents. *J Pediatr.* 2019;204:203–207. https://doi.org/10.1016/j.jpeds.2018.07.086
9. American Psychological Association. Addressing racial and ethnic disparities in youth mental health. 2018. Available at: https://www.apa.org/pi/families/resources/disparities-mental-health. Accessed September 1, 2024.
10. Mansour M, Krishnaprasadh D, Lichtenberger J, Teitelbaum J. Implementing the Patient Health Questionnaire modified for adolescents to improve screening for depression among adolescents in a Federally Qualified Health Centre. *BMJ Open Qual.* 2020;9(4):e000751. https://doi.org/10.1136/bmjoq-2019-000751
11. Flanagan BE, Gregory EW, Hallisey EJ, Heitgerd JL, Lewis B. A social vulnerability index for disaster management. *J Homel Secur Emerg Manag.* 2011;8(1):1–22. https://doi.org/10.2202/1547-7355.1792
12. Ibrahim R, Sainbayar E, Pham HN, et al. Social vulnerability index and cardiovascular disease care continuum: a scoping review. *JACC Adv.* 2024;3(7):100858. https://doi.org/10.1016/j.jacadv.2024.100858
13. Lee YC, Chang KY, Mirsaeidi M. Association of county-degree social vulnerability with chronic respiratory disease mortality in the United States. *Ann Am Thorac Soc.* 2023;20(1):47–57. https://doi.org/10.1513/AnnalsATS.202202-136OC
14. Simon TD, Cawthon ML, Stanford S, Center of Excellence on Quality of Care Measures for Children with Complex Needs (COE4CCN) Medical Complexity Working Group, et al. Pediatric medical complexity algorithm: a new method to stratify children by medical complexity. *Pediatrics.* 2014;133(6):e1647–e1654. https://doi.org/10.1542/peds.2013-3875
15. Elliott MN, Morrison PA, Fremont A, McCaffrey DF, Pantoja P, Lurie N. Using the Census Bureau’s surname list to improve estimates of race/ethnicity and associated disparities. *Health Serv Outcomes Res Method.* 2009;9(2):69–83. https://doi.org/10.1007/s10742-009-0047-1
16. US Dept of Agriculture. Food Access Research Atlas. 2015. Available at: https://www.ers.usda.gov/data-products/food-access-research-atlas/download-the-data. Accessed July 15, 2023.
17. McCue Horwitz S, Storfer-Isser A, Kerker BD, et al. Do on-site mental health professionals change pediatricians’ responses to children’s mental health problems? *Acad Pediatr.* 2016;16(7):676–683. https://doi.org/10.1016/j.acap.2016.03.010
18. Upadhyay N, Rowan PJ, Aparasu RR, et al. Impact of geographic access to primary care providers on pediatric behavioral health screening. *Prev Med.* 2021;153:106856. https://doi.org/10.1016/j.ypmed.2021.106856
19. Habayeb S, Onofaro KC, Hawila N, Druskin LR, Godoy L, Long M. Mental health screening in pediatric primary care: factors associated with screening completion and elevated scores. *Clin Pediatr (Phila).* 2023;62(6):584–591. https://doi.org/10.1177/00099228221139983
20. Imfeld SM, Darang DM, Neudecker M, McVoy MK. Primary care pediatrician perceptions towards mental health within the primary care setting. *Pediatr Res.* 2021;90(5):950–956. https://doi.org/10.1038/s41390-020-01349-7
21. Eisner-Fellay T, Suris JC, Barrense-Dias Y. Adolescent behavioural risk screening in primary care: physician’s point of view. *Fam Pract.* 2024;41(2):123–130. https://doi.org/10.1093/fampra/cmad106
22. Bettencourt AF, Ferro RA, Williams JLL, et al. Pediatric primary care provider comfort with mental health practices: a needs assessment of regions with shortages of treatment access. *Acad Psychiatry.* 2021;45(4):429–434. https://doi.org/10.1007/s40596-021-01434-x

Violence and Depression Among Adolescent Boys in Soweto, South Africa, 2020–2023

Elizabeth M. Inman, PhD, Given Leshabane, BA, Alisa Kalegina, MSW, Avy Violari, FCPaed, and Rachel Kidman, PhD

See also Adolescent Mental Health, pp. 1377–1444.

Objectives. To identify if violence is associated with adolescent depression by leveraging data from a longitudinal, repeated measures study among adolescent boys from an underrepresented context.

Methods. South African adolescent boys (n = 498) enrolled between 2020 and 2023. Participants reported lifetime violence exposure and depression symptoms at baseline and 1-year follow-up. Over the study year, participants reported past-week violence exposure and past-24-hour psychological distress in weekly mobile surveys. We used 4 sets of longitudinal analyses to test associations between violence and depression symptoms, examining the influence of violence type and timing.

Results. Participants reported high levels of violence and distress. Lifetime violence exposure was associated with increased distress over the study year. Ongoing, cumulative exposure to violence was associated with distress over time and depression at follow-up. Past-week victimization was associated with immediate increases in distress. Emotional victimization demonstrated particularly strong associations with mental health.

Conclusions. We found evidence of a relationship between violence exposure and depression in adolescent boys. Multilayered interventions to reduce violence in the lives of boys and young men are necessary to address the mental health crisis. (*Am J Public Health*. 2025;115(9):1445–1453. https://doi.org/10.2105/AJPH.2025.308164)

AJPH September 2025, Vol. 115, No. 9

Adolescence is a critical developmental period marked by biological and psychosocial changes, and a time when many people first experience depression. Globally, one fifth of adolescents experience depression, but recent estimates suggest that the prevalence is rising.[1] One correlate of adolescent depression is exposure to violence, including abuse, bullying, and intimate partner violence (IPV).[2] While the evidence base is growing, recent reviews and meta-analyses on violence and adolescent mental health have identified persistent gaps in the literature, which we will discuss in detail.

First, most research on adolescent depression is conducted in high-income countries (HICs), but the majority of the global adolescent population lives in lower- and middle-income countries (LMICs), and the prevalence of psychopathology is higher in LMICs than in HICs.[1,2] Research from HICs does not necessarily generalize to LMICs, as adolescents in LMICs experience both higher levels of the risk factors identified in HICs and unique, context-specific risk factors.[3] For example, South African adolescents report high levels of violence exposure and victimization.[4,5] This is attributable, in part, to systems of economic and political oppression (e.g., apartheid), which have normalized violence as a tool to solve interpersonal and political conflict and protect one's social status.[6] Furthermore, the HIV epidemic has resulted in orphanhood and illness for millions of adolescents, increasing their vulnerability to victimization and depression.[3] Despite these risks, there is limited research on South African adolescents.[7,8]

Second, adolescent boys are underrepresented in the mental health literature, especially in LMICs, despite reporting high adversity and distress.[3,9] Boys in sub-Saharan Africa likely experience higher levels and more types of violence (i.e., polyvictimization) than girls.[7,10] During adolescence, this includes household violence, community violence (e.g., gang involvement), bullying, and IPV.[4,5,11] Furthermore, associations between violence and mental health may be stronger among boys than girls. Among South African adolescents, witnessing community violence was significantly associated with posttraumatic stress disorder symptoms[12] and externalizing behaviors (e.g., aggression)[13] in boys, but not girls. Sex-disaggregated studies are necessary to identify which types of violence are particularly important for boys' mental health and to understand how boys' disproportionately higher levels of victimization affect mental health over time.

Third, there is a need for rigorous study designs to more precisely estimate and establish associations between violence and depression.[14] Adolescent depression has been identified as both an antecedent[12] and consequence[15] of violence. Simple longitudinal designs are a necessary first step to clarify temporal order. However, more complex designs are needed to isolate the timeframe and type of exposure that matter most.[16] In some studies, cumulative lifetime exposure to violence is modeled as the key determinant of adolescent depression.[17] In others, "snapshots" of recent sexual violence are examined.[18] Careful consideration of timing can illuminate whether childhood violence has a lasting effect on mental health or whether interventions should concentrate on recent exposures. To do this, we need to move beyond traditional longitudinal surveys. Repeated-measure surveys collect data on violence exposure over multiple timepoints, in real time, and in the adolescent's natural environment. Importantly, analyses of repeated measures enable researchers to model the cumulative impact of violence on depression and whether exposure to violence triggers an immediate spike in depressive symptoms.[19]

This article addresses all 3 of these gaps in the literature. We situated our study in an LMIC (South Africa), focused on adolescent boys, and used rigorous methods to identify a longitudinal relationship between violence and depression. By combining in-depth surveys with brief repeated measures, we separated the impact of cumulative lifetime violence, cumulative past-year violence, and acute past-week violence on distress. We hypothesized that there would be significant longitudinal associations between violence and depression, and that violence and depression would covary over the study year.

METHODS

This study took place in Soweto, South Africa. Soweto was developed as a township during apartheid to segregate Black Africans and became a hub of protest and political violence. The lasting socioeconomic and political effects of apartheid have contributed to poverty, unemployment, and violence.[6] Adolescents in this area report high levels of childhood adversity, community violence, and IPV.[4,11]

Participant Recruitment and Data Collection

We drew from a larger longitudinal study on violence among adolescent boys living with and without HIV. Participant recruitment and data collection occurred between November 2020 and June 2023. Study staff visited public HIV care clinics to recruit adolescents living with HIV and visited community centers in the Soweto area to recruit adolescents without HIV. Potential participants were screened at the Perinatal HIV Research Unit at the University of the Witwatersrand. Participants were eligible if they were male, aged 15 to 19 years, living in and around Soweto, and in a dating or sexual relationship. For those living with HIV, a final criterion was documented HIV infection before the age of 10 years (i.e., likely perinatal transmission). Participants completed informed consent or assent procedures. Caregivers provided informed consent for those aged younger than 18 years.

At enrollment, participants completed a baseline survey on a tablet in a private room at the clinic, with staff nearby to answer questions. They then received a smartphone and brief training on how to complete mobile surveys. Each week, on their assigned day, participants received a text message with the survey link. Participants received 2 reminders to complete their survey. Those who completed the survey within a 2-day window were compensated with an airtime voucher. Additional detail on the survey methods has been published previously.[20] Participants could communicate with the study team through WhatsApp, a 24-hour hotline, and a contact request button at the end of each mobile survey. Participants who indicated psychological risks (e.g., suicidality) were contacted by a counselor for assessment and referral to care. One year after enrollment, participants returned to the clinic to complete a follow-up survey.

Measures

Participants completed the Adverse Childhood Experiences–International Questionnaire (ACE–IQ).[21] This measure assesses adverse experiences before age 18 years across 13 domains. For this study, we used 7 domains that pertain to violence: physical abuse, emotional abuse, sexual abuse, witnessing household violence, bullying from peers, witnessing community violence, and exposure to collective violence.

Participants completed 2 measures assessing lifetime experiences of IPV victimization. We used the World Health Organization Violence Against Women Assessment[22] to measure participants' experiences of physical, verbal, and sexual violence from a partner. We added 2 questions about sexual IPV from the United Nations Development Program Report on Violence Against Women,[23] adapted to be gender neutral.

We measured depression by using the Beck Depression Inventory,[24] which has been validated among South African young adults.[25] This 21-item measure asks participants to consider their feelings over the past 2 weeks. Following the measure's scoring guidelines, items are summed (0–63), and participants with scores higher than 20 are identified as likely experiencing depression.

Participant recruitment was stratified by HIV status, which was confirmed in person at the clinic. Participants self-reported their age, race, and school enrollment status.

Psychological distress was assessed at each weekly survey with the Screening Tool for Psychological Distress (STOP-D).[26] For this study, we concentrated on the question "In the past 24 h, how much have you been bothered by feeling sad, down, or uninterested in life?" Participants who indicated that they were "moderately" or "severely" bothered were categorized as experiencing distress.

Participants reported their past-week experiences with 4 types of violence. They indicated whether they had experienced any physical, verbal, or sexual violence or had witnessed violence (i.e., had seen someone in the community stabbed, shot, or threatened with a weapon).

Analyses

We created 4 tests of the longitudinal associations between violence and depression symptomology using different combinations of baseline, weekly, and follow-up data. The first approach was the most traditional, as it relied only on the baseline and follow-up data. We used logistic regression to model the association between each type of lifetime violence reported at baseline and depression scores at follow-up. To examine potential dose–response relationships, we also created a composite baseline variable summing the 7 ACE-IQ domains and the 3 IPV variables (0–10 range).

As a second test of longitudinal association, we built a series of mixed-effects logistic regression models, with each baseline violence experience predicting weekly levels of psychological distress over the study year. Once again, we modeled the composite sum to examine dose–response associations.

Third, we tested the cumulative effects of recent violence on later depression. For each of the 4 types of violence measured weekly, we calculated the average level of victimization across the mobile surveys within each participant (e.g., an average of 0.10 represents violence in 10% of a participant's surveys). We also calculated a weekly sum score of violence using all 4 types (0–4 range) for an average of overall victimization across the mobile surveys. We entered these cumulative scores into logistic regressions predicting depression at follow-up; the unit used was 0.10, representing about a standard deviation in average victimization.

Finally, we tested whether violence and distress covaried over time and, thus, whether violence may have an immediate effect on mood, using only the mobile data. We built 5 generalized linear mixed models with each type of violence (i.e., witnessed, physical, verbal, sexual, overall) predicting distress reported that same week. We split each violence score into an interindividual component (i.e., the participant's average level of victimization over the study year; unit = 0.10) and an intraindividual component (i.e., the deviation of a given week's score from the participant's average, indicating a participant's weekly fluctuation from their average; unit = 1.0). We entered both the inter- and intraindividual components into the model as predictors of weekly distress.

We performed analyses in R version 4.4.0 (R Foundation for Statistical Computing, Vienna, Austria). Models controlled for participant age (continuous) and HIV status (dichotomous). Mixed-effects models also controlled for survey week (continuous) and included a random intercept at the participant level.

RESULTS

The baseline survey was completed by 498 participants. Of these, 466 completed at least 1 of the weekly surveys, and 451 completed the follow-up survey. At baseline, the average age of participants was 16.5 years (SD = 1.4), and the majority were enrolled in school (n = 355; 71.3%). Most participants identified as Black African (n = 458; 92.0%). Half were living with HIV (n = 251; 50.4%).

Participants completed a mean of 27 of the 52 weekly mobile surveys. Completion of the weekly surveys differed significantly between participants identified as experiencing depression (mean = 24.8 surveys) and those who were not (mean = 27.7). Similarly, weekly survey completion differed significantly between participants who scored at or below the mean on composite violence (mean = 29.2) and those above the mean (mean = 24.3). To test the potential impact of this missing data, we conducted additional sensitivity analyses. We split the sample into 2 subgroups (i.e., those at or below the mean of survey completion and those above the mean) and reran the models using the mobile survey data in each group. Results from these analyses align with and support the results presented in this article. See the Appendix, available as a supplement to the online version of this article at https://ajph.org for additional information.

Violence Exposure

At baseline, the most commonly reported lifetime violence experience was witnessing community violence (n = 479; 96.2%) and the least commonly reported was physical IPV (n = 178; 35.7%; Table 1). Across the 10 domains, participants reported experiencing a mean of 6 types of violence in their lifetime (SD = 2.4). Only 1 participant reported that they had never experienced any violence. Most violence experiences did not differ by HIV status. Participants living with HIV reported significantly lower household violence, emotional IPV, and physical IPV than HIV-uninfected participants.

At each mobile survey, participants reported whether they had experienced violence in the previous week. The most commonly reported experience was witnessing violence: more than half (n = 280; 60.1%) witnessed violence in their community at least once during the observation year. The least commonly reported experience was sexual violence, which one quarter (n = 117; 25.1%) of participants reported at least once. HIV status was not associated with average weekly reports of verbal or sexual violence. Participants living with HIV reported significantly lower average levels of witnessed violence and physical violence than HIV-uninfected participants.

TABLE 1— Prevalence of Victimization and Depression Symptoms Among Adolescent Boys: Soweto, South Africa, 2020–2023

	No. (%) or Mean ±SD
Lifetime violence exposure at baseline	
Physical abuse	294 (59.0)
Emotional abuse	376 (75.5)
Sexual abuse	200 (40.2)
Witnessed household violence	396 (79.5)
Bullying	313 (62.9)
Witnessed community violence	479 (96.2)
Collective violence[a]	301 (60.4)
Emotional IPV	277 (55.6)
Physical IPV	178 (35.7)
Sexual IPV	185 (37.2)
Global score (0–10)	6.02 ±2.4
Prevalence of violence over the study year	
Witnessed violence	280 (60.1)
Physical victimization	217 (46.6)
Verbal victimization	263 (56.4)
Sexual victimization	117 (25.1)
Overall victimization (0–4)	0.27 ±0.4
Depression prevalence	
Depression at baseline	133 (28.4)
Depression at follow-up	130 (30.8)
Distress over the study year	246 (52.8)

Note. IPV = intimate partner violence. The sample size was n = 498.
[a]Collective violence refers to witnessing or experiencing violence from an organized group (e.g., gangs, militias, police, military forces) and large-scale events such as war, political violence, and terrorism.

Depression Symptomology

At baseline, more than one quarter (n = 133; 28.4%) of the sample scored above the measure cutoff, indicating likely depression. Prevalence was similar at follow-up (n = 130; 30.8%). Depression scores at baseline and follow-up did not significantly differ by HIV status. Using the continuous depression score revealed that scores at baseline (mean = 12.8) and follow-up (mean = 13.7) were stable and significantly correlated ($r = 0.38$; $P < .001$). More than half (n = 246; 52.8%) of the sample reported distress at least once during the observation year (Table 1).

Longitudinal Associations

To investigate prospective associations between lifetime violence at baseline and depression at follow-up, we created a series of logistic regression models. There was a significant association between the global score at baseline and depression at follow-up (odds ratio [OR] = 1.13; 95% confidence interval [CI] = 1.03, 1.23). Among the individual violence domains, only emotional abuse (OR = 1.83; 95% CI = 1.09, 3.16), childhood sexual abuse (OR = 1.53; 95% CI = 1.01, 2.34), and emotional IPV (OR = 1.80; 95% CI = 1.17, 2.80) at baseline were significantly associated with depression at follow-up (Table 2).

We examined the association between lifetime violence at baseline and subsequent distress over the observation year. The global violence score at baseline was significantly associated with higher odds of psychological distress over the study year (OR = 1.25; 95% CI = 1.15, 1.36). Furthermore, 9 of the 10 individual violence domains, including physical abuse (OR = 1.58; 95% CI = 1.05, 2.40) and sexual IPV (OR = 1.69; 95% CI = 1.11, 2.57) were significantly associated with higher odds of distress over the study year (Table 2). Models included a random intercept at the participant level; likelihood ratio tests indicated that model fit was not improved by adding a random slope (e.g., for physical abuse, $\chi^2(2) = 5.1$; $P = .08$). Only witnessing community violence, reported by 96% of participants, was not associated with distress.

Next, we investigated the association between violence over the observation year and depression at follow-up. To capture the cumulative effect of recent violence, we averaged participants' weekly reports of violence over the survey year for each type of violence and overall violence. We used these average exposures in separate logistic regression models predicting participant depression scores at follow-up (Table 3). A 10% increase in the prevalence of overall weekly violence exposure was associated with higher odds of depression at follow-up (OR = 1.13; 95% CI = 1.06, 1.20). Similarly, a 10% increase in the prevalence of all 4 types of weekly violence exposure was associated with higher odds of depression at follow-up, including witnessing violence (OR = 1.23; 95% CI = 1.05, 1.45) and verbal victimization (OR = 1.32; 95% CI = 1.16, 1.53).

Same-Day Associations

Finally, we used the mobile data to separate the cumulative impact of violence from the same-week (immediate) impact of a single event. We built 5 generalized linear mixed models regressing weekly violence exposure on past-24-hour distress.

Participants who reported higher average levels of violence also reported higher odds of distress than their peers over the study year (Table 4). At the interindividual level, a 10% increase in average weekly violence was associated with participant distress for overall violence (OR = 1.14; 95% CI = 1.08, 1.20), witnessing violence (OR = 1.33; 95% CI = 1.14, 1.54), physical victimization (OR = 1.41; 95% CI = 1.20, 1.66), and verbal victimization (OR = 1.49; 95% CI = 1.32, 1.67).

We also found evidence of a more immediate, same-week association. When participants reported higher-than-usual levels of violence in a given

TABLE 2— Longitudinal Associations Between Lifetime Violence Exposure at Baseline and Depression Symptomology Among Adolescent Boys: Soweto, South Africa, 2020–2023

	Outcome: Depression at Follow-Up Survey			Outcome: Distress Over the Observation Year			
	No.	B (SE)	OR (95% CI)	No.	Observations	B (SE)	OR (95% CI)
Physical abuse	414	0.31 (0.22)	1.37 (0.89, 2.11)	458	12 315	0.46 (0.21)	1.58 (1.05, 2.40)
Emotional abuse	414	0.60 (0.27)	1.83 (1.09, 3.16)	458	12 334	0.98 (0.25)	2.67 (1.64, 4.33)
Sexual abuse	420	0.43 (0.21)	1.53 (1.01, 2.34)	464	12 478	0.46 (0.21)	1.59 (1.06, 2.40)
Witnessed household violence	420	0.33 (0.28)	1.40 (0.82, 2.46)	464	12 467	1.12 (0.27)	3.08 (1.81, 5.22)
Bullying	420	0.001 (0.22)	1.00 (0.65, 1.55)	462	12 429	0.74 (0.22)	2.09 (1.37, 3.19)
Witnessed community violence	420	−0.17 (0.56)	0.84 (0.29, 2.76)	463	12 465	−0.22 (0.59)	0.80 (0.25, 2.56)
Collective violence	421	−0.02 (0.22)	0.98 (0.64, 1.50)	464	12 493	0.56 (0.21)	1.74 (1.15, 2.64)
Emotional IPV	418	0.59 (0.22)	1.80 (1.17, 2.80)	460	12 423	0.87 (0.21)	2.38 (1.57, 3.59)
Physical IPV	420	0.36 (0.22)	1.43 (0.93, 2.20)	462	12 446	0.44 (0.22)	1.55 (1.01, 2.36)
Sexual IPV	418	0.38 (0.22)	1.46 (0.94, 2.27)	460	12 411	0.52 (0.22)	1.69 (1.11, 2.57)
Global score (0–10)	422	0.12 (0.05)	1.13 (1.03, 1.23)	466	12 515	0.23 (0.05)	1.25 (1.15, 1.36)

Note. CI = confidence interval; IPV = intimate partner violence; OR = odds ratio. There were separate models for each type of violence. Models controlled for participant age and HIV status. Mixed-effects models also controlled for survey week.

TABLE 3— Associations Between Average Weekly Violence Exposure During Study Year and Depression at Follow-Up Among Adolescent Boys: Soweto, South Africa, 2020–2023

	B (SE)	OR (95% CI)
Witnessed violence	0.21 (0.08)	1.23 (1.05, 1.45)
Physical victimization	0.18 (0.09)	1.20 (1.00, 1.44)
Verbal victimization	0.28 (0.07)	1.32 (1.16, 1.53)
Sexual victimization	0.33 (0.11)	1.39 (1.15, 1.77)
Overall victimization (0–4)	0.12 (0.03)	1.13 (1.06, 1.20)

Note. CI = confidence interval; OR = odds ratio. The sample size was n = 435. There were separate models for each type of violence. Models controlled for participant age and HIV status. Effects represent a 10% increase in average violence exposure.

week, they were also more likely to report past-24-hour distress that same week. At the intraindividual level, overall violence (OR = 1.68; 95% CI = 1.50, 1.88), witnessing violence (OR = 1.78; 95% CI = 1.40, 2.28), physical victimization (OR = 1.71; 95% CI = 1.30, 2.25), and verbal victimization (OR = 3.05; 95% CI = 2.46, 3.78) were associated with participant distress. There were no associations between weekly sexual victimization and distress at the inter- or intraindividual level. Models were fit with a random intercept at the participant level, and likelihood ratio tests did not support improved model fit with a random slope for intraindividual violence (e.g., for witnessing violence, $\chi^2(2) = 3.1$; $P = .21$).

DISCUSSION

In this article, we provide strong evidence that violence is a critical antecedent of depression among boys. Both violence and depression were prevalent: on average, participants reported 6 types of lifetime violence experiences, and almost one third reported likely depression. We triangulated longitudinal and repeated measures analyses to identify the influence of violence type and timing on mental health.

First, previous violence exposure, including experiences in childhood, has a lasting impact on adolescent mental health. Nine of the 10 types of lifetime violence captured at baseline were significantly associated with higher odds of distress throughout the study year. Using the mobile survey to capture distress provided a more robust association with previous violence, compared with depression symptomology

TABLE 4— Associations Between Past-Week Violence Exposure and Past-Day Distress During Study Year Among Adolescent Boys: Soweto, South Africa, 2020–2023

	B (SE)	OR (95% CI)
Witnessed violence (O = 12 438)		
Interindividual component (mean over the study year)	0.28 (0.08)	1.33 (1.14, 1.54)
Intraindividual component (weekly deviation from the mean)	0.58 (0.13)	1.78 (1.40, 2.28)
Physical victimization (O = 12 384)		
Interindividual component (mean over the study year)	0.34 (0.08)	1.41 (1.20, 1.66)
Intraindividual component (weekly deviation from the mean)	0.54 (0.14)	1.71 (1.30, 2.25)
Verbal victimization (O = 12 387)		
Interindividual component (mean over the study year)	0.40 (0.06)	1.49 (1.32, 1.67)
Intraindividual component (weekly deviation from the mean)	1.12 (0.11)	3.05 (2.46, 3.78)
Sexual victimization (O = 12 385)		
Interindividual component (mean over the study year)	0.08 (0.11)	1.08 (0.88, 1.33)
Intraindividual component (weekly deviation from the mean)	0.11 (0.24)	1.11 (0.69, 1.78)
Overall victimization (O = 12 515)		
Interindividual component (mean over the study year)	0.13 (0.03)	1.14 (1.08, 1.20)
Intraindividual component (weekly deviation from the mean)	0.52 (0.06)	1.68 (1.50, 1.88)

Note. CI = confidence interval; O = observations; OR = odds ratio. The sample size was n = 466. Models control for participant age, participant HIV status, and survey week. Interindividual effects represent a 10% increase in average violence exposure. Intraindividual effects represent a 1.0-unit deviation from average violence exposure.

measured at follow-up. This suggests that repeat measures may yield a more accurate picture of mental health and, thus, better illuminate key risk factors.

Second, we found suggestive evidence that ongoing violence exposure during adolescence increases depression. Across various models, higher average violence exposure over the study year increased the odds of both follow-up depression symptomology and weekly distress. Moreover, we observed an immediate effect of violence on distress when both were measured through mobile surveys. Specifically, the intraindividual effects suggest that participants who experience higher-than-usual violence report higher distress in the following days. Over time, this sustained elevated distress can become depression.[19]

Finally, our findings suggest that emotional and verbal violence may be particularly harmful for adolescent boys. Baseline emotional abuse and emotional IPV and weekly verbal victimization demonstrated consistently strong associations with distress and depression. Emotional victimization is often studied as a precursor or correlate to other, more "serious" forms of violence,[27] but recent research indicates that emotional abuse has a particularly severe impact on emotional, cognitive, and neurological development.[28] These findings suggest that emotional violence is a critical determinant of mental health in its own right, particularly in adolescent boys.

Strengths and Limitations

This study had several notable strengths. First, combining traditional longitudinal surveys with repeated-measure mobile surveys provided robust evidence for a longitudinal association. In each set of analyses, violence was collected temporally before depression or distress. Across analyses, we were able to examine the influence of various types of violence and the influence of timing (i.e., lifetime, past-year, and past-week exposure). Second, we recruited a sample from an underrepresented context (i.e., South Africa, an LMIC) where violence and depression are common and shaped by unique sociopolitical and public health stressors. Third, we recruited a sample of adolescent boys. Very few studies on adolescent mental health recruit all-male samples, despite boys reporting high levels of violence and polyvictimization.

There were also limitations to this study. Primarily, our analyses do not rule out the possibility that depression might be a driver of violence, or that there may be a bidirectional relationship between the two. The depression measure and distress question are not intended to provide a clinical diagnosis, but are used to indicate the presence of depression symptoms. Lifetime reports of violence among adolescents may be inconsistent over time and dependent on the adolescent's mood during the survey.[29] In fact, this may be why we report very few longitudinal associations between baseline lifetime reports of violence and later depression. The weekly violence scores were a more reliable measure of participant experiences and exhibited more robust, consistent associations with depression symptoms. Finally, the sexual abuse measure on the ACE–IQ does not specify the perpetrator; therefore, it is possible that some participants' sexual IPV experiences are being counted twice.

Public Health Implications

Adolescent boys are experiencing a dual crisis of depression and violence victimization. Although effective therapies for depression exist, access is limited in LMICs.[30] This is particularly relevant at present, given the increase in adolescent depression during the COVID-19 pandemic.[31] Expanded access to low-cost, effective mental health interventions, such as peer-led counseling programs, can improve depression symptoms among South African adolescents.[32] However, this needs to be paired with interventions that address key drivers. As we have shown, violence from family, peers, partners, and in the community shapes mental health. In South Africa, parenting programs have shown promise in reducing child abuse,[8] while school-based programs may decrease violence from peers.[33] However, there are few interventions that aim to reduce IPV victimization in boys, specifically,[34] and collective violence remains a problem with no clear solution. Moreover, we observed a spike in distress soon after exposure to violence; thus, adolescents need resources that can guide them to process and cope with their emotions in the aftermath of violence. Brief digital interventions may be appealing to adolescents, but more research is needed to evaluate their efficacy.[35]

Conclusions

In this study, we provide evidence of a longitudinal relationship between violence and depression among adolescent boys in an LMIC. Exposure to violence during childhood continues to reverberate in adolescence, with a clear and consistent association with daily distress. Similarly, ongoing exposure to violence throughout adolescence exhibits cumulative and immediate effects on distress. Researchers should consider repeated-measures designs to better understand drivers of adolescent mental health. Multilayered interventions are necessary in LMICs to improve depression symptoms outside of the medical context, reduce violence in multiple domains, and help adolescent boys cope in the immediate aftermath of violence. AJPH

ABOUT THE AUTHORS

Elizabeth M. Inman is with the Program in Public Health, Stony Brook University, Stony Brook, NY. Given Leshabane and Avy Violari are with the Perinatal HIV Research Unit, University of the Witwatersrand, Johannesburg, South Africa. Alisa Kalegina is with the School of Social Welfare, Stony Brook University. Rachel Kidman is with the Program in Public Health and Department of Family, Population, and Preventive Medicine, Stony Brook University.

CORRESPONDENCE

Correspondence should be sent to Elizabeth M. Inman, PhD, Program in Public Health, Stony Brook University, 100 Nicholls Rd, Stony Brook, NY 11794 (e-mail: elizabeth.inman@stonybrookmedicine.edu). Reprints can be ordered at https://ajph.org by clicking the "Reprints" link.

PUBLICATION INFORMATION

Full Citation: Inman EM, Leshabane G, Kalegina A, Violari A, Kidman R. Violence and depression among adolescent boys in Soweto, South Africa, 2020–2023. *Am J Public Health*. 2025;115(9): 1445–1453.

Acceptance Date: April 12, 2025.

DOI: https://doi.org/10.2105/AJPH.2025.308164

ORCID iDs:

Elizabeth M. Inman https://orcid.org/0000-0002-0679-138X

Given Leshabane https://orcid.org/0000-0001-7212-2689

Alisa Kalegina https://orcid.org/0009-0002-1032-3201

Rachel Kidman https://orcid.org/0000-0001-7202-5571

CONTRIBUTORS

E. M. Inman contributed to conceptualization, data analysis, and writing the original draft. G. Leshabane and A. Kalegina contributed to investigation and writing (review and editing). A. Violari contributed to conceptualization, methodology, writing (review and editing), and funding acquisition. R. Kidman contributed to conceptualization, methodology, writing the original draft, and funding acquisition.

ACKNOWLEDGMENTS

Research reported in this publication was supported by the National Institute of Mental Health of the National Institutes of Health under award R01MH119878.

The authors would like to thank the members of the study staff at Perinatal HIV Research Unit and the University of the Witwatersrand, including Janan Dietrich, Phumla Madi, Candice Ramsammy, Stefanie Vermaak, and Busisiwe Nkala-Dlamini. We would also like to thank all participants for their time and effort in this study.

Note. The content is solely the responsibility of the authors and does not necessarily represent the official views of the National Institutes of Health.

CONFLICTS OF INTEREST

The authors declared no potential conflicts of interest with respect to the research, authorship, or publication of this article.

HUMAN PARTICIPANT PROTECTION

Approval was obtained from the ethics committee of the University of the Witwatersrand in South Africa (approval ID: 191001) and by Stony Brook University in the United States (approval ID: FWA#00000125, IRB2019-00567).

REFERENCES

1. Shorey S, Ng ED, Wong CH. Global prevalence of depression and elevated depressive symptoms among adolescents: a systematic review and meta-analysis. *Br J Clin Psychol*. 2022;61(2):287–305. https://doi.org/10.1111/bjc.12333
2. Thapar A, Eyre O, Patel V, Brent D. Depression in young people. *Lancet*. 2022;400(10352):617–631. https://doi.org/10.1016/S0140-6736(22)01012-1
3. Jörns-Presentati A, Napp A-K, Dessauvagie AS, et al. The prevalence of mental health problems in sub-Saharan adolescents: a systematic review. *PLoS One*. 2021;16(5):e0251689. https://doi.org/10.1371/journal.pone.0251689
4. Otwombe KN, Dietrich J, Sikkema KJ, et al. Exposure to and experiences of violence among adolescents in lower socio-economic groups in Johannesburg, South Africa. *BMC Public Health*. 2015;15(1): 450–411. https://doi.org/10.1186/s12889-015-1780-8
5. Meinck F, Cluver LD, Boyes ME, Loening-Voysey H. Physical, emotional and sexual adolescent abuse victimisation in South Africa: prevalence, incidence, perpetrators and locations. *J Epidemiol Community Health*. 2016;70(9):910–916. https://doi.org/10.1136/jech-2015-205860
6. Hoosen P, Adams S, Tiliouine H, Savahl S. Youth and adolescents' perceptions of violence in post-apartheid South Africa: a systematic review of the literature. *Child Indic Res*. 2022;15(3): 885–911. https://doi.org/10.1007/s12187-021-09890-5
7. Stansfeld SA, Rothon C, Das-Munshi J, et al. Exposure to violence and mental health of adolescents: South African Health and Well-Being Study. *BJPsych Open*. 2017;3(5):257–264. https://doi.org/10.1192/bjpo.bp.117.004861
8. Ward CL, Artz L, Leoschut L, Kassanjee R, Burton P. Sexual violence against children in South Africa: a nationally representative cross-sectional study of prevalence and correlates. *Lancet Glob Health*. 2018;6(4):e460–e468. https://doi.org/10.1016/S2214-109X(18)30060-3
9. Infurna MR, Reichl C, Parzer P, Schimmenti A, Bifulco A, Kaess M. Associations between depression and specific childhood experiences of abuse and neglect: a meta-analysis. *J Affect Disord*. 2016;190:47–55. https://doi.org/10.1016/j.jad.2015.09.006
10. Miedema SS, Stamatakis C, Tracy A, et al. Patterns of adverse childhood experiences and their associations with mental distress, substance use and sexual risk behaviors in sub-Saharan Africa. *Child Abuse Negl*. 2024;150:106494. https://doi.org/10.1016/j.chiabu.2023.106494
11. Pengpid S, Peltzer K. Intimate partner violence victimization and associated factors among male and female university students in 22 countries in Africa, Asia and the Americas. *Afr J Reprod Health*. 2016;20(1):29–39. https://doi.org/10.29063/ajrh2016/v20i1.3
12. Schwartz B, Kaminer D, Hardy A, Nöthling J, Seedat S. Gender differences in the violence exposure types that predict PTSD and depression in adolescents. *J Interpers Violence*. 2021; 36(17–18):8358–8381. https://doi.org/10.1177/0886260519849691
13. North A, Donenberg G, Vermaak R, et al. Pathways from witnessing community violence to mental health problems among South African adolescents. *S Afr Med J*. 2020;110(2):145–153. https://doi.org/10.7196/SAMJ.2020.v110i2.13929
14. Radtke SR, Wretman CJ, Fraga Rizo C, et al. A systematic review of conceptualizations and operationalizations of youth polyvictimization. *Trauma Violence Abuse*. 2024;25(4):2721–2734. https://doi.org/10.1177/15248380231224026
15. Kennedy AC, Bybee D, Sullivan CM, Greeson M. The impact of family and community violence on children's depression trajectories: examining the interactions of violence exposure, family social support, and gender. *J Fam Psychol*. 2010;24(2): 197–207. https://doi.org/10.1037/a0018787
16. Juen F, Hecker T, Hermenau K, et al. Child maltreatment in a high adversity context: associations of age, type and timing of exposure with psychopathology in middle childhood. *Child Abuse Negl*. 2024;157:107060. https://doi.org/10.1016/j.chiabu.2024.107060
17. Lee KS, Wolke D, Bärnighausen T, Ouermi L, Bountogo M, Harling G. Sexual victimisation, peer victimisation, and mental health outcomes among adolescents in Burkina Faso: a prospective cohort study. *Lancet Psychiatry*. 2024;11(2): 134–142. https://doi.org/10.1016/S2215-0366(23)00399-1
18. Richter LM, Mathews S, Nonterah F, Masilela L. A longitudinal perspective on boys as victims of childhood sexual abuse in South Africa: consequences for adult mental health. *Child Abuse Negl*. 2018;84:1–10. https://doi.org/10.1016/j.chiabu.2018.07.016
19. Odgers CL, Russell MA. Violence exposure is associated with adolescents' same-and next-day mental health symptoms. *J Child Psychol Psychiatry*. 2017;58(12):1310–1318. https://doi.org/10.1111/jcpp.12763
20. Dietrich JJ, Hornschuh S, Madi P, et al. Implementing ecological momentary assessments to

measure violence and adolescent HIV transmission risk: lessons from Johannesburg, South Africa. *PLOS Digit Health.* 2024;3(2):e0000283. https://doi.org/10.1371/journal.pdig.0000283

21. Adverse Childhood Experiences International Questionnaire (ACE-IQ)—rationale for ACE-IQ. Geneva, Switzerland: World Health Organization; 2012.
22. García-Moreno C, Jansen HA, Ellsberg M, Heise L, Watts C. *WHO Multi-country Study on Women's Health and Domestic Violence Against Women.* Geneva, Switzerland: World Health Organization; 2005.
23. Fulu E, Jewkes R, Roselli T, Garcia-Moreno C, UN Multi-country Cross-sectional Study on Men and Violence research team. Prevalence of and factors associated with male perpetration of intimate partner violence: findings from the UN Multi-country Cross-sectional Study on Men and Violence in Asia and the Pacific. *Lancet Glob Health.* 2013;1(4):e187–e207. https://doi.org/10.1016/S2214-109X(13)70074-3
24. Beck AT, Ward CH, Mendelson M, Mock J, Erbaugh J. An inventory for measuring depression. *Arch Gen Psychiatry.* 1961;4(6):561–571 https://doi.org/10.1001/archpsyc.1961.01710120031004
25. Dolle K, Schulte-Körne G, O'Leary AM, von Hofacker N, Izat Y, Allgaier A-K. The Beck Depression Inventory-II in adolescent mental health patients: cut-off scores for detecting depression and rating severity. *Psychiatry Res.* 2012;200(2–3):843–848. https://doi.org/10.1016/j.psychres.2012.05.011
26. Young Q-R, Ignaszewski A, Fofonoff D, Kaan A. Brief screen to identify 5 of the most common forms of psychosocial distress in cardiac patients: validation of the screening tool for psychological distress. *J Cardiovasc Nurs.* 2007;22(6):525–534. https://doi.org/10.1097/01.JCN.0000297383.29250.14
27. Berzenski SR, Yates TM. A developmental process analysis of the contribution of childhood emotional abuse to relationship violence. In: Reyome N, ed. *The Effect of Childhood Emotional Maltreatment on Later Intimate Relationships.* London, England: Routledge; 2019:180–203.
28. Dye HL. Is emotional abuse as harmful as physical and/or sexual abuse? *J Child Adolesc Trauma.* 2020;13(4):399–407. https://doi.org/10.1007/s40653-019-00292-y
29. Breton E, Kidman R, Behrman J, Mwera J, Kohler H-P. Longitudinal consistency of self-reports of adverse childhood experiences among adolescents in a low-income setting. *SSM Popul Health.* 2022;19:101205. https://doi.org/10.1016/j.ssmph.2022.101205
30. Docrat S, Besada D, Cleary S, Daviaud E, Lund C. Mental health system costs, resources and constraints in South Africa: a national survey. *Health Policy Plan.* 2019;34(9):706–719. https://doi.org/10.1093/heapol/czz085
31. Pillay J. Difficulties experienced by South African adolescents during COVID-19 lockdown: implications for early mental health interventions. *S Afr J Psychol.* 2023;53(2):211–224. https://doi.org/10.1177/00812463221133964
32. Chibanda D. Reducing the treatment gap for mental, neurological and substance use disorders in Africa: lessons from the Friendship Bench in Zimbabwe. *Epidemiol Psychiatr Sci.* 2017;26(4):342–347. https://doi.org/10.1017/S2045796016001128
33. Ngidi LZ, Kaye SB. Reducing school violence: a peace education project in KwaZulu-Natal, South Africa. *S Afr J Educ.* 2022;42(2):1–14. https://doi.org/10.15700/saje.v42n2a1989
34. Reyes HLM, Graham LM, Chen MS, et al. Adolescent dating violence prevention programmes: a global systematic review of evaluation studies. *Lancet Child Adolesc Health.* 2021;5(3):223–232. https://doi.org/10.1016/S2352-4642(20)30276-5
35. Osborn TL, Rodriguez M, Wasil AR, et al. Single-session digital intervention for adolescent depression, anxiety, and well-being: outcomes of a randomized controlled trial with Kenyan adolescents. *J Consult Clin Psychol.* 2020;88(7):657–668. https://doi.org/10.1037/ccp0000505

Effects of Medicaid Expansion on HPV Vaccination Uptake Among Adolescents in the United States: Difference-in-Differences Analyses From 2011 to 2022

Angela W. Chen, MSc, Taryn L. Amberson, RN-BC, MPH, Harriet Fridah Adhiambo, RN, MSN, and Bradley H. Wagenaar, PhD, MPH

See also Brandt, p. 1346.

AJPH September 2025, Vol. 115, No. 9

Objectives. To determine if Medicaid expansion was associated with increased human papillomavirus (HPV) vaccination among adolescents in the United States.

Methods. We conducted a quasi-experimental study using generalized difference-in-differences on National Immunization Survey–Teen data from 2011 to 2022 among adolescents aged 13 to 17 years, comparing HPV vaccination in Medicaid expansion states to nonexpansion states by sex and race/ethnicity subgroups.

Results. There was a significant 10.1-percentage-point increase in HPV vaccination among male adolescents in expansion states (95% confidence interval [CI] = 8.9, 12.4; $P < .001$). Significant increases in HPV vaccination were observed among all male racial subgroups, with largest effects among Black, Latino, and other or multiple races. No effect was observed among female adolescents or any racial subgroup.

Conclusions. Medicaid expansion was associated with significant increases in HPV vaccination among male adolescents, with no effects observed among female adolescents. All male race/ethnicity subgroups showed increases, with Black, Latino, and other or multiple race/ethnicity male adolescents having the largest effect.

Public Health Implications. Medicaid expansion is an appropriate and effective policy for increasing HPV vaccination uptake for priority populations, including historically marginalized racial/ethnic groups and male adolescents. (*Am J Public Health*. 2025;115(9):1454–1462. https://doi.org/10.2105/AJPH.2025.308165)

Human papillomavirus (HPV) is the most common sexually transmitted infection (STI) in the United States, with an approximate lifetime infection rate of 90%.[1] It is associated with 6 types of cancer: cervical, penile, anal, vaginal, vulvar, and oropharyngeal.[2] Several types of HPV vaccines have been licensed for use in the United States: the quadrivalent, approved in 2006; the bivalent, approved in 2009; and the nonavalent, approved in 2014 and the only vaccine used in the United States as of 2016.[3] Despite the proven safety and effectiveness of the HPV vaccine at preventing up to 90% of HPV-related cancers,[2] vaccination rates in the United States remain suboptimal.[4]

Two doses of the vaccine are recommended for individuals aged 9 to 14 years; 3 doses are recommended for individuals aged 15 to 26 years.[3] However, as of 2021, only 58% of adolescents aged 13 to 15 years had received the recommended doses for their age, below the Healthy People 2030 target of 80% for this demographic.[4] HPV vaccination rates are lower than other routinely recommended vaccinations for adolescents; rates are approximately 90% for tetanus/diphtheria/acellular pertussis (TdaP) and 61% for 2 doses of meningococcal conjugate (MenACWY).[5] Reasons for this include lack of strong provider recommendations, stigma associated with sex and STIs, religious beliefs, and vaccine hesitancy.[6,7]

HPV vaccination rates differ by sex, as initial clinical trials and subsequent Food and Drug Administration (FDA) approval focused on cervical cancer prevention in females.[8] As of 2022, among individuals aged 9 to 17 years, only 35% of males, compared with 43% of females, had received at least 1 dose.[9] The Advisory Committee on Immunization Practices recommended routine HPV vaccination for girls aged 11 or 12 years in 2006, but did not do so for boys aged 11 or 12 years until 2011.[6] Current sex differences in vaccination may be partially attributed to timing, as well as other factors, such as providers being more likely to recommend HPV vaccination for females.[10]

Racialized disparities also exist in HPV vaccination and vary by insurance type. A 2019 meta-analysis found minoritized racial/ethnic adolescents aged 13 to 17 years to be more likely to initiate, but less likely to complete, HPV vaccination.[11] National Immunization Survey–Teen (NIS–Teen) data from 2009 to 2016 showed that Hispanic female adolescents were most likely to initiate and complete HPV vaccination compared with non-Hispanic Black, White, and multiracial adolescents.[12]

As a part of the Affordable Care Act, Medicaid expansion allowed for the enrollment of individuals under 138% of the federal poverty level.[13] This expansion has been associated with increased access to care and utilization of preventive care measures, particularly among traditionally difficult-to-reach subpopulations,[14,15] as well as increased influenza and pneumonia vaccination rates in adults.[14] Recent evidence suggests Medicaid expansion improved HPV vaccination among adolescent females but not until 3 years after expansion.[16]

Expanded Medicaid coverage could be associated with reduced disparities in HPV vaccination rates, as vaccination initiation varies by health insurance coverage: 42% for privately insured children, 37% for those on Medicaid, and only 21% for uninsured children.[9] Before Medicaid expansion, approximately 59% of Medicaid enrollees identified as belonging to a non-White racial/ethnic subgroup.[17] Consequently, expanded Medicaid coverage could have a positive impact on HPV vaccination, particularly among racialized subgroups given their overrepresentation in Medicaid enrollment.

Given this evidence on differential HPV vaccination rates, studies informing evidence-based strategies to increase vaccination are important. We used a quasi-experimental difference-in-differences with multiple time periods approach to assess the impact of Medicaid expansion on HPV vaccination initiation in adolescents aged 13 to 17 years, with particular emphasis on subgroups for sex and race/ethnicity.

METHODS

We followed the Strengthening the Reporting of Observational Studies in Epidemiology (STROBE) reporting guidelines for cross-sectional studies.[18]

Study Objectives

We investigated several hypotheses: Our first hypothesis was that Medicaid expansion results in increases in HPV vaccination initiation among adolescents. Our second hypothesis was that Medicaid expansion results in greater HPV vaccination initiation among male adolescents. Our third hypothesis was that the effects of Medicaid expansion are higher among racialized groups.

Data Source

We used NIS–Teen data from 2011 to 2022, collected by the Centers for Disease Control and Prevention. NIS–Teen is an annual, national, repeated cross-sectional survey of the civilian US population conducted via random-digit-dialing telephone survey to parents and guardians of adolescents aged 13 to 17 years to monitor vaccination coverage. Information is collected on immunization history and self-reported demographic and socioeconomic information. After obtaining parental or guardian consent, mailed immunization forms are sent to providers for verification of vaccination status. For our study, we excluded adolescents who did not have provider-verified information.

We used Kaiser Family Foundation documentation to define the occurrence of Medicaid expansion for each state and year.[19]

Measures

The primary outcome was provider-verified vaccination status of at least 1 HPV dose received, coded as a binary variable. While other provider-verified HPV vaccination status variables were also captured in NIS–Teen, such as 2 doses received or at least 1 dose received by age 13, we chose to include a broader measure focused on vaccination initiation at the time of the survey. Our choice allowed for the full range of adolescents to be included, rather than restricting the data to subsets of the eligible population.

Our intervention variable was coded as a binary variable indicating Medicaid expansion. To date, a total of 41 states (including the District of Columbia) have expanded Medicaid coverage[19]; our model included states as having expanded Medicaid based on their specific expansion year (Table A, available as a supplement to the online version of this article at https://ajph.org). Because NIS–Teen data are currently available until 2022, we excluded states that expanded in 2023 and included them in our control group of nonexpansion states.

We included the following covariates: age (continuous), sex (binary), medical visit in the past year (binary), poverty level, maternal education level, and race/ethnicity. We coded maternal education categorically as less than 12 years, 12 years, greater than 12 years without a college degree, and college graduate. We coded poverty level categorically as below poverty (based on 2020 US Census poverty thresholds), below poverty (≤ $75 000), and above poverty (> $75 000). We coded race/ethnicity categorically into the following mutually exclusive categories: White, Black, Latino, and other or multiple races. Our choice of covariates was informed by previous studies examining Medicaid expansion and HPV vaccination and other studies on factors influencing HPV vaccination.[16,20,21]

Statistical Analyses

To estimate the association between Medicaid expansion and HPV vaccination uptake, we estimated generalized difference-in-differences models. We compared changes in HPV vaccination initiation for adolescents living in expansion states to those in nonexpansion states. Our equation is defined as

$$Y_{ist} = \beta_0 + \beta_1(Medicaid\ Expansion_{st}) + \beta_2(X_{it}) + State_s + Year_t + \varepsilon_{ist} \quad (1)$$

Our outcome *Y* represents HPV vaccination initiation; *Medicaid expansion* represents the policy indicator for Medicaid expansion, with the variable changing from being coded 0 to 1 in the calendar year that a particular state expanded and remains 1 in subsequent years; *X* represents individual covariates; *State* represents state fixed effects; *Year* represents yearly fixed effects; and ε is the error term. The subscripts *i*, *s*, and *t* represent individuals, states, and time in years, respectively. The β1 is our parameter of interest and could be interpreted as the estimated effect of Medicaid expansion on HPV vaccination initiation under the assumption that the change in HPV vaccination in expansion states would have been the same as the change for nonexpansion states in the absence of expansion.

We assessed whether overall trends in HPV vaccination before Medicaid expansion differed in states that expanded coverage versus those that did not to determine the plausibility of the parallel trends assumption. To assess parallel trends, we graphed trends in HPV vaccination in expansion and nonexpansion states before initial Medicaid expansion in 2014 (Figure 1) and also for each year of Medicaid expansion in separate graphs (Figure A, available as a supplement to the online

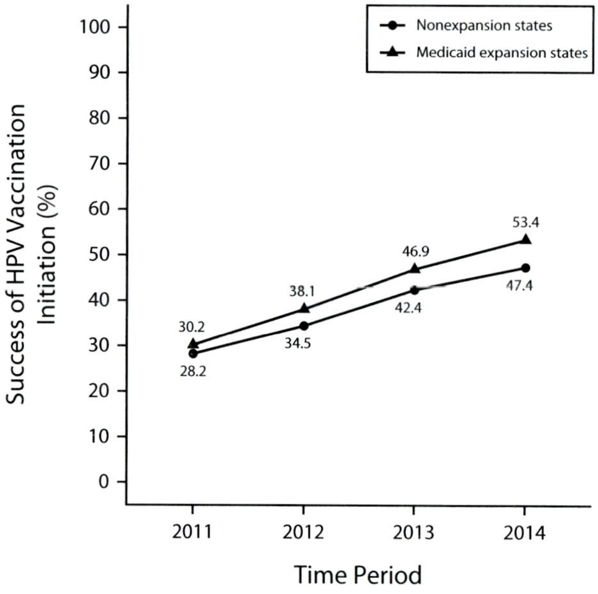

FIGURE 1— HPV Vaccination Initiation Among Adolescents Before Medicaid Expansion by Expansion and Nonexpansion States: United States, 2011–2014

Note. Unadjusted human papillomavirus (HPV) vaccination initiation trends before the Affordable Care Act's Medicaid Expansion in 2014. HPV vaccination initiation indicates the percentage of adolescents aged 13 to 17 years who received at least 1 dose of the HPV vaccine. Data for this figure come from the National Immunization Survey–Teen, 2011–2014. Medicaid expansion states are defined as states that expanded in 2014. Nonexpansion states include data from all states that did not expand Medicaid in 2014.

version of this article at https://ajph.org), with expansion states including states that expanded Medicaid up to that specific year and nonexpansion states including states that did not expand up to that specific year. In addition, we formally tested the parallel trends assumption for each expansion year using a Wald test to assess if expansion and nonexpansion states would have had similar trends if Medicaid expansion had not been implemented (Table B, available as a supplement to the online version of this article at https://ajph.org).[22] All Wald tests were not statistically significant; in all instances, we found no evidence of differential trends in HPV vaccination initiation in the preperiod between expansion and nonexpansion states.

We estimated difference-in-differences using linear probability models for several reasons. First, there are documented shortcomings with nonlinear fixed-effects models.[23] Second, linear probability models allow for the interpretation of coefficient estimates as percentage-point changes in the likelihood of HPV vaccination uptake. This provides a more intuitive interpretation of absolute percentage changes rather than odds ratios on a multiplicative scale from a binomial model, which may be more difficult to interpret.

In our models, we included fixed time effects to account for any trends across years and state fixed effects to account for fixed differences between states, such as political, cultural, or educational differences. We calculated Huber–White standard errors robust to heteroscedasticity and clustered by state. We estimated a crude model and an adjusted model for the full study sample, both with state and year fixed effects, and adjusted for age, race/ethnicity, sex, maternal education, poverty level, and receipt of health care in the past year. In addition, we estimated separate adjusted models by sex and race/ethnicity to investigate effect heterogeneity.

We weighted all analyses to account for the complex sampling design and to ensure a nationally representative sample. We conducted data analyses from April to June 2024, using R statistical software, version 4.2.1 (R Core Team, R Foundation for Statistical Computing, Vienna, Austria). Tests were 2-sided, and we defined statistical significance as $P < .05$.

Sensitivity Analysis

We conducted several analyses to test model assumptions and evaluate the robustness of our results to alternative model specifications. We estimated logistic regression models for our binary outcome. In light of recent discussions surrounding difference-in-differences estimation when treatment timing varies,[24] we tested the robustness of the observed effect from our model comparing expansion states to nonexpansion states with different timings (Table C, available as a supplement to the online version of this article at https://ajph.org). We ran 4 alternative models with variations in treatment timing: comparing early expansion states (defined as 2014–2018) with later expansion states (defined as 2019–2022); comparing early expansion states to nonexpansion states (excluding late expansion states); leveraging only states that expanded in 2014 and considering the rest as nonexpansion states; and excluding expansion states that did not expand in 2014.

RESULTS

From 2011 to 2022, in NIS–Teen, 227 133 adolescents had provider-verified HPV vaccination information. Of these adolescents, 46.6% (105 908) lived in a Medicaid expansion state while 53.3% (121 225) lived in a nonexpansion state. In both groups, the average age was 15 years. Before Medicaid expansion, HPV vaccination initiation in expansion states was 37.2% compared with 33.1% in nonexpansion states. Adolescents in both groups were similar in terms of sex, race/ethnicity, health care visits, and maternal education (Table 1).

After Medicaid expansion, HPV vaccination initiation in expansion states was higher than in nonexpansion states (68.6% vs 60.6%; Figure 2). Table 2 presents difference-in-differences linear regression estimates that are percentage-point differences between changes in HPV vaccination initiation comparing expansion states with nonexpansion states during the period after Medicaid expansion relative to the period before expansion.

The overall adjusted model found that Medicaid expansion produced a significant 5.4 (95% confidence interval [CI] = 4.1, 6.7) percentage-point increase in HPV vaccination initiation ($P < .001$). No statistically significant effect was observed among female adolescents overall (95% CI = −2.0, 1.8; $P < .92$). Among male adolescents overall, Medicaid expansion was associated with a statistically significant 10.1 (95% CI = 8.9, 12.4) percentage-point increase in HPV vaccination uptake ($P < .001$).

By race/ethnicity–level subgroups, Medicaid expansion was associated with statistically significant increases in HPV vaccination initiation among all race/ethnicity subgroups. Among White adolescents, expansion was associated with a 4.8 (95% CI = 3.3, 6.2) percentage-point increase ($P < .001$). The largest association was observed among Black adolescents, with a

TABLE 1— Baseline Characteristics of Adolescents According to State Medicaid Expansion Status: United States, 2011–2022

Characteristic	Nonexpansion States (n = 121 225), Mean (SD) or %	Expansion States (n = 105 908), Mean (SD) or %
Age, y	15.0 (1.4)	15.0 (1.4)
Sex		
Male	51.2	51.0
Female	48.8	49.0
Race/ethnicity		
White	53.1	53.5
Black	16.2	11.0
Latino	22.0	23.6
Other or multiple	8.7	11.9
Health care visit in past year	83.6	84.9
Poverty level[a]		
Below poverty	23.0	19.6
≤ $75 000	38.3	32.0
> $75 000	38.7	48.3
Maternal education		
< 12 y	12.4	11.9
12 y	23.4	21.4
> 12 y, but no college degree	26.3	23.6
College degree or more	37.9	43.1

Note. Weighted baseline characteristics were estimated with the use of pooled National Immunization Survey–Teen data from 2011 to 2022. The sample included data only for respondents for whom there was provider-verified human papillomavirus (HPV) vaccination information. HPV vaccination initiation was defined as provider-verified minimum 1 dose of HPV vaccine at the time of the survey. The numbers are unweighted and represent the actual numbers of individuals in our baseline sample.
[a]Based on 2020 US Census poverty thresholds.

7.7 (95% CI = 4.0, 11.4) percentage-point increase (P < .001). Among Latinos, Medicaid expansion was associated with a 4.6 (95% CI = 1.0, 8.2) percentage-point increase (P < .001). For adolescents of other or multiple races/ethnicities, Medicaid expansion was associated with a 5.2 (95% CI = 1.1, 9.3) percentage-point increase (P < .001).

Looking at race/ethnicity subgroups by sex, Medicaid expansion was associated with significant increases in HPV vaccination among male adolescents for all racial/ethnic subgroups. The smallest association was observed among White male adolescents, with an 8.8 (95% CI = 6.9, 10.7) percentage-point increase (P < .001). The largest association was observed among Latino males with a 13.4-percentage-point increase (95% CI = 8.4, 18.4; P < .001). Among Black male adolescents, Medicaid expansion was associated with an 11-percentage-point increase (95% CI = 5.8, 16.1; P < .001). Among male adolescents of other and multiple races/ethnicities, Medicaid expansion was associated with a 12.2-percentage-point increase (95% CI = 6.7, 17.8; P < .001). No statistically significant effects were observed among any female race/ethnicity subgroups.

Our logistic regression models produced results similar to our linear models, serving as confirmation that our models are not dependent on the assumptions of a linear probability model (Table D, available as a supplement to the online version of this article at https://ajph.org). The alternative models we ran to assess variations in treatment timing produced results consistent with our main analysis and prespecified subgroup analyses (Table C, available as a supplement to the online version of this article at https://ajph.org).

DISCUSSION

We conducted a quasi-experimental study using a difference-in-differences with multiple time periods approach with NIS–Teen data from 2011 to 2022, comparing states that expanded Medicaid to those that did not. We found that Medicaid expansion was associated with statistically significant increases in HPV vaccination initiation among adolescents in the United States. This overall effect was maintained across all racial/ethnic subgroups, with the largest effect observed among Black adolescents. However, from our prespecified subgroup analyses, when looking at differences by sex, the increase in HPV vaccination was confined to male adolescents, with female adolescents having no significant changes in vaccination. In the subgroup analyses, our findings were consistent across all subgroups of race/ethnicity by sex, with significant observed effects for all race/ethnicity subgroups among male adolescents and no observed effects among female adolescents of any race/ethnicity subgroups. Our findings were consistent and robust to different sensitivity analyses.

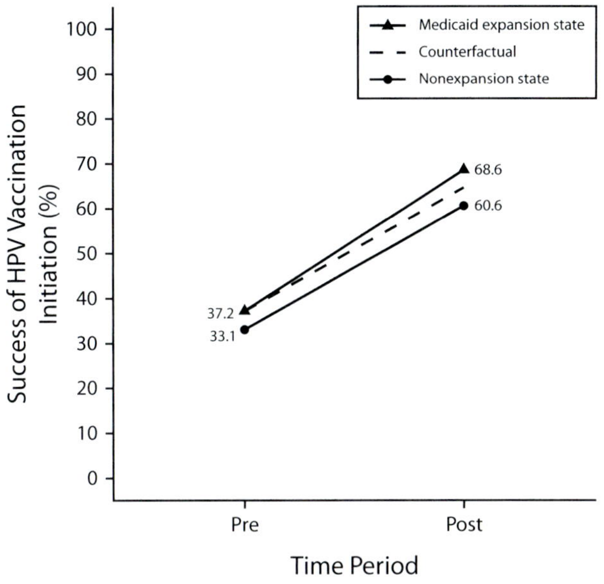

FIGURE 2— HPV Vaccination Initiation Among Adolescents Before and After Medicaid Expansion by Expansion and Nonexpansion States: United States, 2011–2022

Note. Unadjusted human papillomavirus (HPV) vaccination initiation trends before and after the Affordable Care Act's Medicaid Expansion in 2014. HPV vaccination initiation indicates the percentage of adolescents aged 13 to 17 years who received at least 1 dose of the HPV vaccine. Data for this figure come from the National Immunization Survey–Teen, 2011–2022. The "pre" time period includes 2011 to 2014, and the "post" time period includes 2015 to 2022. Medicaid expansion states include data from all states that passed Medicaid expansion from 2014 to 2022. Nonexpansion states include data from all states that did not expand Medicaid and states that expanded in 2023 because of a lack of data for analyses. The dashed black line represents the counterfactual line of what HPV vaccination initiation trends would have been observed among Medicaid expansion states had Medicaid expansion not occurred. The HPV vaccination initiation percentages for the counterfactual line are as follows: pre = 37.2; post = 64.7.

To the best of our knowledge, this study is the first analytical assessment to consider the impacts of Medicaid expansion for both sexes and race/ethnicity subgroups. The few studies that previously examined the association between Medicaid expansion and HPV vaccination focused on the overall impact of Medicaid expansion,[25] income levels,[21] or only females.[16,26] Our findings are consistent with previous studies in that Medicaid expansion was positively associated with HPV vaccination overall and among lower-income individuals.[21,25] This analysis contributes robust evidence to understanding the effects of Medicaid expansion on HPV vaccination, particularly among priority populations previously not considered.

In our study, we observed a statistically significant increase in HPV vaccination initiation after expansion among male adolescents in expansion states compared with those in nonexpansion states, but not among female adolescents. The statistically insignificant slight decrease among female adolescents, both overall and among female race/ethnicity subgroups, suggests that being in a Medicaid expansion state does not significantly impact the likelihood of HPV vaccination initiation compared with being in a nonexpansion state. However, it is important to note that this does not indicate that HPV vaccination initiation among female adolescents was not increasing overall.

The differences in HPV vaccination initiation rates observed between male and female adolescents are likely attributable to existing gendered HPV vaccination disparities.[8] While males in heterosexual relationships are more likely to have and receive HPV in their lifetime,[27] the long-standing attribution of HPV and HPV vaccination as female-specific has adversely impacted males, resulting in HPV vaccination rates that have been lower than expected.[8] Long-held gender biases have increased stigma and imposed a burden of sexual responsibility on females, who are seen as both the carriers and receivers of HPV.[8] Early public health campaigns focused on females, likely explaining why evidence shows females have greater knowledge of the HPV vaccine compared with males[8] and why females did not experience significant increases in HPV vaccination with Medicaid expansion. In addition, females have received more consistent and extensive health care provider recommendations for HPV vaccination compared with males,[28,29] likely contributing to their higher likelihood of vaccination, regardless of Medicaid expansion; this is especially concerning for males given the reliance in the United States on providers for achieving vaccination uptake.[6,7] Finally, the lack of HPV screening available for males has reinforced the traditional cultural narrative of female sexual responsibility, whereby females are responsible for both the screening and treatment of HPV-related diseases, and males ultimately fail to receive important care for the screening and prevention of HPV-related diseases.[8]

The misguided approach of achieving high HPV vaccination among females has resulted in lower vaccination rates among males.[8] However, given changing attitudes and awareness surrounding HPV vaccination and its importance for all young people, there have been

TABLE 2— Medicaid Expansion Effects on Provider-Verified HPV Vaccination Initiation

	No.	Percentage Point Change (95% CI)	P
Overall, crude	227 133	5.8 (4.4, 7.1)	.001
Overall, adjusted	227 133	5.4 (4.10, 6.67)	.001
Sex			
Male	119 175	10.1 (8.9, 12.4)	.001
White	76 384	8.8 (6.9, 10.7)	.001
Black	10 713	11.0 (5.8, 16.1)	.001
Latino	19 610	13.4 (8.4, 18.4)	.001
Other or multiple	12 468	12.2 (6.7, 17.8)	.001
Female	107 958	−0.001 (−2.0, 1.8)	.92
White	68 263	0.6 (−1.6, 2.7)	.6
Black	9 922	4.1 (−1.0, 9.1)	.12
Latino	17 868	−4.6 (−8.7, 1.0)	.07
Other or multiple	11 905	−1.6 (−7.6, 4.4)	.6
Race/ethnicity			
White	144 647	4.8 (3.3, 6.2)	.001
Black	20 635	7.7 (4.0, 11.4)	.001
Latino	37 478	4.6 (1.0, 8.2)	.01
Other or multiple	24 373	5.2 (1.1, 9.3)	.01

Note. CI = confidence interval; HPV = human papillomavirus. Each row represents a separate adjusted regression model. Covariates include age, sex, race/ethnicity, maternal education, income, and health care visit in the past year. Models include year fixed effects and state fixed effects. The overall crude model was unadjusted. National Immunization Survey–Teen pooled data from 2011 to 2022. Survey weights were applied to the pooled data. HPV vaccination initiation was defined as provider-verified minimum 1 dose of HPV vaccine at the time of the survey.

increased efforts to promote HPV vaccination as gender neutral and to increase vaccination rates among males.[8] Providers have increased emphasis on male HPV vaccination, and the push for promotion of HPV vaccination among males in the last decade has coincided with Medicaid expansion, which likely helped increase HPV vaccination rates among males more substantially than for females.[30]

Our findings highlight the effects Medicaid expansion has in increasing HPV vaccination initiation among all racial/ethnic subgroups. We observed notable percentage point increases, with the most significant impacts observed among traditionally underserved populations, such as Black adolescents and Latino male adolescents. These findings underscore the potential of policy initiatives such as Medicaid expansion to mitigate health care disparities and enhance population health outcomes within historically marginalized communities.[31,32] States yet to adopt Medicaid expansion should consider these findings when evaluating their health policy.

The 5-percentage-point increase in HPV vaccination initiation overall and the 10-percentage-point increase among male adolescents are large effects, particularly given that adolescents were not directly impacted by Medicaid expansion. Medicaid expansion likely facilitated higher HPV vaccination uptake through reduced financial barriers, enhanced engagement, and increased access.[13,14] In addition, Medicaid expansion likely had positive spillover effects from adolescents' parents' enrollment and coverage that positively influenced HPV vaccination among their children through increased visits to providers and access to care. Other spillover effects of Medicaid expansion have been documented, including increased Supplemental Nutrition Assistance Program participation,[33] decreased household purchases of sugar-sweetened beverages,[34] and increased annual well-child visits.[35] These findings underscore the importance for nonexpansion states to consider the benefits of expanding Medicaid. States that have chosen not to expand Medicaid have delayed their progress toward greater and more equitable HPV vaccination coverage.

Limitations

Our study had several limitations. First, because of the large time period and nature of our data, we were unable to definitively disregard the possibility that a change unrelated to Medicaid expansion, such as changes in provider recommendations[8,30] or shifts in vaccination guidelines, occurred during the same period that could have influenced HPV vaccination uptake.[6] Second, there may be uncaptured confounders that are correlated with both Medicaid expansion and HPV vaccination that could have biased our analysis. While we attempted to adjust for such confounders, we cannot definitively exclude the possibility of residual bias. Third, our study was limited to adolescents aged 13 to 17 years, and the effects of Medicaid expansion may be different for others in the 9- to 26-year age range for whom HPV vaccination is recommended. Fourth, though we would have liked to analyze the data among additional racial/ethnic groups, our analysis was restricted to the limited categories that NIS–Teen utilizes. We advocate for greater data disaggregation efforts of race/ethnicity data to inform future research more accurately. Fifth, our study was not designed to follow individuals over time, and we do not have information on individual-level changes to Medicaid enrollment or eligibility, an area for future research. Consequently, results should be interpreted within the context of our limitations.

Despite these limitations, our study had some notable strengths. We analyzed NIS–Teen data using robust statistical methods to evaluate the effect of Medicaid expansion on HPV vaccination initiation. Moreover, our study included 12 years of nationally representative data, resulting in more than 225 000 observations and allowing for analysis of Medicaid expansion beyond the initial years and at the subgroup levels for sex and race/ethnicity. We used provider-verified HPV vaccination initiation information, compared with other studies that used self-reported HPV vaccination information, whose estimates may not be as reliable.

Public Health Implications

The findings of our study indicate that Medicaid expansion had a positive effect on increasing HPV vaccination initiation among adolescents, particularly among historically marginalized racial/ethnic subgroups and male adolescents. By extending coverage to a larger segment of eligible individuals, Medicaid expansion has served as an important strategy for increasing HPV vaccination. Our results lend support for the consideration of other near-universal policies that have the ability to indiscriminately reach large demographics, including priority populations with lower vaccination rates. Implementation of further evidence-based policies could contribute to advancing optimal and equitable HPV vaccination coverage. AJPH

ABOUT THE AUTHORS

Angela W. Chen is with the Department of Health Systems and Population Health at the University of Washington School of Public Health, Seattle. Taryn L. Amberson is a PhD candidate with the Department of Health Systems and Population Health at the University of Washington School of Public Health. Harriet Fridah Adhiambo was a PhD candidate with the Department of Child, Family, and Population Health Nursing at the University of Washington School of Nursing at the time of this study. Bradley H. Wagenaar is with the Department of Global Health and Department of Epidemiology at the University of Washington School of Public Health.

CORRESPONDENCE

Correspondence should be sent to Angela W. Chen, MSc, UW Department of Health Systems and Population Health, 1959 NE Pacific Street, H-wing, Sixth Floor, Box 357660, Seattle, WA 98195 (e-mail: achen88@uw.edu). Reprints can be ordered at https://ajph.org by clicking the "Reprints" link.

PUBLICATION INFORMATION

Full Citation: Chen AW, Amberson TL, Adhiambo HF, Wagenaar BH. Effects of Medicaid expansion on HPV vaccination uptake among adolescents in the United States: difference-in-differences analyses from 2011 to 2022. *Am J Public Health*. 2025; 115(9):1454–1462.

Acceptance Date: April 12, 2025.

DOI: https://doi.org/10.2105/AJPH.2025.308165

ORCID iDs:

Angela W. Chen https://orcid.org/0000-0001-6656-128X

Harriet Fridah Adhiambo https://orcid.org/0000-0002-5323-5474

Bradley H. Wagenaar https://orcid.org/0000-0002-3351-7175

CONTRIBUTORS

A. W. Chen originated the project, obtained the data, performed the analysis, designed the figures, and took the lead in writing the article. T. L. Amberson and H. F. Adhiambo were involved in the planning of the study, contributed to the interpretation of the results, and assisted in drafting the article. B. H. Wagenaar supervised the project. All authors provided critical feedback on the article and project.

ACKNOWLEDGMENTS

A. W. Chen was supported by grant T32HS013853 from the Agency for Healthcare Research and Quality (AHRQ). T. L. Amberson was supported by the National Institute for Occupational Safety and Health (NIOSH) under Federal Training Grant T42OH008433.

The authors thank Mohamed Albirair, PhD-c, MPH, MBBS, for his support and teaching assistance of the advanced methods coursework that facilitated the analysis behind this study.

Note. The content is solely the responsibility of the authors and does not necessarily represent the official views of AHRQ or NIOSH.

CONFLICTS OF INTEREST

The authors declare no conflicts of interest.

HUMAN PARTICIPANT PROTECTION

We used de-identified, publicly available data; therefore, this study did not meet the definition of human participant research outlined by the Revised Common Rule (45 CFR §46).

REFERENCES

1. Chesson HW, Dunne EF, Hariri S, Markowitz LE. The estimated lifetime probability of acquiring human papillomavirus in the United States. *Sex Transm Dis*. 2014;41(11):660–664. https://doi.org/10.1097/OLQ.0000000000000193
2. National Cancer Institute. HPV and cancer. National Institutes of Health. 2023. Available at: https://www.cancer.gov/about-cancer/causes-prevention/risk/infectious-agents/hpv-and-cancer. Accessed January 6, 2025.
3. US Food and Drug Administration. Human papillomavirus vaccine. 2024. Available at: https://www.fda.gov/vaccines-blood-biologics/human-papillomavirus-vaccine. Accessed January 6, 2025.
4. US Department of Health and Human Services. Increase the proportion of adolescents who get recommended doses of the HPV vaccine—IID-08. Available at: https://health.gov/healthypeople/objectives-and-data/browse-objectives/vaccination/increase-proportion-adolescents-who-get-recommended-doses-hpv-vaccine-iid-08. Accessed April 29, 2024.
5. Pingali C, Yankey D, Elam-Evans LD, et al. National vaccination coverage among adolescents aged 13–17 years—National Immunization Survey–Teen, United States, 2021. *MMWR Morb Mortal Wkly Rep*. 2022;71(35):1101–1108. https://doi.org/10.15585/mmwr.mm7135a1
6. Markowitz LE, Dunne EF, Saraiya M, et al. Human papillomavirus vaccination: recommendations of the Advisory Committee on Immunization Practices (ACIP) [erratum in *MMWR Recomm Rep*. 2014;63(49):1182]. *MMWR Recomm Rep*. 2014;63(RR-05):1–30.
7. Bartlett JA, Peterson JA. The uptake of human papillomavirus (HPV) vaccine among adolescent females in the United States: a review of the literature. *J Sch Nurs*. 2011;27(6):434–446. https://doi.org/10.1177/1059840511415861
8. Daley EM, Vamos CA, Thompson EL, et al. The feminization of HPV: how science, politics, economics and gender norms shaped US HPV

vaccine implementation. *Papillomavirus Res.* 2017;3:142–148. https://doi.org/10.1016/J.PVR.2017.04.004

9. Villarroel M, Galinksy A, Lu P-J, Pingali C, Valenzuela C. Human papillomavirus vaccination coverage in children ages 9–17 years: United States, 2022. *NCHS Data Brief.* 2024;(495):1–8. https://doi.org/10.15620/CDC:145593
10. Kong WY, Bustamante G, Pallotto IK, et al. Disparities in healthcare providers' recommendation of HPV vaccination for US adolescents: a systematic review. *Cancer Epidemiol Biomarkers Prev.* 2021;30(11):1981–1992. https://doi.org/10.1158/1055-9965.EPI-21-0733
11. Spencer JC, Calo WA, Brewer NT. Disparities and reverse disparities in HPV vaccination: a systematic review and meta-analysis. *Prev Med.* 2019;123:197–203. https://doi.org/10.1016/J.YPMED.2019.03.037
12. Hirth J. Disparities in HPV vaccination rates and HPV prevalence in the United States: a review of the literature. *Hum Vaccin Immunother.* 2019;15(1):146–155. https://doi.org/10.1080/21645515.2018.1512453
13. Access to preventive services without cost-sharing: evidence from the Affordable Care Act. Issue Brief No. HP-202201. Washington, DC: Office of the Assistant Secretary for Planning and Evaluation, US Department of Health and Human Services; January 2022.
14. Tummalapalli SL, Keyhani S. Changes in preventative health care after Medicaid expansion. *Med Care.* 2020;58(6):549–556. https://doi.org/10.1097/MLR.0000000000001307
15. Miller S, Wherry LR. Health and access to care during the first 2 years of the ACA Medicaid expansions. *N Engl J Med.* 2017;376(10):947–956. https://doi.org/10.1056/NEJMSA1612890
16. Agénor M, Unger ES, McConnell MA, et al. Affordable Care Act state Medicaid expansion and human papillomavirus vaccination among adolescent and young adult US women: a national study. *Health Serv Res.* 2023;58(4):792–799. https://doi.org/10.1111/1475-6773.14133
17. Kaiser Family Foundation. Distribution of the nonelderly with Medicaid by race/ethnicity. 2024. Available at: https://www.kff.org/medicaid/state-indicator/medicaid-distribution-nonelderly-by-raceethnicity/?currentTimeframe=7&sortModel=%7B%22colId%22:%22Location%22,%22sort%22:%22asc%22%7D. Accessed May 12, 2024.
18. Von Elm E, Altman DG, Egger M, Pocock SJ, Gøtzsche PC, Vandenbroucke JP, STROBE Initiative. The Strengthening the Reporting of Observational Studies in Epidemiology (STROBE) statement: guidelines for reporting observational studies. *Ann Intern Med.* 2007;147(8):573–577. https://doi.org/10.7326/0003-4819-147-8-200710160-00010
19. Kaiser Family Foundation. Status of state Medicaid expansion decisions: interactive map. 2024. Available at: https://www.kff.org/affordable-care-act/issue-brief/status-of-state-medicaid-expansion-decisions-interactive-map. Accessed April 28, 2024.
20. Dang JHT, Stewart SL, Blumberg DA, Rodriguez HP, Chen MS. Patient and clinician factors associated with uptake of the human papillomavirus (HPV) vaccine among adolescent patients of a primary care network. *Vaccine.* 2021;39(26):3528–3535. https://doi.org/10.1016/J.VACCINE.2021.04.055
21. Hoff BM, Livingston MD, Thompson EL. The association between state Medicaid expansion and human papillomavirus vaccination. *Vaccine.* 2020;38(38):5963–5965. https://doi.org/10.1016/J.VACCINE.2020.07.024
22. de Chaisemartin C, D'Haultfœuille X. Two-way fixed effects and differences-in-differences with heterogeneous treatment effects: a survey. *Econom J.* 2023;26(3):C1–C30. https://doi.org/10.1093/ECTJ/UTAC017
23. Greene W. The behaviour of the maximum likelihood estimator of limited dependent variable models in the presence of fixed effects. *Econometrics J.* 2004;7(1):98–119. https://doi.org/10.1111/J.1368-423X.2004.00123.X
24. Goodman-Bacon A. Difference-in-differences with variation in treatment timing. *J Econom.* 2021;225(2):254–277. https://doi.org/10.1016/J.JECONOM.2021.03.014
25. Churchill BF. Insurance coverage, provider contact, and take-up of the HPV vaccine. *Am J Health Econ.* 2021;7(2). https://doi.org/10.1086/713037
26. Lipton BJ, Decker SL. ACA provisions associated with increase in percentage of young adult women initiating and completing the HPV vaccine. *Health Aff (Millwood).* 2015;34(5):757–764. https://doi.org/10.1377/HLTHAFF.2014.1302
27. Giuliano AR, Nyitray AG, Kreimer AR, et al. EUROGIN 2014 roadmap: differences in HPV infection natural history, transmission, and HPV-related cancer incidence by gender and anatomic site of infection. *Int J Cancer.* 2015;136(12):2752–2760. https://doi.org/10.1002/IJC.29082
28. Lindley MC, Jeyarajah J, Yankey D, Curtis CR, Markowitz LE, Stokley S. Comparing human papillomavirus vaccine knowledge and intentions among parents of boys and girls. *Hum Vaccin Immunother.* 2016;12(6):1519–1527. https://doi.org/10.1080/21645515.2016.1157673
29. Gilkey MB, Moss JL, McRee AL, Brewer NT. Do correlates of HPV vaccine initiation differ between adolescent boys and girls? *Vaccine.* 2012;30(41):5928–5934. https://doi.org/10.1016/J.VACCINE.2012.07.045
30. Lu PJ, Yankey D, Fredua B, et al. Association of provider recommendation and human papillomavirus vaccination initiation among male adolescents aged 13–17 Years—United States. *J Pediatr.* 2019;206:33–41.e1. https://doi.org/10.1016/J.JPEDS.2018.10.034
31. Sonawane K, Garg A, Meissner EG, et al. Human papillomavirus vaccination among young adults before and during the COVID-19 pandemic. *JAMA Netw Open.* 2024;7(2):e2356875. https://doi.org/10.1001/JAMANETWORKOPEN.2023.56875
32. Spencer JC, Brewer NT, Coyne-Beasley T, Trogdon JG, Weinberger M, Wheeler SB. Reducing poverty-related disparities in cervical cancer: the role of HPV vaccination. *Cancer Epidemiol Biomarkers Prev.* 2021;30(10):1895–1903. https://doi.org/10.1158/1055-9965.EPI-21-0307
33. Cha P, Escarce JJ. The Affordable Care Act Medicaid expansion: a difference-in-differences study of spillover participation in SNAP. *PLoS One.* 2022;17(5):e0267244. https://doi.org/10.1371/JOURNAL.PONE.0267244
34. He X, Lopez RA, Boehm R. Medicaid expansion and non-alcoholic beverage choices by low-income households. *Health Econ.* 2020;29(11):1327–1342. https://doi.org/10.1002/HEC.4133
35. Venkataramani M, Pollack CE, Roberts ET. Spillover effects of adult Medicaid expansions on children's use of preventive services. *Pediatrics.* 2017;140(6):e20170953. https://doi.org/10.1542/PEDS.2017-0953/38165

Advancing a Measure of Sexual and Reproductive Well-Being Aligned With Core Values of Reproductive Justice and Human Rights

Christine Dehlendorf, MD, MAS, Sheila Desai, DrPH, MPH, Jessica Danaux, MPH, Carmen Green, MPH, Shashi Sarnaik, MPH, MID, Joia Crear-Perry, MD, and Jamie Hart, PhD, MPH

See also Higgins et al., p. 1349.

Sexuality and reproduction are central to people's life experiences and their ability to thrive. Existing frameworks and measurements related to sexuality and reproduction are predominantly focused on the presence or absence of adverse outcomes, neglecting the critical question of whether people experience positive outcomes and have the sexual and reproductive lives they wish to have. The increased attention to well-being in economic, political, and health spheres presents an opportunity to define and measure the holistic construct of sexual and reproductive well-being.

To this end, we engaged in an 18-month collaborative process to develop a definition of sexual and reproductive well-being, with the ultimate goal of informing the development of a measure that would be self-reported and assessed at the population level.

The resulting draft definition and measure development approach will serve as the foundation for subsequent measure development. This values-driven process of defining sexual and reproductive well-being will contribute to developing a reproductive justice– and human rights–aligned measure that can illuminate the extent to which structures and systems enable optimal sexual and reproductive experiences. (*Am J Public Health*. 2025;115(9):1463–1471. https://doi.org/10.2105/AJPH.2025.308119)

AJPH September 2025, Vol. 115, No. 9

Sexuality and reproduction are core dimensions of the human experience that have wide-ranging impacts across the life course, including on physical and mental health,[1,2] and are central components of life satisfaction.[3,4] The World Health Organization has recognized the centrality of these experiences with a published working definition for sexuality as "a central aspect of being human throughout life [that] encompasses sex, gender identities and roles, sexual orientation, eroticism, pleasure, intimacy and reproduction."[5] In the United States, the reproductive justice movement was borne out of and has foregrounded a recognition that reproduction and, more recently, sexuality are central to people's lives; this recognition includes the "human right to maintain personal bodily autonomy, have children, not have children, and parent those children we have in safe and sustainable communities."[6] The movement has emphasized how inequities in access to desired reproductive and sexual experiences are injustices and violations of human rights.

The increasing traction of and attention to how people's holistic and interconnected experiences of sexuality and reproduction relate to human rights and to social justice have led to a shift among clinical and public health organizations toward calls for reproductive justice.[7–9] However, this shift has not permeated deeply into programs and policies, with ongoing siloes in sexual and reproductive health (SRH) between those, for example, engaged in pregnancy prevention, in sexually transmitted infection prevention and treatment, and in pregnancy-related care. Furthermore, SRH policies and programs in the United States continue to be entrenched in a deficit perspective focused on avoiding adverse outcomes, as opposed to emphasizing positive experiences, as evidenced by the lack of attention on a national level to positive sexuality and support and services for those unable to achieve desired pregnancies owing to infertility.[4,10–12]

One barrier to breaking through these siloes and moving toward a holistic, positive frame with respect to sexuality and reproduction is the lack of availability of metrics that reflect a more aspirational vision. In the United States, the state of the population's SRH is tracked using disparate measures, including the rates of unintended pregnancy, abortion, and contraceptive continuation.[13–15] These measures are influential tools that guide much of the conversation (and funding) related to sexuality and reproduction. However, these metrics were not developed from the framework of seeking to understand and support people's sexual and reproductive lives from a holistic and positive perspective and have been criticized from both conceptual and methodological standpoints.[16] This has included questioning the extent to which "intention" truly measures the acceptability of a pregnancy to an individual and whether decreases in abortion rates should be interpreted as representing a decreased need for this care as opposed to decreased access.[17–20] Rates of contraceptive continuation and the use of long-acting reversible contraceptive methods—other commonly used metrics—are also problematic, as they do not center people's needs, values, and preferences with respect to contraceptive use, while they perpetuate stigmatizing and oppressive narratives of reproduction.[21–23]

The prioritization of measures related to pregnancy intention and contraceptive use stems from prescriptive ideas about what reproductive behaviors and outcomes are desirable and therefore does not reflect a focus on person centeredness or reproductive autonomy.[16,24] The emphasis on these measures in public health and clinical research has the potential to incentivize programs and policies away from what people care about, including by encouraging directive contraceptive counseling.[25] Furthermore, the degree to which people achieve the pregnancies they wish to have and their experiences of sexuality are neglected.

Existing measures used in the United States are therefore ill-suited to support the clinical and public health communities as they move toward a focus on people's holistic lived experience of sex and reproduction owing to their fragmented approach and the notable gaps in the outcomes that are included. Of note, there have been recent innovations in measurement that are moving in the direction of centering human rights in SRH programs. This includes, both in the United States[26,27] and globally,[28,29] increasing focus on measures of person-centered reproductive health care. Furthermore, in the global context, measures have been developed to capture constructs such as contraceptive agency,[30] contraceptive autonomy,[31] and preference-aligned fertility management.[32] However, this type of innovation has not been prominent in the United States, and even these measures do not fully capture people's experiences, as they are focused on specific aspects of sexual and reproductive lives and are generally focused on pregnancy prevention, as opposed to, for example, obtaining desired fertility. New measures that more holistically reflect people's sexual and reproductive experiences—and those that align with values of justice, equity, autonomy, human rights, and person-centeredness—are sorely needed to inform policy and programmatic priorities in the United States.[33,34]

SEXUAL AND REPRODUCTIVE WELL-BEING

In economic and political spaces, there has been increasing recognition of the value of prioritizing and measuring well-being as a means of determining how well people's health and social needs are met. Well-being—defined as what is "non-instrumentally good for a person"—is a positively framed outcome that represents whether people are able to thrive in their lives.[35] This shift in focus—in geographies as varied as Iceland,[36] Scotland,[37] and Bhutan[38]—stems from a recognition that the success of programs and policies does not depend only on individual- or population-level financial statistics, such as that captured with gross domestic product, but also on other components of the lived experiences of populations. Jacinda Ardern, former prime minister of New Zealand, verbalized this perspective: "We need to address the societal well-being of our nation, not just the economic well-being."[39]

Aspects of people's lives that are included in measures of well-being include the work environment, leisure activities, mental and physical health, and interpersonal relationships. To date, however, well-being measures used in these political and economic contexts have neglected the experiences of sexuality and reproduction, despite their central salience to the human experience.

Applying a frame of well-being to SRH and to measurement in SRH research and practice provides an opportunity to advance work both in well-being and in SRH. From the perspective of SRH, applying the well-being framework is consistent with the reproductive justice framework because they both focus on people's experience of sexuality and reproduction holistically and comprehensively.

Creating a valid measure of sexual and reproductive well-being (SRWB) would be a critical step toward addressing the gaps in the measurement landscape because it would move us away from a deficit approach and capture the ultimate outcome of interest: whether people are living the sexual and reproductive lives they wish to. In economics and policy contexts, attending to and measuring SRWB offer a mechanism for tracking this important component of lived experience, both in general and in response to policy interventions. This is particularly critical because the importance of sexuality and reproduction in people's lived experience is frequently neglected or minimized in policy spheres, owing at least in part to the gendered nature of reproduction as well as the stigma of and discomfort with discussing issues related to sexual experience and pleasure.[40] Well-being as a measure of a society's success must include consideration of people's sexual and reproductive experiences if we are to understand how to undertake evidence-based policy interventions to improve SRWB and well-being overall.

We note that globally, and most prominently in Northern Europe, there has been increasing attention to the concept of sexual well-being, including the development of measures that capture this construct.[41] This work is an important departure from stigmatizing narratives on sexuality and has already had consequences for policy and practice that incorporate positive sexuality[42–44]; it has not, however, had substantial impact in the United States.[45] Our interest in a measure of SRWB for the United States is informed by this work and is distinct in incorporating experiences of reproduction to consider sexuality and reproduction holistically to align with reproductive justice. In addition, our conceptualization of well-being is as the ultimate aspirational outcome related to sexuality and reproduction. By contrast, most recent definitions of sexual well-being, including that of the United Kingdom's National Survey of Sexual Attitudes and Lifestyles, consider sexual well-being as coexisting with, and not including, other components of sexuality, such as sexual health and sexual pleasure.[4,46] Our framing of SRWB as the ultimate end goal is aligned with how well-being is defined in economic and policy spheres and is consistent with the rights-based reproductive justice framework.

TOWARD A SEXUAL AND REPRODUCTIVE WELL-BEING MEASURE

To move forward with applying the construct of well-being to measurement in SRH, the Coalition to Expand Contraceptive Access, the Person-Centered Reproductive Health Program at the University of California, San Francisco, and the National Birth Equity Collaborative engaged in a collaborative process to develop a definition of SRWB, with the ultimate goal of informing the development of a measure of this construct that would be self-reported and assessed at the population level.

Recognizing that measure development work, particularly in SRH, is often limited by a lack of intentional framing and defining of the construct of interest—which can result in imprecise measures without broad acceptability—this work was intentionally collaborative and longitudinal, with the goal of ensuring careful and inclusive consideration of the definition of SRWB before moving to the measure development process. By engaging in an intensive, 18-month foundational process, the team showed their commitment to avoiding the errors of many previous efforts at developing measures of sexuality and reproduction, which have been siloed by discipline and have not engaged consistently or rigorously with the lived realities of the populations whose experiences are being measured. We acknowledged the reality of stratified reproduction, in which people from minoritized groups—including individuals with disabilities, gender-expansive individuals, and people of color—have their reproduction devalued in formal and informal ways.[47] In doing this, we worked to ensure that our definition and measure development approach incorporated this reality to consider the full range of influences on SRWB.

To initiate this process, we convened a working group of experts in reproductive epidemiology, maternal and child health, reproductive health care, economics, and reproductive justice in a series of virtual meetings; our goal was to produce and disseminate a definition of SRWB and create a strategy to develop and validate a SRWB measure. This group was intentionally diverse with respect to discipline, gender, race/ethnicity, and region of the country.

Aligning Measures With Values

In the expert working group's early engagements, concern and skepticism about previous measurement efforts in SRH was evident, as we recognized the potential harm of these measures and how public health and clinical priorities, as opposed to reproductive rights and justice, have been foregrounded. There was a demonstrated need for a common foundation and understanding for conducting this work to provide a touchpoint and an accountability mechanism throughout the process. To this end, the working group developed a collaborative set of principles to ground the work. Recognizing how process and output are intricately interrelated, these principles were intended to capture the underlying goal of this work—to develop a subjectively defined, holistic, and positively framed measure—and process considerations such as centering values and engaging with communities.

The principles we developed are as follows:

1. Center values of reproductive justice throughout this process. Root this measure and the process in concrete values and goals from conceptualization through implementation.
2. Define SRWB "in the eye of the beholder." Everyone has different lived experiences and desires, impacted differently by policy and structural contexts. Prioritize how individuals understand and define their subjective well-being across the life course.
3. Rely on diverse community engagement. Measure developers alone should not define well-being for all individuals. The development process must engage in an inclusive process that is informed by community feedback and qualitative information gathering conducted throughout measure development and validation.
4. Move away from negative definitions and toward a positive framing. Many existing health-related measures are defined in the negative, including by the absence of illness or problem. Focus the SRWB measure on positive elements, emphasizing the outcome of well-being and key components along the pathway to achieving well-being.
5. Reiterate the importance and unique contribution of holistic measures, such as that of SRWB. Frame why a SRWB measure is needed and its intended use as part of this process to emphasize the potential positive impacts and promote culture shift.
6. Build on, but do not be constrained by, previous measurement approaches. Measures have their limitations and can be used inappropriately. It is important to consider both traditional and innovative approaches to measure development to learn from and reimagine their value and utility and not re-create previous harms.

An additional consideration that arose from conversations among the working group was the need for explicit grounding of SRWB in the structures and systems that influence people's ability to achieve this aspirational outcome. We identified this step as an essential component of developing any robust measure to ensure that this process was contextualized and not performed in isolation without considering oppressive factors.

We developed a conceptual model that proposed the socioecological factors and context that constitute SRWB and influence people's ability to achieve SRWB (Figure 1). The graphic is an adaptation of a model developed by Braveman et al. for the Robert Wood Johnson Foundation[48] and illustrates how structural, social, and individual determinants directly and indirectly shape the outcome of SRWB. The social determinants of health equity are intentionally illustrated as a "sea" in which this model "swims" to demonstrate how systems of power and history pervade all societal structures, policies, practices, values, choices, and, ultimately, SRWB.[49–50] Being explicit about the relationship between SRWB and these social determinants of health equity and the socioecological determinants included in the model helps ensure that the continued development of the SRWB measure, including the definition of SRWB, will be informed by contextual factors.

Defining Sexual and Reproductive Well-Being

With a foundation for measure development shaped by reproductive justice and a contextual understanding of the construct of interest, we collaboratively defined the concept of SRWB (Box 1) based on the conceptual model; evidence about people's experiences, and insights into their SRWB; existing SRH definitions and measures; expert working group discussions; and reproductive justice. Our definition articulates the key concepts and overarching domains of the construct, identifying the ultimate health and social outcomes as well as essential factors along the pathway to achieving those outcomes. Throughout the process of

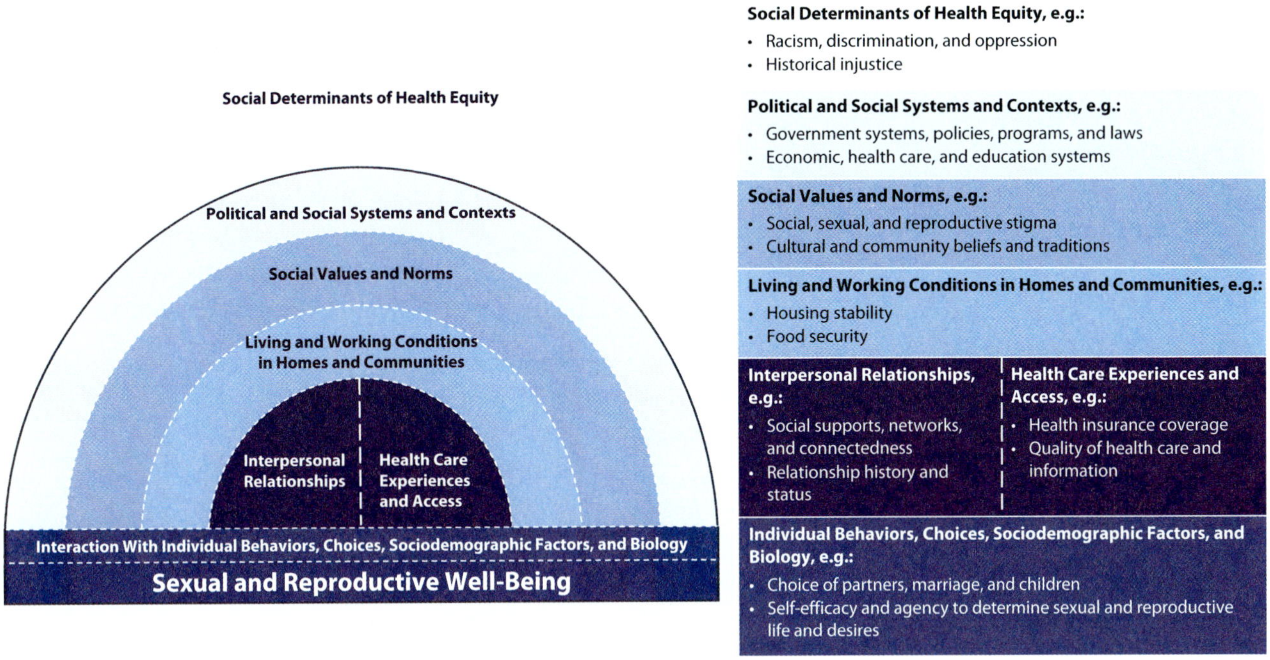

FIGURE 1— Socioecological Determinants of Sexual and Reproductive Well-Being

Source. Adapted from Braveman et al.[48] for the Robert Wood Johnson Foundation; Commission to Build a Healthier America, www.commissiononhealth.org for the Sexual and Reproductive Wellbeing Measure Planning Project, January 2023.
Note. See additional examples at each socioecological level in Figure A (available as a supplement to the online version of this article at http://www.ajph.org).

AJPH September 2025, Vol. 115, No. 9

developing the definition, we ensured attention to inclusivity and worked to develop a broad definition that is applicable to people across the life course regardless of context, preference, or specific sexual and reproductive experiences.

In framing this definition, we intentionally moved beyond health outcomes being considered equivalent to well-being and recognized how experiences in the process of achieving these health outcomes also contribute to achieving well-being. As an evocative example, we considered how someone who has the number of children they wish but experiences a lack of agency in their sexual relationships or abusive or disrespectful health care could not be considered to have achieved SRWB. Rather, SRWB occurs when someone has good SRH outcomes, the family size they desire, positive sexuality, and experiences agency and quality care in the process of achieving those outcomes.

BOX 1— Draft Definition of Sexual and Reproductive Well-Being

Sexual and reproductive well-being is a state of complete physical, mental, and social fulfillment in all matters related to sex and reproduction free of injustice, oppression, coercion, violence, and stigma and their consequences. This includes having the following:

- Freedom and ability to control, act on, and not act on one's sexual and reproductive decisions, desires, goals, and identities, including having comprehensive information, services, and supports and not being hindered or harmed
- Access to and experience of holistic and high-quality care for one's sexuality and reproduction, free of judgement, bias, and coercion, that prioritizes personal needs and desires
- Optimal sexual and reproductive outcomes in accordance with one's needs and desires:
  - Attaining one's ideal state of sexual and reproductive health
  - Choosing if, when, and how to become a parent, and the ability and resources to do so
  - Having a pleasurable and safe sex life

Developing a Measurement Strategy

To move toward a measurement for this definition, the project team, in consultation with the working group, developed an initial measurement framework of SRWB drawing from the draft definition. The initial measurement framework distills the conceptual definition into initial proposed measurement domains to guide measure development, including item generation. These domains were as follows:

1. Agency, autonomy, and freedom from oppression in matters related to sexuality and reproduction;
2. Experience of SRH care;
3. One's ideal state of SRH;
4. The choice of if, when, and how to become a parent and the ability and resources to do so; and
5. A pleasurable and safe sex life.

We next considered with the working group how to use this draft definition and measurement framework as a foundation for the process of measure development, including ensuring continued adherence to the core identified values and to scientific rigor. Specifically, we considered the importance of centering the perspectives and expertise of the population for whom the measure is designed and developed a plan for prioritizing community voices through the measure development process, building on principles of cocreation.[51] This includes extensive qualitative work and community consultation in each stage of the measure development process, including in refining the definition of SRWB. By contrast to the common strategy of item generation occurring through consultation between researchers, we intentionally planned for exploration of item wording through the first stage of our qualitative work.[52] The proposed steps for measure development, with attention to how community voices will be included in this process, were as follows:

- Step 1. Refine the definition and measurement framework through interviews and other stakeholder discussions
  - Ensure intentionality in the inclusion of diverse communities and perspectives
  - Iteratively explore the wording and interpretation of the domains and questions
- Step 2. Draft a preliminary instrument and conduct cognitive interviews with a representative sample of different populations
  - Based on the results of step 1 and reviews of qualitative and quantitative research on sexual and reproductive experiences in the United States and globally, develop a preliminary set of survey items
  - Learn from participants' impressions and experiences about the items to refine and revise them to best represent the perspectives of diverse communities
- Step 3. Rigorously test and refine the instrument and develop recommendations for use
  - Evaluate validity and reliability to determine whether the measure accurately represents the construct of SRWB
  - Ensure that testing represents and is relevant for diverse communities
  - Conduct a stakeholder-engaged consensus-building process to develop appropriate implementation and interpretation guidance that optimizes impact

Having laid the groundwork for a values-driven and rights-based measure development process of SRWB, we now look forward to the next steps: operationalizing this strategy and achieving the goal of a valid and reliable measure of the degree to which people are living the sexual and reproductive lives they wish to. In doing so, we will benefit from the work that has already been done in developing measures of several domains included in this definition, such as experience of care and agency.[27,30] However, recognizing that our ultimate goal is a concise measure appropriate for use in demographic monitoring, it will be necessary to modify existing items or develop new items to more concisely capture these constructs with wording that is universally relevant and understood across contexts, preferences, and experiences. Although this will be challenging, this difficulty cannot and should not stand in the way of working to measure what we actually care about, rather than continuing to measure things that are more easily quantifiable but do not adequately capture the realities of people's lives.

Having a population-level measure of SRWB would mark a fundamental shift in how SRH is measured. Through tracking SRWB over time and in response to policies and programs, we can see how factors such as contraceptive and abortion access, paid family leave policies, and economic supports can influence people's holistic experience of their sexuality and reproduction. Furthermore, by stratifying the measure by age, sexual orientation, race, and gender, inequities in this outcome can be identified and mitigated.

In addition to these practical implications, the availability of metrics drives what is prioritized, as laid out in the frequently used adage "What gets measured gets done." The currently available SRH metrics—including unintended pregnancy rates, abortion rates, and metrics of sexually transmitted infections (with a notable lack of focus on people's ability to achieve desired fertility)—drive a fragmented policy and programmatic agenda that seeks to address individual negative outcomes, without attending to the bigger picture of people's lives. Furthermore, these metrics are disconnected from a human rights–based framework that centers people's right to optimal SRH and experiences. As a result, the SRH narrative tends to focus on risks and challenges rather than on supporting people in achieving their optimal sexual and reproductive lives. A SRWB measure can help to shift the narrative for SRH with respect to clinical care, public health, and policy interventions so that the guiding light is not focused on specific deficit-framed metrics but on a vision of the world as we want it to be and, ultimately, on reproductive justice.

Importantly, a SRWB measure alone will not address the inability of our current measurement approach to help us understand how to improve people's sexual and reproductive lives. Nevertheless, as the ultimate aspirational measure, the SRWB measure would provide a critical shift in focus and ability to track this population-level outcome over time. Results of this measure would by necessity have to be interpreted in the context of both more detailed measures (e.g., existing measures and those to be developed that capture experiences with abortion, obstetrics, or gender-affirming care; sexual pleasure; and reproductive services access) and contextual measures (e.g., those related to policy environments). The development and dissemination of a SRWB measure would provide a critical foundation for an evolving measurement approach that centers people, their experiences, and how systems and structures can best support them.

More broadly, we recognize that the opportunity to engage in an extended, iterative process with a diverse working group to define the construct of interest before beginning measure development is uncommon in measurement work. This process was instrumental in our effort to ensure that our definition and the measure that will ultimately be created reflect people's lived experiences. In SRH and beyond there is an unrealized need for metrics that reflect values related to person centeredness and autonomy. Efforts to develop these metrics will benefit from an intentional approach to community engagement and explicit grounding in principles and values from the outset. Doing this will ensure that the too often siloed and unrepresentative measure development processes of the past, which have resulted in measures that do not capture what people themselves care about, are not reproduced.

CONCLUSIONS

A move toward values-aligned, holistic, and person-centered metrics such as SRWB can help center our focus on achieving positive outcomes for people's SRH and beyond. Our process of defining SRWB in an intentional and collaborative manner will contribute to our ultimate work to develop a reproductive justice–aligned measure that can inform an understanding of how much structures, systems, and policies enable optimal sexual and reproductive experiences and promote sexual and reproductive equity. AJPH

ABOUT THE AUTHORS

Christine Dehlendorf and Shashi Sarnaik are with the Person-Centered Reproductive Health Program, Department of Family and Community Medicine, University of California, San Francisco. Sheila Desai, Jessica Danaux, and Jamie Hart are with the Coalition to Expand Contraceptive Access, Sacramento, CA. Carmen Green is with the Department of Social and Behavioral Sciences, University of California, San Francisco. Joia Crear-Perry is with the National Birth Equity Collaborative.

CORRESPONDENCE

Correspondence should be sent to Christine Dehlendorf, 2540 23rd St, #5702, San Francisco CA 94110 (e-mail: christine.dehlendorf@ucsf.edu). Reprints can be ordered at https://www.ajph.org by clicking the "Reprints" link.

PUBLICATION INFORMATION

Full Citation: Dehlendorf C, Desai S, Danaux J, et al. Advancing a measure of sexual and reproductive well-being aligned with core values of reproductive justice and human rights. *Am J Public Health*. 2025;115(9):1463–1471.

Acceptance Date: March 14, 2025.

https://doi.org/10.2105/AJPH.2025.308119

ORCID iDs:

Jessica Danaux https://orcid.org/0009-0002-1130-8601

Shashi Sarnaik https://orcid.org/0000-0002-1108-4348

CONTRIBUTORS

C. Dehlendorf, S. Desai, J. Danaux, and J. Hart wrote the original draft of the essay. C. Dehlendorf, C. Green, and J. Hart facilitated expert working group meetings. C. Dehlendorf, J. Crear-Perry, and J. Hart conceptualized the study and developed the methodology. C. Dehlendorf and J. Hart secured funding. S. Desai, J. Danaux, and S. Sarnaik administered the project. S. Sarnaik, C. Green, and J. C. Crear-Perry helped write and edited the essay. All authors reviewed and approved the final version.

ACKNOWLEDGMENTS

This work was made possible by an anonymous foundation through the Coalition to Expand Contraceptive Access.

The authors would like to thank the expert panel—Angela Aina, Anu Manchikanti Gómez, Arik Marcell, Celia Karp, David Bell, Dionna Cheatham, Elle Lett, Gillian Sealy, Jamila Taylor, Jamila Perritt, Jeannette Wade, June Gipson, Kathryn Kost, Kelly Jones, Kelsey Holt, Milan Spencer, Miriam Yeung, Monica McLemore, Natalie Hernandez, Shay-Akil McLean, Sonya Borrero, Ushma Upadhyay, and Whitney Rice—for their support and oversight. We also thank Alyssa Lindsey for support with essay preparation and submission.

CONFLICTS OF INTEREST

The authors have no conflicts of interest to disclose.

HUMAN PARTICIPANT PROTECTION

No protocol approval was necessary because no human participants were involved in this study.

REFERENCES

1. Diamond LM, Huebner DM. Is good sex good for you? Rethinking sexuality and health. *Soc Personal Psychol Compass.* 2012;6(1):54–69. https://doi.org/10.1111/j.1751-9004.2011.00408.x
2. Anderson RM. Positive sexuality and its impact on overall well-being. *Bundesgesundheitsblatt Gesundheitsforschung Gesundheitsschutz.* 2013;56(2):208–214. https://doi.org/10.1007/s00103-012-1607-z
3. Laumann EO, Paik A, Glasser DB, et al. A cross-national study of subjective sexual well-being among older women and men: findings from the Global Study of Sexual Attitudes and Behaviors. *Arch Sex Behav.* 2006;35(2):143–159. https://doi.org/10.1007/s10508-005-9005-3
4. Mitchell KR, Lewis R, O'Sullivan LF, Fortenberry JD. What is sexual wellbeing and why does it matter for public health? *Lancet Public Health.* 2021;6(8):e608–e613. https://doi.org/10.1016/S2468-2667(21)00099-2
5. World Health Organization. Defining sexual health. 2006. Available at: https://www.who.int/teams/sexual-and-reproductive-health-and-research/key-areas-of-work/sexual-health/defining-sexual-health. Accessed January 28, 2022.
6. SisterSong. Reproductive justice. Available at: https://sistersong.net/reproductive-justice. Accessed December 2, 2023.
7. Hart J, Crear-Perry J, Stern L. US sexual and reproductive health policy: which frameworks are needed now, and next steps forward. *Am J Public Health.* 2022;112(suppl 5):S518–S522. https://doi.org/10.2105/AJPH.2022.306929
8. Gilliam ML, Neustadt A, Gordon R. A call to incorporate a reproductive justice agenda into reproductive health clinical practice and policy. *Contraception.* 2009;79(4):243–246. https://doi.org/10.1016/j.contraception.2008.12.004
9. Cohen RE, Wilkinson TA, Staples-Horne M. The need for reproductive justice in pediatrics. *JAMA Pediatr.* 2021;175(12):1207–1208. https://doi.org/10.1001/jamapediatrics.2021.2978
10. Kantor LM, Lindberg L. Pleasure and sex education: the need for broadening both content and measurement. *Am J Public Health.* 2020;110(2):145 148. https://doi.org/10.2105/AJPH.2019.305320
11. Öztürk R, Herbell K, Morton J, Bloom T. "The worst time of my life": treatment-related stress and unmet needs of women living with infertility. *J Community Psychol.* 2021;49(5):1121–1133. https://doi.org/10.1002/jcop.22527
12. Donchin A. In whose interest? Policy and politics in assisted reproduction. *Bioethics.* 2011;25(2):92–101. https://doi.org/10.1111/j.1467-8519.2010.01869.x
13. Jones RK, Jerman J. Population group abortion rates and lifetime incidence of abortion: United States, 2008–2014. *Am J Public Health.* 2022;112(9):1284–1296. https://doi.org/10.2105/AJPH.2017.304042
14. US Centers for Disease Control and Prevention. Unintended pregnancy. May 15, 2024. Available at: https://cdc.gov/reproductive-health/hcp/unintended-pregnancy/index.html. Accessed November 21, 2024.
15. Peipert JF, Zhao Q, Allsworth JE, et al. Continuation and satisfaction of reversible contraception. *Obstet Gynecol.* 2011;117(5):1105–1113. https://doi.org/10.1097/AOG.0b013e31821188ad
16. Dehlendorf C, Reed R, Fox E, Seidman D, Hall C, Steinauer J. Ensuring our research reflects our values: the role of family planning research in advancing reproductive autonomy. *Contraception.* 2018;98(1):4–7. https://doi.org/10.1016/j.contraception.2018.03.015
17. Gomez AM, Arteaga S, Ingraham N, Arcara J, Villaseñor E. It's not planned, but is it okay? The acceptability of unplanned pregnancy among young people. *Womens Health Issues.* 2018;28(5):408–414. https://doi.org/10.1016/j.whi.2018.07.001
18. Borrero S, Nikolajski C, Steinberg JR, et al. "It just happens": a qualitative study exploring low-income women's perspectives on pregnancy intention and planning. *Contraception.* 2015;91(2):150–156. https://doi.org/10.1016/j.contraception.2014.09.014
19. Aiken ARA, Borrero S, Callegari LS, Dehlendorf C. Rethinking the pregnancy planning paradigm: unintended conceptions or unrepresentative concepts? *Perspect Sex Reprod Health.* 2016;48(3):147–151. https://doi.org/10.1363/48e10316
20. Dehlendorf C, Weitz T. Access to abortion services: a neglected health disparity. *J Health Care Poor Underserved.* 2011;22(2):415–421. https://doi.org/10.1353/hpu.2011.0064
21. Gomez AM, Fuentes L, Allina A. Women or LARC first? Reproductive autonomy and the promotion of long-acting reversible contraceptive methods. *Perspect Sex Reprod Health.* 2014;46(3):171–175. https://doi.org/10.1363/46e1614
22. Higgins JA. Celebration meets caution: LARC's boons, potential busts, and the benefits of a reproductive justice approach. *Contraception.* 2014;89(4):237–241. https://doi.org/10.1016/j.contraception.2014.01.027
23. Romero D, Agénor M. US fertility prevention as poverty prevention: an empirical question and social justice issue. *Womens Health Issues.* 2009;19(6):355–364. https://doi.org/10.1016/j.whi.2009.08.004
24. Dehlendorf C, Bellanca H, Policar M. Performance measures for contraceptive care: what are we actually trying to measure? *Contraception.* 2015;91(6):433–437. https://doi.org/10.1016/j.contraception.2015.02.002
25. Brandi K, Fuentes L. The history of tiered-effectiveness contraceptive counseling and the importance of patient-centered family planning care. *Am J Obstet Gynecol.* 2020;222(suppl 4):S873–S877. https://doi.org/10.1016/j.ajog.2019.11.1271
26. Afulani PA, Coleman-Phox K, Leon-Martinez D, et al. Psychometric assessment of the US person-centered prenatal and maternity care scales in a low-income predominantly Latinx population in California. *BMC Womens Health.* 2023;23(1):616. https://doi.org/10.1186/s12905-023-02721-5
27. Dehlendorf C, Fox E, Silverstein IA, et al. Development of the Person-Centered Contraceptive Counseling scale (PCCC), a short form of the Interpersonal Quality of Family Planning care scale. *Contraception.* 2021;103(5):310–315. https://doi.org/10.1016/j.contraception.2021.01.008
28. Afulani PA, Nakphong MK, Sudhinaraset M. Person-centred sexual and reproductive health: a call for standardized measurement. *Health Expect.* 2023;26(4):1384–1390. https://doi.org/10.1111/hex.13781
29. Holt K, Gebrehanna E, Sarnaik S, et al. Adaptation and validation of the quality of contraceptive counseling (QCC) scale for use in Ethiopia and India. *PLoS One.* 2023;18(3):e0283925. https://doi.org/10.1371/journal.pone.0283925
30. Holt K, Challa S, Alitubeera P, et al. Conceptualizing contraceptive agency: a critical step to enable human rights-based family planning programs and measurement. *Glob Health Sci Pract.* 2024;12(1):e2300299. https://doi.org/10.9745/GHSP-D-23-00299
31. Senderowicz L, Bullington BW, Sawadogo N, et al. Measuring contraceptive autonomy at two sites in Burkina Faso: a first attempt to measure a novel family planning indicator. *Stud Fam Plann.* 2023;54(1):201–230. https://doi.org/10.1111/sifp.12224
32. Rothschild CW, Bulama A, Odeh R, et al. Preference-aligned fertility management among married adolescent girls in Northern Nigeria: assessing a new measure of contraceptive autonomy. *BMJ Glob Health.* 2024;9(5):e013902. https://doi.org/10.1136/bmjgh-2023-013902
33. Dehlendorf C, Akers AY, Borrero S, et al. Evolving the preconception health framework: a call for reproductive and sexual health equity. *Obstet Gynecol.* 2021;137(2):234–239. https://doi.org/10.1097/AOG.0000000000004255
34. Potter JE, Stevenson AJ, Coleman-Minahan K, et al. Challenging unintended pregnancy as an indicator of reproductive autonomy. *Contraception.* 2019;100(1):1–4. https://doi.org/10.1016/j.contraception.2019.02.005
35. Crisp R. Well-Being. Stanford Encyclopedia of Philosophy Archive. September 15, 2021. Available at: https://plato.stanford.edu/archives/win2021/entries/well-being. Accessed December 2, 2023.
36. Government of Iceland. Well-Being. Available at: https://www.government.is/topics/sustainable-iceland/well-being. Accessed December 2, 2023.
37. Scottish Government. Wellbeing Economy Governments (WEGo). Available at: https://www.gov.scot/groups/wellbeing-economy-governments-wego. Accessed December 2, 2023.
38. Sithey G, Thow AM, Li M. Gross national happiness and health: lessons from Bhutan. *Bull World Health Organ.* 2015;93(8):514. https://doi.org/10.2471/BLT.15.160754
39. Parker C. New Zealand will have a new "well-being budget," says Jacinda Ardern. January 23, 2019. Available at: https://www.weforum.org/agenda/2019/01/new-zealand-s-new-well-being-budget-will-fix-broken-politics-says-jacinda-ardern. Accessed December 2, 2023.
40. Ford JV, Corona Vargas E, Finotelli I Jr, et al. Why pleasure matters: its global relevance for sexual health, sexual rights and wellbeing. *Int J Sex Health.* 2019;31(3):217–230. https://doi.org/10.1080/19317611.2019.1654587
41. Sundgren M, Damiris I, Stallman H, et al. Investigating psychometric measures of sexual wellbeing: a systematic review. *Sex Relatsh Ther.* 2024;39(4):1492–1517. https://doi.org/10.1080/14681994.2022.2033967
42. Scottish Government. Sexual health and blood borne virus action plan: 2023 to 2026. November 28, 2023. Available at: https://www.gov.scot/publications/sexual-health-blood-borne-virus-action-plan-2023-2026/documents. Accessed November 13, 2024.
43. International Planned Parenthood Federation. Putting sexuality back into comprehensive sexuality education: making the case for a rights-based, sex-positive approach. Available at:

https://www.ippf.org/sites/default/files/2016-10/Putting%20Sexuality%20back%20into%20Comprehensive%20Sexuality%20Education_0.pdf. Accessed November 13, 2024.

44. Ford JV, Corona-Vargas E, Cruz M, et al. The World Association for Sexual Health's declaration on sexual pleasure: a technical guide. *Int J Sex Health*. 2022;33(4):612–642. https://doi.org/10.1080/19317611.2021.2023718

45. Ford JV, Ivankovich MB, Coleman E. Sexual health indicators for the United States: measuring progress and documenting public health needs. *Front Public Health*. 2023;10:1040097. https://doi.org/10.3389/fpubh.2022.1040097

46. Mitchell KR, Palmer MJ, Lewis R, et al. Development and validation of a brief measure of sexual wellbeing for population surveys: the Natsal Sexual Wellbeing Measure (Natsal-SW). *J Sex Res*. 2025;62(1)1–11. https://doi.org/10.1080/00224499.2022.2035663

47. Harris LH, Wolfe T. Stratified reproduction, family planning care and the double edge of history. *Curr Opin Obstet Gynecol*. 2014;26(6):539–544. https://doi.org/10.1097/GCO.0000000000000121

48. Braveman PA, Egerter SA, Mockenhaupt RE. Broadening the focus: the need to address the social determinants of health. *Am J Prev Med*. 2011;40(suppl 1):S4–S18. https://doi.org/10.1016/j.amepre.2010.10.002

49. Jones CP. Systems of power, axes of inequity: parallels, intersections, braiding the strands. *Med Care*. 2014;52(Supplement 3):S71–S75. https://doi.org/10.1097/MLR.0000000000000216

50. Crear-Perry J, Correa-de-Araujo R, Lewis Johnson T, McLemore MR, Neilson E, Wallace M. Social and structural determinants of health inequities in maternal health. *J Womens Health (Larchmt)*. 2021;30(2):230–235. https://doi.org/10.1089/jwh.2020.8882

51. Leask CF, Sandlund M, Skelton DA, et al. Framework, principles and recommendations for utilising participatory methodologies in the co-creation and evaluation of public health interventions. *Res Involv Engagem*. 2019;5(1):2. https://doi.org/10.1186/s40900-018-0136-9

52. Boateng GO, Neilands TB, Frongillo EA, Melgar-Quiñonez HR, Young SL. Best practices for developing and validating scales for health, social, and behavioral research: a primer. *Front Public Health*. 2018;6:149. https://doi.org/10.3389/fpubh.2018.00149

Public Firearms Carriage and Public Opinion, National Gun Policy Survey, 2023

Cassandra K. Crifasi, PhD, MPH, Kelly E. W. Roskam, JD, and Alex D. McCourt, JD, PhD, MPH

See also Klarevas, p. 1352.

Objectives. To examine US public opinion on whether people should be allowed to carry firearms in "sensitive locations" (i.e., where firearm carry is not allowed, even for those with valid concealed carry permits).

Methods. We used data from the 2023 National Gun Policy Survey to understand attitudes on gun carrying in potentially sensitive places. Respondents were asked to respond yes or no to allowing people to carry in various locations. We generated weighted proportions for prohibiting carry overall and by gun ownership among gun owners and among those who affirmed feeling safer if more people could legally carry guns.

Results. More than 70% of respondents said guns should not be carried at bars, sports stadiums, or protests or rallies. Among gun owners, there was broad support for prohibiting gun carrying in these locations, even among those who would feel safer if more people could legally carry guns.

Conclusions. Prohibiting gun carrying where alcohol is served or where there is a greater perception of conflict is broadly supported.

Public Health Implications. These findings can inform evidence-based strategies to reduce firearm-related harm in sensitive public settings. (*Am J Public Health*. 2025;115(9):1472–1479. https://doi.org/10.2105/AJPH.2025.308152)

AJPH September 2025, Vol. 115, No. 9

Over the past 40 years, there has been an immense shift in the way US states have regulated the public's concealed carry of firearms.[1] In the 1980s, most states either did not allow concealed carry or did so under a "may issue" system that generally required an individual to meet a set of objective criteria (e.g., background check, safety training, accuracy requirements) and have a good and substantial need to carry a concealed handgun in public spaces (i.e., subjective requirements at the discretion of law enforcement). The shift toward "shall issue" systems began in the 1990s and 2000s whereby states retained at least some objective criteria but offered little to no discretion to law enforcement to deny applicants based on dangerousness. As of the writing of this article, more than half of states have eliminated the concealed carry licensing requirement entirely through so-called permitless carry, thereby allowing anyone not legally prohibited from owning a gun to carry a gun concealed in public (Figure 1).

Previous research has found that this shift to relaxed regulations for concealed carry is associated with increases in firearm violence. Research by Donohue et al. found that violent crime increased in states that shifted to "right to carry" (i.e., shall issue or permitless) in the 10 years following the law change.[2] Gun theft in cities was also higher when states shifted to right to carry.[3] Increases in firearm homicide in large, urban counties[4,5] and in the workplace[6] have also been associated with states shifting from may issue to right to carry. The passage of shall issue laws that removed prohibitions on those previously convicted of a violent misdemeanor was associated with increases in rates of firearm assaults,[7] and the adoption of permitless carry laws was associated with increased rates of injurious shootings by police.[8] Although most research has focused on changes to the concealed carry licensing requirements,

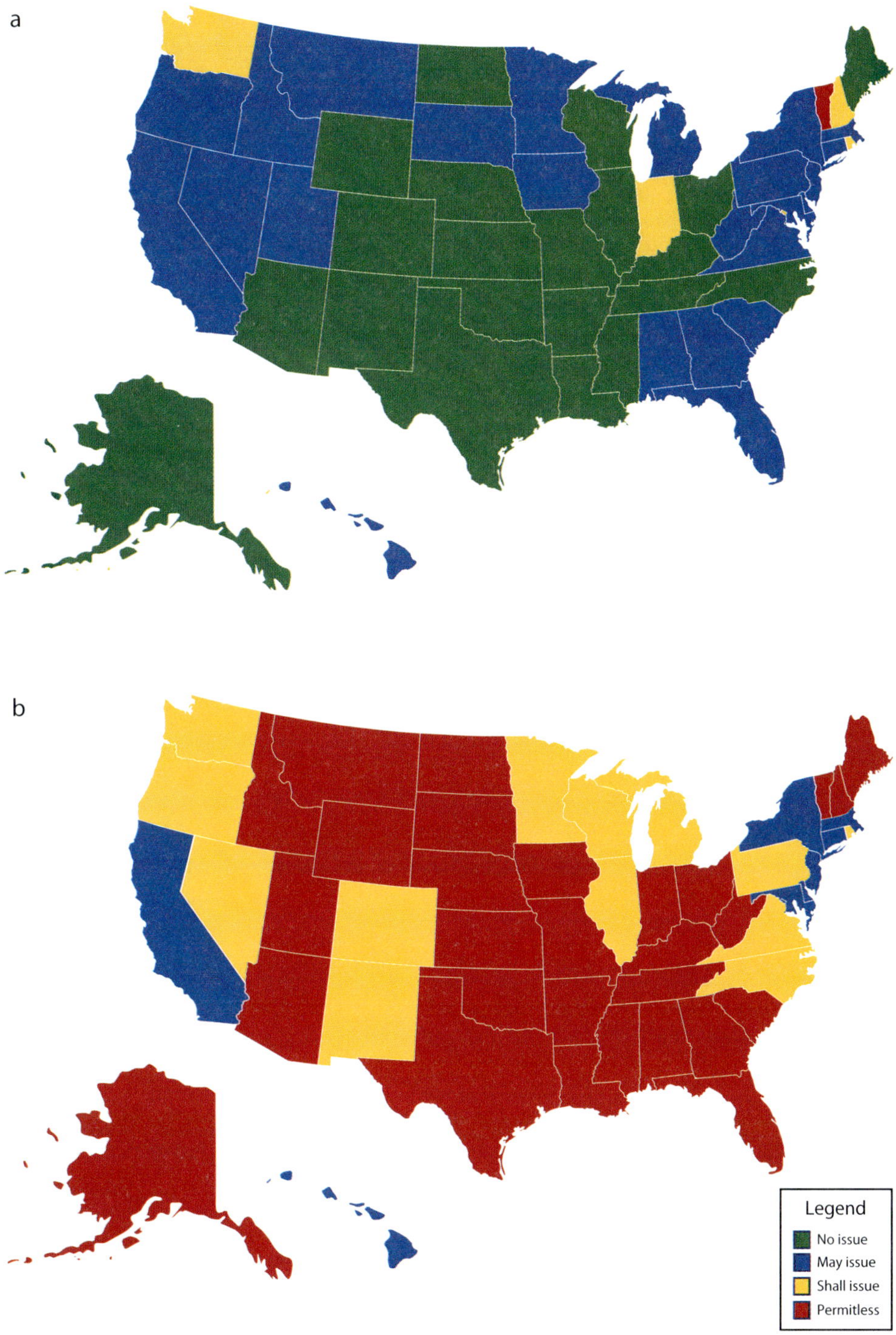

FIGURE 1— Variation in State Concealed Carry Policies in (a) 1980 and (b) 2024: Johns Hopkins Center for Gun Violence Solutions, United States

Note. States with no issue laws do not allow concealed carry and do not issue permits to carry. States with may issue laws allow concealed carry but require a permit and afford law enforcement some discretion when evaluating permit applications. States with shall issue laws allow concealed carry but require a permit and allow law enforcement little to no discretion when evaluating permit applications. States with permitless laws allow concealed carry but do not require a permit.

another important feature of regulating concealed carry, and public carry more broadly, focuses on where individuals can lawfully carry their firearms. For this reason, it is important to understand public opinions on where individuals should and should not be allowed to carry loaded, concealed handguns.

In 2008, in its landmark Second Amendment decision, *District of Columbia v Heller* (hereafter *Heller*), the US Supreme Court held for the first time that the Second Amendment protects an individual right to possess an operable handgun in the home for the purpose of self-defense.[9] The court also identified "sensitive places" (e.g., schools, government buildings) where the prohibition of carrying firearms was "presumptively lawful" but provided no explanation for lower courts to identify additional sensitive places.[9] In June 2022, in *New York State Rifle and Pistol Association v Bruen* (hereafter *Bruen*), the Supreme Court struck down a provision of New York's public carry licensing law The court also dramatically altered the way courts are required to evaluate Second Amendment challenges, abandoning balancing how closely the law was fit to achieve an important government interest in favor of a history-focused test.[10] However, the court also referred to *Heller*'s discussion of the longstanding regulations on sensitive places. Once more, the court articulated a nonexhaustive list of sensitive places and instructed that lower courts may identify new sensitive places by analogizing to these historical locations.[10] It did not explain what characteristics of these historically sensitive places were relevant for analogizing to new locations.

In the absence of Supreme Court guidance, courts have reasoned that the sensitivity of a place is related to the people who congregate there (e.g., children and other vulnerable populations) or the activities that occur there (e.g., governmental functions) or to people's reasonable expectation of safety in those locations.[11,12] Additionally, legal scholars have asserted that sensitive locations are those where constitutional rights may come into conflict, where there is a high likelihood of conflict, or "where the presence of weapons is incompatible with the actual functioning of the place itself."[11,13,14(p1)]

As legislatures and courts wrestle with identifying sensitive places where firearms should be prohibited, survey data on Americans' attitudes regarding where public carry should be allowed may be particularly relevant in determining whether these public safety laws are consistent with constitutional principles.

Previous research has explored public opinions on firearm carry in certain locations. In 2015, Wolfson et al. examined attitudes on carrying firearms in locations such as schools, bars, and sports stadiums and found overall support to be low—although support was higher among gun owners.[15] Support for allowing concealed carry on college campuses and K–12 school grounds remained low in 2021[16] and 2023.[17] However, more work is needed to understand how the public, including firearm owners, thinks about concealed carry in various locations and whether an individual's perceptions of safety if more people could legally carry firearms in public spaces affects their support for carrying in those locations. Additionally, given the differences in victimization and perpetration of gun violence across racial and ethnic groups[18] and the diversification of gun ownership,[19,20] understanding the perspectives on gun carrying among racial and ethnic subgroups of gun owners will further improve our understanding of perspectives on this pressing issue.

Given the attention on firearm carrying generally, and sensitive places specifically, we sought to examine levels of support for some places that may be deemed sensitive as well as whether support for prohibiting firearm carrying varied by firearm ownership or race and ethnicity.

METHODS

The 2023 National Survey of Gun Policy was fielded in the United States from January 4 through February 6, 2023. We used NORC's AmeriSpeak panel to obtain a nationally representative sample of US adults.[21] Surveys could be completed online or by telephone in English or Spanish. There was an oversample of gun owners and Black Americans, Hispanic Americans, and Asian Americans to allow analyses among demographic subgroups. We determined personal gun ownership by a yes answer to 2 questions: "Do you happen to have in your home or garage any guns or revolvers?" and "Do any of these guns personally belong to you?" We identified new gun owners as those who reported buying their first gun after January 1, 2020. Race and ethnicity were self-reported as part of the AmeriSpeak demographic panel: non-Hispanic White, non-Hispanic Black, non-Hispanic Asian, non-Hispanic other race, or Hispanic of any race. Because of an issue with sample size, we excluded respondents who reported their race as "other" from the stratified analyses. The survey completion rate was 76.5% for a total of 3096 respondents including 1002 gun owners. Specific details on the overall sample in this survey are available elsewhere.[17,20]

For this study, we focused on the responses to questions specific to gun carrying in various places that might be considered sensitive other than school settings. Respondents were presented with the following prompt: "Many people are authorized to carry firearms, either openly or concealed on their person. Other than law enforcement, do you think that people who are authorized to carry firearms in your community should or should not be allowed to bring their guns into the following places?" They were then presented response options of yes or no and a list of locations: restaurants, bars, sports stadiums, retail stores, protests and political rallies, service settings (hair salons, barbershops, etc.), and places of worship (churches, synagogues, mosques, etc.). Respondents were also asked to respond on a 5-point Likert scale from strongly agree to strongly disagree to the following statement: "I would feel safer if more people were allowed to legally carry guns."

We applied survey weights provided by NORC to weight the sample to be nationally representative of US gun owners and used the svy command in Stata version 17.1 (StataCorp LP, College Station, TX). We generated survey-weighted proportions overall and stratified by gun ownership of those who responded no to whether people should or should not be allowed to bring guns into certain places. Among gun owners, we stratified responses by race and ethnicity categories as well as by new gun owners. Finally, we assessed support for gun carrying in certain locations among those who affirmed feeling safer if more people could legally carry guns overall and among gun owners. The survey-weighted proportions are presented as percentages along with 95% confidence intervals (Table 1).

RESULTS

Responses to allowing gun carrying in specified locations overall as well as stratified by gun ownership are presented in Table 1. Although there were significant differences between gun owners and nonowners across all locations, we focused on policies with majority support across both groups to inform ongoing policy discourse on sensitive place restrictions. Overall, more than 70% of respondents said guns should not be carried at bars (75%), sports stadiums (71%), and protests or rallies (71%). For places of worship, 61% said no. Support for prohibiting gun carrying was lowest for service settings (50%), retail stores (49%), and restaurants (49%). Compared with nonowners, there were lower levels of support for prohibiting gun carrying at each location. However, there was still broad support for restrictions at bars (70%), sports stadiums (61%), and protests or rallies (59%).

Responses to allowing gun carrying at specified locations among gun owners stratified by race and ethnicity are presented in Table 2. Among gun owners, support for prohibiting gun carrying was highest for Black and Asian respondents. Support for prohibiting gun carrying in these locations was lowest among new gun owners (i.e., those who reported that their first gun purchase was after January 1, 2020). Despite differences among gun owners, there was consistently high support for prohibiting gun carrying at bars in particular, ranging from 62% among new gun owners to 77% of Black gun owners.

Responses to allowing gun carrying at specific locations among those who

TABLE 1— Percentage Supporting Prohibiting Gun Carrying in Certain Locations: National Gun Policy Survey, United States, 2023

Location	Overall (n = 3063), Prohibit % (95% CI)	All Gun Owners (n = 1002), Prohibit % (95% CI)	Nonowners[a] (n = 2061), Prohibit % (95% CI)
Restaurants	49 (46, 51)	31 (27, 35)	57 (54, 60)
Bars	75 (73, 77)	70 (66, 73)	77 (74, 80)
Sports stadiums	71 (70, 73)	61 (57, 65)	76 (73, 78)
Retail stores	49 (46, 51)	30 (26, 34)	58 (55, 61)
Protests or rallies	71 (69, 73)	59 (55, 63)	77 (75, 80)
Service settings	50 (47, 53)	32 (28, 36)	59 (56, 62)
Places of worship	61 (58, 63)	42 (38, 46)	70 (67, 73)

Note. Data are presented as weighted percentages from a survey of a nationally representative sample of US adults using NORC's AmeriSpeak panel fielded in 2023.

[a]Difference compared with gun owners was statistically significant at $P < .05$.

AJPH September 2025, Vol. 115, No. 9

TABLE 2— Percentage of Gun Owners Supporting Prohibiting Gun Carrying in Certain Locations, Stratified by Race and Ethnicity: National Gun Policy Survey, United States, 2023

Location	All Gun Owners (n = 1002), Prohibit % (95% CI)	Non-Hispanic White (n = 597), Prohibit % (95% CI)	Non-Hispanic Black (n = 177), Prohibit % (95% CI)	Hispanic (n = 153), Prohibit % (95% CI)	Asian (n = 42), Prohibit % (95% CI)	New Owners (n = 102), Prohibit % (95% CI)
Restaurants	31 (27, 35)	28 (24, 33)	44 (35, 54)[a]	30 (21, 41)	50 (31, 69)[a]	20 (12, 32)
Bars	70 (66, 73)	69 (64, 73)	77 (68, 84)	69 (57, 79)	73 (54, 86)	62 (48, 74)
Sports stadiums	61 (57, 65)	58 (53, 63)	71 (62, 79)[a]	63 (52, 73)	71 (52, 85)	54 (40, 67)
Retail stores	30 (26, 34)	26 (22, 30)	51 (41, 60)[a]	30 (21, 41)	47 (28, 66)[a]	20 (12, 32)
Protests or rallies	59 (55, 63)	58 (54, 63)	68 (59, 77)	56 (44, 66)	63 (44, 78)	45 (32, 58)[b]
Service settings	32 (28, 36)	29 (24, 33)	46 (37, 56)[a]	31 (22, 41)	47 (28, 66)	20 (12, 31)[b]
Places of worship	42 (38, 46)	38 (33, 43)	60 (50, 69)[a]	43 (33, 55)	59 (40, 75)[a]	34 (32, 48)

Note. Data are presented as weighted percentages from a survey of a nationally representative sample of US adults using NORC's AmeriSpeak panel fielded in 2023.
[a]Difference compared with non-Hispanic White gun owners was statistically significant at $P < .05$.
[b]Difference between new (first gun purchased after January 1, 2020) compared with previous gun owners was statistically significant at $P < .05$.

somewhat or strongly agreed that they would feel safer if more people could legally carry guns are presented in Table 3. Although there was lower support among this group, 51% of these respondents overall and 53% of these respondents who personally own guns supported prohibiting gun carrying at bars.

DISCUSSION

Although more work is needed to understand support for gun carrying in various locations that may be deemed sensitive, our study adds to knowledge regarding support for prohibiting gun carrying among those who own guns or would feel safer if more people carried guns in public. We consistently found at least majority support for prohibiting gun carrying at bars, a location where gun carrying may be less supported because of the presence of alcohol and the related potential increased risk of physical conflict. Previous research has found that approximately one third of gun homicide perpetrators drank

TABLE 3— Percentage Supporting Prohibiting Gun Carrying in Certain Locations Among Those Who Would Feel Safer if More People Could Legally Carry Guns: National Gun Policy Survey, United States, 2023

Location	Overall (n = 3063), Prohibit % (95% CI)	Feel Safer if More People Could Legally Carry Guns,[a] Overall (n = 821), Prohibit % (95% CI)	Feel Safer if More People Could Legally Carry Guns,[a] Gun Owners (n = 429), Prohibit % (95% CI)
Restaurants	49 (46, 51)	19 (15, 22)	14 (10, 18)
Bars	75 (73, 77)	51 (47, 56)	53 (47, 59)
Sports stadiums	71 (70, 73)	45 (40, 49)	42 (36, 48)
Retail stores	49 (46, 51)	19 (15, 22)	13 (10, 18)
Protests or rallies	71 (69, 73)	43 (39, 48)	38 (32, 43)
Service settings	50 (47, 53)	21 (17, 25)	15 (11, 20)
Places of worship	61 (58, 63)	29 (25, 33)	22 (18, 28)

Note. Data are presented as weighted percentages from a survey of a nationally representative sample of US adults using NORC's AmeriSpeak panel fielded in 2023.
[a]Difference compared with those who did not report feeling safer if more people could legally carry guns was statistically significant at $P < .05$.

heavily before committing the homicide.[22,23] The COVID-19 pandemic appears to have exacerbated problem drinking,[24,25] and gun purchasing[19,26,27] along with gun homicides[28,29] increased substantially during the pandemic. Based on this evidence, the Consortium for Risk-Based Firearm Policy issued a recommendation in their 2023 report "Alcohol Misuse and Gun Violence" to limit access to guns when and where alcohol is consumed.[30]

There was also generally broad support for prohibiting carrying guns at sports stadiums, where there is potential for conflict to occur, for example, between fans of opposing teams. For sports stadiums, there is the added dimension of being a location where alcohol is available, whether brought by attendees for tailgate parties or sold inside the venue.[31,32] The intersection of alcohol and potential conflict at sports stadiums may contribute to broader support for prohibiting gun carrying in these locations. During oral arguments in the *Bruen* case, Supreme Court justices seemed particularly concerned about guns in settings where alcohol is served and sports stadiums. This concern, in conjunction with public support and the link between alcohol and violence, supports the notion that these locations remain sensitive places.[33]

Prohibiting gun carrying at protests or rallies may indicate a particular situation in which rights may come into conflict (e.g., between police and participants or between participants with different perspectives at protests or rallies), where the presence of guns might chill otherwise protected First Amendment rights.[11] There have been several high-profile incidents of gun violence at protests, including a 2020 case in Kenosha, Wisconsin, where a young man brought a semiautomatic rifle to a demonstration and fatally shot individuals during the civil unrest following a police shooting.[34,35] Protests or rallies where guns were present have been associated with a more than 6-fold increase in violence or destructive behavior compared with those where firearms were not obviously present.[36] More research is needed to understand if or how the presence of guns might affect individuals' decisions to engage in various democratic processes; however, public opinion indicates fairly broad support for prohibiting gun carrying at these types of events.

Differences in support for prohibiting gun carrying in certain locations among gun owners again demonstrate that gun owners are not a monolith.[16] Support for carrying restrictions at each of the locations assessed was lowest among new gun owners. This may be related to different reasons for gun ownership overall[20] or differences in what motivated their first gun purchase: previous research found that new gun owners were significantly more likely to report that concerns of racial or political violence motivated their purchase.[17] This may influence their perceptions of restricting gun carrying. It is necessary to engage with gun owners across a range of identities to craft solutions that are both effective at reducing violence and supported by community members.

These survey data may be especially relevant for Second Amendment litigation. Although the Supreme Court has repeatedly indicated that laws prohibiting carrying guns in sensitive places are presumptively lawful, it has failed to adequately define a "sensitive place" and has not provided guardrails for lower courts seeking to rule on this issue. Since *Bruen*, courts must start their analysis of new place-based firearm prohibitions by seeking to find historical analogues: historical laws that prohibited guns in a similar location or for similar reasons. As they analyze these historical analogies, courts may identify historical principles that governed whether firearms were allowed in certain places. For example, courts may determine that firearms have traditionally been prohibited in places where people enjoy a reasonable expectation of safety, where conflict is likely, and where the presence of guns is incompatible with the primary function of the place.

Public perception of a place may be a critical piece of this analysis. To determine whether a place is one where people enjoy a reasonable expectation of safety, for instance, it may be necessary to understand how people view that space and what they think about the presence of firearms in that space. For this reason, survey results such as those we present here may be essential to future Second Amendment litigation on place-specific gun-carrying prohibitions. We examined a limited number of locations that one might consider sensitive. As conversations on the history, tradition, and utility of gun carry restrictions in sensitive places progress, future research should explore support for other locations.

This study is not without limitations. As with any survey, sampling biases may have affected our results. However, the use of NORC's AmeriSpeak panel helped minimize these biases through their probability-based sampling. Despite a large overall sample, the sample sizes for some intersectional groups were small; therefore, we restricted our analysis to look at race and ethnicity strata among gun owners to ensure that we had sufficient power. Our question regarding support for gun carrying did not differentiate between open versus concealed carry. Future research should examine whether support for restricting gun carrying at these locations differs for open versus concealed carry to better inform policy discussions.

Despite these limitations, our study makes an important contribution to the understanding of support for restricting gun carrying in various places that might be deemed sensitive. There was broad and consistent support for prohibiting gun carrying at places where conflict may occur, such as protests or rallies, or where alcohol may be served, such as bars or sports stadiums. AJPH

ABOUT THE AUTHORS

All authors are with the Center for Gun Violence Solutions, Department of Health Policy and Management, Johns Hopkins Bloomberg School of Public Health, Baltimore, MD.

CORRESPONDENCE

Correspondence should be sent to Cassandra K. Crifasi, PhD, MPH, 750 E Pratt St, 15th Floor, Baltimore, MD 21202 (e-mail: crifasi@jhu.edu). Reprints can be ordered at http://www.ajph.org by clicking the "Reprints" link.

PUBLICATION INFORMATION

Full Citation: Crifasi CK, Roskam KEW, McCourt AD. Public firearms carriage and public opinion, National Gun Policy Survey, 2023. *Am J Public Health*. 2025;115(9):1472–1479.

Acceptance Date: April 9, 2025.

DOI: https://doi.org/10.2105/AJPH.2025.308152

ORCID iDs:

Cassandra K. Crifasi https://orcid.org/0000-0001-6748-5389

Kelly E. W. Roskam https://orcid.org/0009-0004-8327-2112

Alex D. McCourt https://orcid.org/0000-0002-3524-3454

CONTRIBUTORS

C. K. Crifasi conceptualized the study and conducted data analysis. All authors interpreted the data, drafted and revised the article, reviewed and approved the final version for publication, and agreed to be accountable for the work.

ACKNOWLEDGMENTS

We would like to acknowledge the Robert Wood Johnson Foundation for funding the survey data presented in this article.

Note. The contents of this article are solely the responsibility of the authors and do not necessarily represent the official views of the funder. The funder had no role in the study design, statistical analysis, interpretation of the data, or drafting of this article.

CONFLICTS OF INTEREST

The authors have no conflicts of interest to disclose.

HUMAN PARTICIPATION PROTECTION

This study was reviewed by the Johns Hopkins Bloomberg School of Public Health institutional review board and deemed not human participant research.

REFERENCES

1. Johns Hopkins Bloomberg School of Health. Regulation of public carry of firearms. 2024. Available at: https://publichealth.jhu.edu/center-for-gun-violence-solutions/solutions/regulation-of-public-carry-of-firearms. Accessed November 6, 2024.
2. Donohue JJ, Aneja A, Weber KD. Right-to-carry laws and violent crime: a comprehensive assessment using panel data and a state-level synthetic control analysis. *J Empir Leg Stud.* 2019;16(2):198–247. https://doi.org/10.1111/jels.12219
3. Donohue JJ, Cai SV, Bondy MV, Cook PJ. *More Guns, More Unintended Consequences: The Effects of right-to-carry on Criminal Behavior and Policing in US Cities.* Cambridge, MA: National Bureau of Economic Research; 2022. NBER working paper 30190. https://doi.org/10.3386/w30190
4. Crifasi CK, Merrill-Francis M, McCourt A, Vernick JS, Wintemute GJ, Webster DW. Association between firearm laws and homicide in urban counties. *J Urban Health.* 2018;95(3):383–390. https://doi.org/10.1007/s11524-018-0273-3
5. Crifasi CK, Merrill-Francis M, McCourt A, Vernick JS, Wintemute GJ, Webster DW. Correction to: Association between firearm laws and homicide in urban counties. *J Urban Health.* 2018;95(5):773–776. https://doi.org/10.1007/s11524-018-0306-y
6. Doucette ML, Crifasi CK, Frattaroli S. Right-to-carry laws and firearm workplace homicides: a longitudinal analysis (1992–2017). *Am J Public Health.* 2019;109(12):1747–1753. https://doi.org/10.2105/AJPH.2019.305307
7. Doucette ML, McCourt AD, Crifasi CK, Webster DW. Impact of changes to concealed-carry weapons laws on fatal and nonfatal violent crime, 1980–2019. *Am J Epidemiol.* 2023;192(3):342–355. https://doi.org/10.1093/aje/kwac160
8. Doucette ML, Ward JA, McCourt AD, Webster D, Crifasi CK. Officer-involved shootings and concealed carry weapons permitting laws: analysis of Gun Violence Archive data, 2014–2020. *J Urban Health.* 2022;99(3):373–384. https://doi.org/10.1007/s11524-022-00627-5
9. *District of Columbia v Heller*, 554 US 570, 128 S. Ct. 2783, 171 L. Ed. 2d 637 (2008).
10. *New York State Rifle & Pistol Ass'n v Bruen*, 597 US 1, 142 S. Ct. 2111, 213 L. Ed. 2d 387 (2022).
11. Miller DAH. Constitutional conflict and sensitive places. *Wm & Mary Bill Rts J.* 2019;28(2):459–487. Available at: https://scholarship.law.wm.edu/cgi/viewcontent.cgi?article=1929&context=wmborj. Accessed June 5, 2025.
12. Hesse J, Schascheck K II. The expansive "sensitive places" doctrine: the limited right to "keep and bear" arms outside the home. SSRN. July 4, 2023. Available at: https://ssrn.com/abstract=4500140. Accessed June 5, 2025.
13. Blocher J, Siegel RB. Guided by history: protecting the public sphere from weapons threats under *Bruen. NYUL Rev.* 2023;98(6):1795–1830. https://doi.org/10.2139/ssrn.4355024
14. Heniford K, Still K. Panic! at the ballroom: the 1804 New Orleans ballroom weapons ban in a post-*Bruen* context. *Buffalo Law Rev.* [Preprint: September 4, 2024]. https://doi.org/10.2139/ssrn.4946772
15. Wolfson JA, Teret SP, Azrael D, Miller M. US public opinion on carrying firearms in public places. *Am J Public Health.* 2017;107(6):929–937. https://doi.org/10.2105/AJPH.2017.303712
16. Crifasi CK, Ward JA, McGinty EE, Barry CL, Webster DW. Public opinion on laws regulating public gun carrying. *Prev Med.* 2022;159:107067. https://doi.org/10.1016/j.ypmed.2022.107067
17. Valek R, Ward JA, Jones V, Crifasi CK. Political violence, racial violence, and new gun ownership: results from the 2023 National Survey of Gun Policy. *Inj Epidemiol.* 2024;11(1):48. https://doi.org/10.1186/s40621-024-00527-z
18. Centers for Disease Control and Prevention. WISQARS—Leading causes of death visualization tool. Available at: https://wisqars-viz.cdc.gov/lcd/?o=LCD&y1=2023&y2=2023&ct=10&cc=ALL&g=00&s=0&r=0&ry=2&e=0&ar=lcd1age&at=groups&ag=lcd1age&a1=0&a2=199. Accessed March 3, 2025.
19. Miller M, Zhang W, Azrael D. Firearm purchasing during the COVID-19 pandemic: results from the 2021 National Firearms Survey. *Ann Intern Med.* 2022;175(2):219–225. https://doi.org/10.7326/M21-3423
20. Ward JA, Valek RA, Jones VC, Crifasi CK. Reasons for gun ownership among demographically diverse new and prior gun owners. *Am J Prev Med.* 2024;67(5):730–739. https://doi.org/10.1016/j.amepre.2024.06.026
21. NORC. AmeriSpeak. NORC at the University of Chicago's panel-based research platform. Available at: https://amerispeak.norc.org. Accessed June 5, 2025.
22. Branas CC, Han S, Wiebe DJ. Alcohol use and firearm violence. *Epidemiol Rev.* 2016;38(1):32–45. https://doi.org/10.1093/epirev/mxv010
23. Kuhns JB, Exum ML, Clodfelter TA, Bottia MC. The prevalence of alcohol-involved homicide offending: a meta-analytic review. *Homicide Stud.* 2014;18(3):251–270. https://doi.org/10.1177/1088767913493629
24. Barbosa C, Cowell AJ, Dowd WN. Alcohol consumption in response to the COVID-19 pandemic in the United States. *J Addict Med.* 2021;15(4):341–344. https://doi.org/10.1097/ADM.0000000000000767
25. Grossman ER, Benjamin-Neelon SE, Sonnenschein S. Alcohol consumption during the COVID-19 pandemic: a cross-sectional survey of US adults. *Int J Environ Res Public Health.* 2020;17(24):9189. https://doi.org/10.3390/ijerph17249189
26. Lyons VH, Haviland MJ, Azrael D, et al. Firearm purchasing and storage during the COVID-19 pandemic. *Inj Prev.* 2021;27(1):87–92. https://doi.org/10.1136/injuryprev-2020-043872

27. Crifasi CK, Ward JA, McGinty EE, Webster DW, Barry CL. Gun purchasing behaviours during the initial phase of the COVID-19 pandemic, March to mid-July 2020. *Int Rev Psychiatry*. 2021;33(7): 593–597. https://doi.org/10.1080/09540261.2021.1901669
28. Davis A, Geller L, Kim R, et al. A year in review: 2020 gun deaths in the US. April 28, 2022. Available at: https://publichealth.jhu.edu/sites/default/files/2022-05/2020-gun-deaths-in-the-us-4-28-2022-b.pdf. Accessed June 5, 2025.
29. Davis A, Kim R, Crifasi C. US gun violence in 2021: an accounting of a public health crisis. June 2023. Available at: https://publichealth.jhu.edu/sites/default/files/2024-01/2023-june-cgvs-u-s-gun-violence-in-2021-v3.pdf. Accessed June 5, 2025.
30. Villarreal S, Barnhorst A, Bonnie RJ, et al. Alcohol misuse and gun violence: an evidence-based approach for state policy. May 5, 2023. Available at: https://publichealth.jhu.edu/sites/default/files/2023-05/2023-may-cgvs-alcohol-misuse-and-gun-violence.pdf. Accessed June 5, 2025.
31. Lenk KM, Toomey TL, Erickson DJ. Alcohol-related problems and enforcement at professional sports stadiums. *Drugs Educ Prev Policy*. 2009;16(5): 451–462. https://doi.org/10.1080/09687630802278478
32. Menaker BE, Chaney BH. College football game day stadium incidents: policy and environmental effects on alcohol-related ejections and crime. *J Policy Res Tour Leis Events*. 2014;6(2):119–134. https://doi.org/10.1080/19407963.2014.895286
33. *New York State Rifle & Pistol Association, Inc., et al. v. Kevin P. Bruen, et al.* 597 US 1, 142 S. Ct. 2111, 213 L. Ed. 2d 387 (2022). Available at: https://www.supremecourt.gov/oral_arguments/argument_transcripts/2021/20-843_7m5e.pdf. Accessed June 5, 2025.
34. Morales C. What we know about the shooting of Jacob Blake. *New York Times*. November 16, 2021. Available at: https://www.nytimes.com/article/jacob-blake-shooting-kenosha.html. Accessed June 5, 2025.
35. Givetash L, Romero D, Zadrozy B. 2 dead, 1 injured, in Wisconsin protests over shooting of Jacob Blake. NBC News. August 25, 2020. Available at: https://www.nbcnews.com/news/us-news/wisconsin-braces-more-outrage-protests-wake-jacob-blake-shooting-n1238102. Accessed June 5, 2025.
36. Armed Conflict Location & Event Data Project. Updated armed demonstration data released a year after the 6 January insurrection show new trends. January 5, 2022. Available at: https://acleddata.com/2022/01/05/updated-armed-demonstration-data-released-a-year-after-the-6-january-insurrection-show-new-trends. Accessed June 5, 2025.

HIV Care Linkage and Initial Viral Suppression Among Persons Newly Diagnosed With HIV in North Carolina Before and After the Start of the COVID-19 Pandemic

Courtney N. Maierhofer, PhD, Brian W. Pence, PhD, Erika Samoff, PhD, Abigail N. Turner, PhD, Victoria Mobley, MD, Jason Maxwell, William C. Miller, MD, PhD, and Kimberly A. Powers, PhD

See also Nijhawan, p. 1354.

Objectives. To examine changes to HIV care outcomes during the COVID-19 pandemic.

Methods. We used North Carolina HIV surveillance data between 2018 and 2022 to calculate cumulative incidence differences (CIDs) and subdistribution hazard ratios (sdHRs) for (1) 30-day initial HIV care linkage, (2) 150-day stable linkage, and (3) 180-day viral suppression, comparing persons diagnosed with HIV during (starting March 1, 2020) versus before the pandemic. We defined a notable decrease as CID of −0.05 or less or an sdHR of 0.95 or less.

Results. Overall, there were no notable decreases in linkage and viral suppression during the pandemic. In subgroup analyses, Black, Hispanic, and transgender persons had higher rates of initial linkage and unchanged or lower rates of stable linkage during versus before the pandemic. Hispanic persons had progressively lower viral suppression incidence during the pandemic.

Conclusions. The North Carolina HIV care system appeared robust to pandemic harms overall; however, we observed notable differences in some subpopulations and pandemic subintervals.

Public Health Implications. Statewide programs will need to build on past successes while strengthening current efforts to meet national HIV goals, particularly in groups experiencing pandemic harms to care. (*Am J Public Health*. 2025;115(9):1480–1489. https://doi.org/10.2105/AJPH.2025.308108)

AJPH September 2025, Vol. 115, No. 9

Timely HIV care linkage and viral suppression through antiretroviral therapy (ART) are critical to improving health and preventing onward HIV transmission among persons with HIV (PWH).[1] A key component of the US initiative for Ending the HIV Epidemic (EHE)[2] is to treat PWH rapidly and effectively to induce sustained viral suppression, with the ultimate goal of reducing new HIV infections in the United States by at least 90% by 2030. EHE targets for 2025 include having 95% of all people with HIV aware of their status, 95% of newly diagnosed persons linked to HIV care within 30 days of diagnosis, and 95% of diagnosed persons virally suppressed.[2] However, population levels of HIV care linkage, retention, and viral suppression are below national targets,[3] with the largest disparities affecting communities of color and young persons. Delayed care initiation and inadequate retention present considerable barriers to reaching the goals set forth in the national initiative, particularly in subpopulations who disproportionately experience social and structural barriers to HIV care (e.g., discrimination based on race, gender, or sexual orientation; HIV-related stigma; or lack of financial resources).[4]

The COVID-19 pandemic substantially affected HIV services throughout the United States.[5] To comply with pandemic-related physical distancing standards in early 2020,[6] HIV clinics were compelled to rearrange care delivery, resulting in clinic closures, visit delays, and migration from in-person to virtual care.[7,8] These disruptions to the care system, coupled with pandemic-induced challenges in other aspects of daily life, likely impacted HIV care engagement in myriad ways.[5] Assessing COVID-19–related impacts on HIV care outcomes during the initial pandemic years can help to identify subpopulations or aspects of HIV care delivery that may require concerted efforts to rectify ongoing COVID-19 effects or safeguard against future pandemic threats.

Existing knowledge about COVID-19 impacts on HIV care indicators is largely limited to the earliest months of the pandemic or confined to single clinics or clinical networks.[9–11] In addition, although pre- and early pandemic sociodemographic disparities across the HIV care continuum are well documented,[10–12] we do not have a comprehensive understanding of how these disparities may have changed over the long course of the pandemic. To address these knowledge gaps, we used statewide HIV surveillance data to assess COVID-19 pandemic impacts on HIV care linkage and initial viral suppression among persons newly diagnosed with HIV in North Carolina (NC), overall and according to key covariates.

METHODS

We conducted a retrospective cohort study using statewide HIV surveillance data from the North Carolina Electronic Disease Surveillance System (NCEDSS)[13] between January 1, 2018, and February 28, 2022. The database includes patient-level data on all new HIV diagnoses and all HIV RNA and CD4-positive cell count tests performed in NC, each of which is reportable by law to the surveillance system.[14] NCEDSS also includes patient-level demographics, clinical characteristics, transmission-relevant behaviors, relocation out of NC, and vital statistics.

The study population included all persons in NCEDSS who were newly HIV-diagnosed in NC between January 1, 2018, and August 31, 2021, and who were aged at least 13 years and living in NC at the time of diagnosis. The end of this diagnosis period was chosen to allow 6 months of follow-up time in the full study population.

Measures and Follow-Up

Outcomes. Consistent with Centers for Disease Control and Prevention (CDC) recommendations and previous surveillance-based studies of HIV care engagement,[15,16] we used HIV laboratory records as proxies for HIV primary care visits. We followed persons from the date of HIV diagnosis for 2 separate outcomes: (1) initial HIV care linkage, defined as the first HIV RNA or CD4 record, and (2) initial HIV viral suppression, defined as the first HIV RNA record with fewer than 200 HIV copies per milliliter of blood (cp/mL) more than 14 days after HIV diagnosis. Persons were followed separately for each outcome, a competing event (all-cause mortality or relocation out of NC), or administrative censoring (30 days for linkage, 180 days for suppression), whichever was earliest. To evaluate key HIV care metrics aligned with national HIV prevention and care objectives (Table A, available as a supplement to the online version of this article at https://ajph.org),[3] we based the 30-day window for initial linkage on the EHE initiative and the CDC care continuum measure[2,15] and the 180-day window for initial viral suppression on CDC metrics and previous literature.[15–17] Standard in surveillance-based analyses of HIV care engagement,[16,18] people without an HIV RNA or CD4 record in the 30-day window were classified as not experiencing the linkage outcome, and persons without an HIV RNA record between 14 and 180 days of diagnosis were classified as having no evidence of viral suppression (i.e., missing values during the defined follow-up period represent absence of the outcome during that period).

We also followed persons who were initially linked to HIV care for an additional outcome of stable HIV care linkage, since some initial HIV laboratory records following diagnosis may be related to diagnostic or routine tests for those seeking emergency services and not necessarily reflective of true HIV care entry.[16,18] We defined stable linkage as the first HIV RNA or CD4 record 30 days or more after initial linkage, following persons for the first of the outcome, a competing event, or administrative censoring at 150 days after initial linkage. This outcome was chosen in light of clinical and laboratory monitoring guidelines indicating that all persons should initiate ART at or soon after diagnosis, with HIV RNA and CD4 measurement at ART initiation and additional HIV RNA measurement 4 to 8 weeks and 3 months after initiation.[19] Under these guidelines, all persons meeting our initial linkage definition would be expected to have at least 1 additional laboratory record within 5 to

6 months of diagnosis. For those whose first laboratory measures represented "true linkage," additional measures would be consistent with ART initiation or monitoring. For those whose first laboratory measures were obtained at or near diagnosis without "true linkage," we considered additional measures to be suggestive of true care entry.

Exposures. The first severe acute respiratory coronavirus 2 (SARS-CoV-2) infection on the East Coast of the United States was identified on February 29, 2020, and reported on March 1, 2020.[20,21] The first NC case was reported on March 3, 2020,[22] followed by a series of statewide emergency prevention responses (Figure A, available as a supplement to the online version of this article at https://ajph.org).[23] Thus, our first main exposure was a dichotomous variable representing the pandemic period of HIV diagnosis, where the prepandemic period included persons diagnosed between January 1, 2018, and February 29, 2020, and the overall pandemic period included persons diagnosed between March 1, 2020, and August 31, 2021.

For greater temporal granularity, we defined a second exposure with a 3-level variable, where the (1) prepandemic included (as before) persons diagnosed between January 1, 2018, and February 29, 2020; (2) early pandemic included persons diagnosed between March 1, 2020, and February 28, 2021; and (3) late pandemic included persons diagnosed between March 1, 2021, and August 31, 2021. The distinction between early and late pandemic periods was based on the public availability of COVID-19 vaccines and the lifting of "stay at home" orders in late February 2021.[23]

Covariates. Consistent with selected characteristics in CDC's National HIV Surveillance Report,[3] baseline covariates of interest included race and ethnicity (non-Hispanic Black, non-Hispanic White, Hispanic, Asian or Pacific Islander, American Indian or Alaska Native, and multiple races), gender (cisgender male, cisgender female, transgender female, transgender male), age in years (continuous), HIV exposure category (male–male sexual contact, male–female sexual contact, injection drug use, other [hemophilia, blood transfusion, perinatal exposure, or unknown]), and rurality of residence (urban or rural based on NC Department of Health and Human Services Office of Rural Health County classifications[24]). Additional variables of descriptive interest included HIV RNA level (cp/mL) and CD4 cell count at the first documented laboratory record after HIV diagnosis and within 14 days of initial linkage among those linked within 30 days of diagnosis.

Statistical Analyses

We summarized baseline characteristics of the study population, and CD4 and RNA levels for those initially linked within 30 days, using counts and percentages, overall and according to pandemic period of HIV diagnosis. We calculated the frequency of outcome events, competing events, and administrative censoring, as well as the total person-days of follow-up, overall and by each outcome and exposure of interest.

Given the competing events of all-cause mortality and relocation out of NC, we used the Aalen–Johansen estimator of the cumulative incidence function (CIF)[25] to separately estimate the cumulative incidence of initial and stable linkage and initial viral suppression, overall and by pandemic exposure period (see additional details in Supplementary Text, available as a supplement to the online version of this article at https://ajph.org). We estimated CIF differences (CIDs) and 95% confidence intervals (CIs) using robust variance estimators for initial linkage at 30 days, stable linkage at 150 days, and initial viral suppression at 180 days, comparing prepandemic and pandemic periods.

We used unadjusted Fine and Gray subdistribution proportional hazard models,[25] accounting for competing events, to estimate subdistribution hazard ratios (sdHRs) and 95% CIs for each outcome of interest, comparing the pandemic period to the prepandemic period for the dichotomous exposure and comparing each pandemic exposure group (early and late) to the prepandemic period, separately, for the multiperiod exposure. We used the Efron method[26] to handle tied event times in all models. We assessed the proportional hazards assumption evaluating the log(-log) transformation of the nonparametric CIF estimators stratified by main exposure variables, assessing whether the step function curves were separated by a constant difference.[25]

We stratified all analyses by key covariates to examine pandemic impacts on subpopulations. Stratified analyses were not adjusted for additional covariates. We considered only non-Hispanic Black, non-Hispanic White, and Hispanic groups for race and ethnicity because of small sample sizes of the remaining race groups, choosing not to combine these groups to avoid masking heterogeneity. We considered only male–female sexual contact, any male–male sexual contact, and injection drug use only for HIV exposure categories, while choosing not to report the other HIV exposure category given its potentially heterogeneous nature. We combined transgender men and transgender women as 1 category to improve precision from small sample sizes and to reflect the shared experience of stigma and discrimination in health care settings among transgender persons,[27] and we categorized age as 13 to 24 years, 25 to 44 years, and 45 years or older.

In interpreting our results, we focused on substantive significance of a clinically relevant and notably negative effect (vs no negative effect), rather than statistical significance based on a *P* value. For absolute and relative measures of association, respectively, we defined estimates with an absolute difference of at least 5 percentage points and at least 5% relative effect in a negative direction (i.e., CID ≤ −0.05 and sdHR ≤ 0.95) as a notable decrease, while considering all other estimates to be not a notable decrease. These thresholds represent rates of change in a negative direction that are similar in magnitude to the changes in a beneficial direction required to meet 2025 National HIV/AIDS Strategy goals[28] (see Supplementary Text). We also reported the corresponding 95% CI as a measure of precision.

Sensitivity Analysis

Because a small proportion of persons diagnosed before the pandemic experienced person-time in both prepandemic and pandemic periods during follow-up for initial care linkage and viral suppression, we repeated analyses for these outcomes with a time-varying pandemic period exposure. In these analyses, days living with diagnosed HIV between January 1, 2018, and February 29, 2020, were classified as prepandemic person-days, and days living with diagnosed HIV between March 1, 2020, and August 31, 2021, were classified as pandemic person-days.

All statistical analyses were performed in SAS version 9.4 (SAS Institute, Cary, NC).

RESULTS

Overall, 4402 persons were newly HIV-diagnosed in NC between January 1, 2018, and August 31, 2021: 61% (n = 2700) in the prepandemic period and 39% (n = 1702) in the pandemic period (Tables B and C, available as supplements to the online version of this article at https://ajph.org). Baseline characteristics were similar across pandemic periods—most persons were cisgender male, non-Hispanic Black, aged younger than 35 years, and urban residents. HIV exposure category distributions were also similar across periods, with slightly more than half of new diagnoses being attributed to male–male sexual contact. Among persons who were initially linked within 30 days (n = 3200; 72.7%), higher proportions of persons diagnosed during versus before the pandemic had HIV RNA greater than 500 000 cp/mL (21.0% vs 18.2%; *P* = .03) and CD4 cell count less than 200 cells per microliter (25.1% vs 20.6%; *P* < .01) at the time of linkage, both overall and in most subgroups (Tables D and E, available as supplements to the online version of this article at https://ajph.org).

Baseline characteristics were similarly distributed by the multiperiod pandemic exposure (Table F, available as a supplement to the online version of this article at https://ajph.org).

Initial HIV Care Linkage

We did not find notable decreases overall in initial linkage, which improved in persons diagnosed with HIV during the overall (CID = 0.05 [95% CI = 0.01, 0.09]; sdHR = 1.14 [95% CI = 1.06, 1.22]), early (CID = 0.05 [95% CI = 0.01, 0.08]; sdHR = 1.13 [95% CI = 1.04, 1.23]), and late (CID = 0.05 [95% CI = 0.00, 0.10]; sdHR = 1.15 [95% CI = 1.04, 1.26]) pandemic compared with those diagnosed before (Figures 1 and 2; and Figure B and Table G, available as supplements to the online version of this article at https://ajph.org). Most stratum-specific estimates were similar when we compared each pandemic period with the prepandemic period; however, we observed notable decreases in initial linkage for persons who inject drugs (CID = −0.07 [95% CI = –0.24, 0.10]; sdHR = 1.01 [95% CI = 0.52, 2.00]) and Hispanic persons (CID = −0.04 [95% CI = –0.10, 0.02]; sdHR = 0.94 [95% CI = 0.73, 1.22]) diagnosed in the late pandemic period.

Stable HIV Care Linkage

Among persons initially linked to care within 30 days, we observed no changes in stable linkage overall during the pandemic versus before (Figures 2 and 3 and Figure C and Table H, available as supplements to the online version of this article at https://ajph.org), but certain subgroups experienced decreases. Hispanic persons had notably lower stable linkage during all pandemic periods compared with the prepandemic period (overall: CID = −0.05 [95% CI = –0.08, −0.03]; sdHR = 0.85 [95% CI = 0.68, 1.05]; early: CID = −0.06 [95% CI = –0.12, 0.01]; sdHR = 0.86 [95% CI = 0.67, 1.10]; late: CID = −0.05 [95% CI = –0.20, 0.09]; sdHR = 0.83 [95% CI = 0.62, 1.10]). Persons with male–female sexual exposure had notable decreases in stable

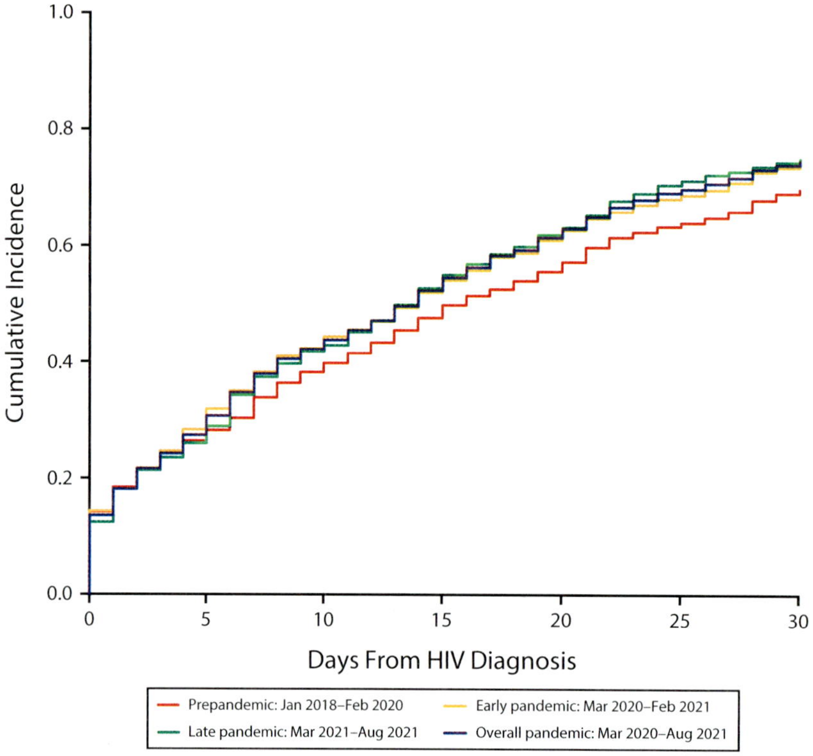

FIGURE 1— Cumulative Incidence Curves for Overall Initial HIV Care Linkage by COVID-19 Pandemic Period: North Carolina, 2018–2022

Note. Initial HIV care linkage = first CD4 or HIV RNA laboratory record within 30 days of HIV diagnosis.

linkage during the overall pandemic period versus the prepandemic period (CID = −0.07 [95% CI = -0.15, 0.00]; sdHR = 0.87 [95% CI = 0.65, 1.16]), with a notable decrease in the early period (CID = −0.10 [95% CI = -0.22, 0.03]; sdHR = 0.78 [95% CI = 0.57, 1.09]) that became attenuated as the pandemic progressed into the late period (CID = −0.03 [95% CI = -0.28, 0.22]; sdHR = 1.09 [95% CI = 0.68, 1.76]). We observed notably lower hazards of stable linkage in the overall and early pandemic periods among non-Hispanic Black (overall sdHR = 0.94 [95% CI = 0.85, 1.04]; early sdHR = 0.91 [95% CI = 0.80, 1.04]) and transgender persons (overall sdHR = 0.87 [95% CI = 0.39, 1.95]; early sdHR = 0.57 [95% CI = 0.20, 1.68]).

Initial HIV Viral Suppression

We did not observe notable decreases in initial viral suppression during versus before the pandemic overall or in most subgroups, with a few exceptions (Figures 2 and 4 and Figure D and Table I, available as supplements to the online version of this article at https://ajph.org). Hispanic persons had notably lower viral suppression during the overall pandemic (CID = −0.11 [95% CI = -0.15, −0.06]; sdHR = 0.79 [95% CI = 0.64, 0.97]), with progressively decreasing viral suppression as the pandemic advanced (early: CID = −0.05 [95% CI = -0.14, 0.04]; sdHR = 0.92 [95% CI = 0.73, 1.16]; late: CID = −0.20 [95% CI = -0.41, 0.01]; sdHR = 0.62 [95% CI = 0.46, 0.84]). Although transgender persons had a notably lower hazard of viral suppression in the overall pandemic versus before (sdHR = 0.90; 95% CI = 0.46, 1.74), we observed a much lower hazard early in the pandemic and a higher hazard later in the pandemic (early sdHR = 0.65 [95% CI = 0.28, 1.50]; late sdHR = 1.28 [95% CI = 0.59, 2.80]), with similar patterns for CIDs.

A summary of key findings from these results can be found in Table J (available as a supplement to the online version of this article at https://ajph.org).

Sensitivity Analysis

With only slight variations relative to the main analysis in the strength of associations between our time-varying

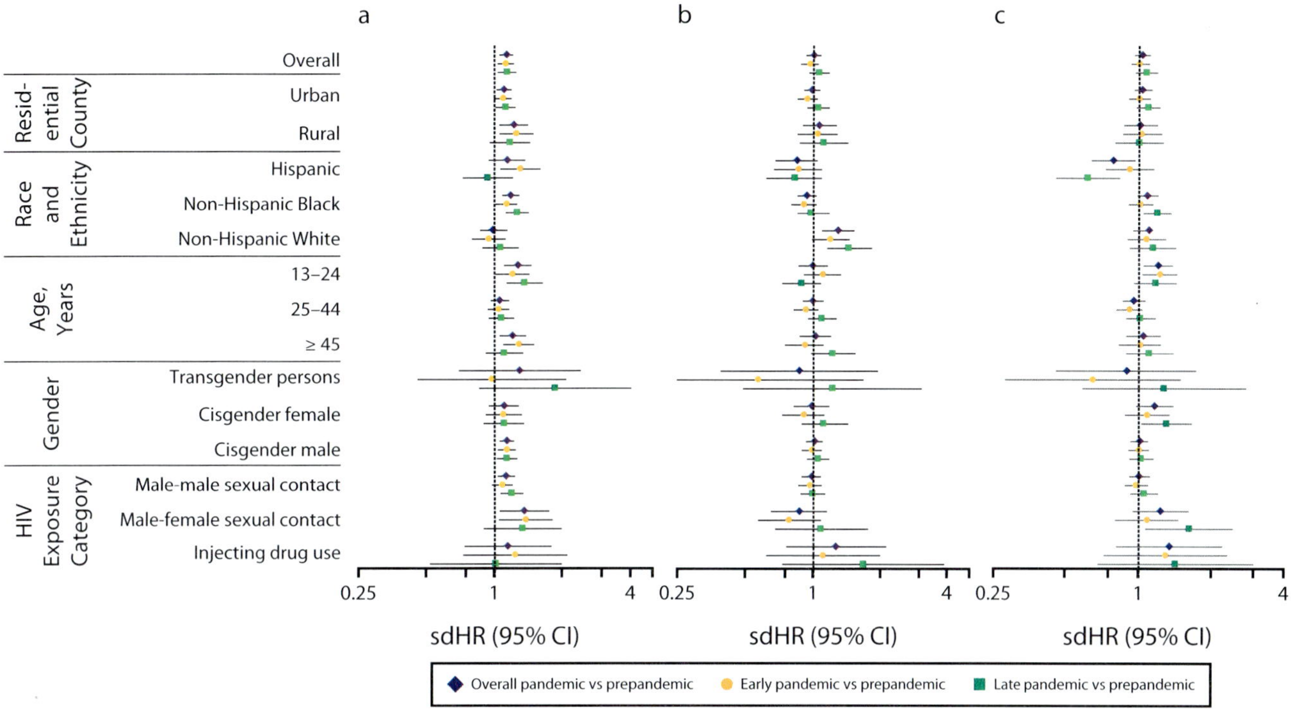

FIGURE 2— Associations by COVID-19 Pandemic Period for (a) Initial HIV Care Linkage, (b) Stable HIV Care Linkage, and (c) Initial HIV Viral Suppression: North Carolina, 2018–2022

Note. CI = confidence interval; sdHR = subdistribution hazard ratio. Numerical estimates for the sdHRs and 95% CIs are presented in Tables G, H, and I (available as supplements to the online version of this article at https://ajph.org). Initial HIV care linkage = first CD4 or HIV RNA laboratory record within 30 days of HIV diagnosis; stable HIV care linkage = additional CD4 or HIV RNA laboratory record between 30 and 150 days after initial HIV care linkage; initial HIV viral suppression = HIV RNA laboratory record less than 200 copies per milliliter of blood between 15 and 180 days after HIV diagnosis.

exposure and both initial linkage and viral suppression, our main conclusions were unchanged in sensitivity analyses (Figure E and Tables K and L, available as supplements to the online version of this article at https://ajph.org).

DISCUSSION

In our surveillance-based analysis of persons newly diagnosed with HIV in NC, we unexpectedly found slight improvements in overall rates of initial HIV care linkage and no overall changes in stable linkage and initial viral suppression during the COVID-19 pandemic. Although our findings are reflective of an HIV care system that was robust to pandemic harms overall, HIV care linkage and viral suppression remain below EHE goals, with notable differences across some subpopulations and pandemic subintervals. While we observed no notable decreases in initial care linkage among Black and transgender persons overall, we observed lower stable linkage during the pandemic. Among Hispanic persons, an increase in initial linkage during the early pandemic was followed by a subsequent decrease as the pandemic evolved, and stable linkage was consistently lower during all pandemic periods. Viral suppression rates progressively decreased among Hispanic persons over the course of the pandemic, while remaining unchanged or slightly higher among Black and White persons.

Our finding of increased initial HIV care linkage overall during the pandemic may be related to underlying differences between persons presenting for HIV testing during versus before the pandemic. Because only positive HIV test results are reportable to NCEDSS, we were unable to examine changes across pandemic periods in persons presenting for testing, and although RNA and CD4 levels are not routinely assessed at diagnosis (but instead at linkage), we found that those diagnosed during the pandemic presented with higher HIV RNA levels and lower CD4 counts on average at the first documented laboratory record (i.e., our definition for initial care linkage) than did those diagnosed before the pandemic. It may

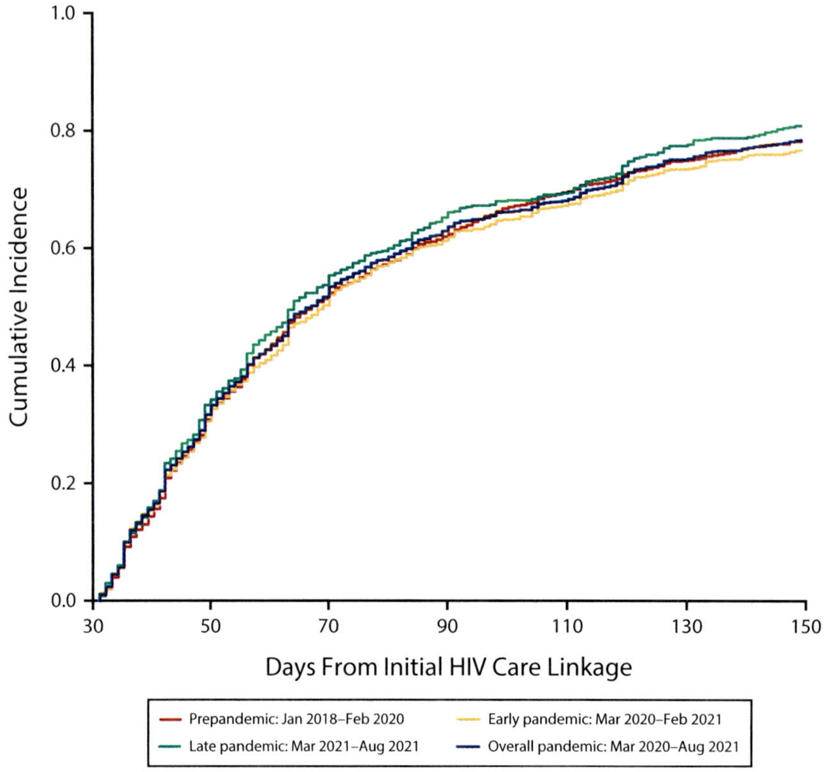

FIGURE 3— Cumulative Incidence Curves for Overall Stable HIV Care Linkage Among Those With Initial Linkage by COVID-19 Pandemic Period: North Carolina, 2018–2022

Note. Stable HIV care linkage = additional CD4 or HIV RNA laboratory record between 30 and 150 days after initial HIV care linkage.

be that amid pandemic disruptions, people experiencing symptoms of acute retroviral syndrome or late-stage HIV infection were more likely to overcome SARS-CoV-2 exposure fears or other barriers to seek HIV testing and care.[7] It is also possible that, because many local HIV testing facilities closed early in the pandemic,[8] people may have sought testing or care for associated symptoms at emergency departments, potentially leading to more rapid linkage to co-located HIV services than might be achievable at stand-alone testing sites. Our finding that stable linkage was similar overall among those linked within 30 days before and during the pandemic, despite some differences in initial linkage, is consistent with these possibilities and previous observations that immediate "linkages" may not represent true entry into HIV care.[16,18]

The observed improvements in initial linkage among Black and Hispanic persons diagnosed with HIV during the pandemic appear inconsistent with widespread evidence of the disproportionate experience of social and structural barriers to HIV care[4,29] and higher risk of COVID-19 disease severity[30,31] in these populations. If, however, the increase in pandemic-era initial HIV linkage was driven by disproportionate presentation of persons with symptomatic infection for testing, followed by rapid linkage for urgent clinical needs, then increased initial linkage rates among Black and Hispanic persons during the pandemic may reflect longstanding racial health disparities. This possibility is consistent with the lower estimated proportions of Black and Hispanic (vs White) persons diagnosed within 9 months of HIV acquisition between 2018 and 2021 in NC, along with longer estimated delays between HIV acquisition and diagnosis in 2021 versus 2020 for persons of color, but not White persons.[32]

If pandemic disruptions led to disproportionate HIV testing among those urgently needing immediate care, then a higher prevalence of late-stage infection among persons with undiagnosed HIV in communities of color and gender minorities could result in the initial linkage increases we saw in these groups–but not among White and cisgender people––during the pandemic.[33] Furthermore, although

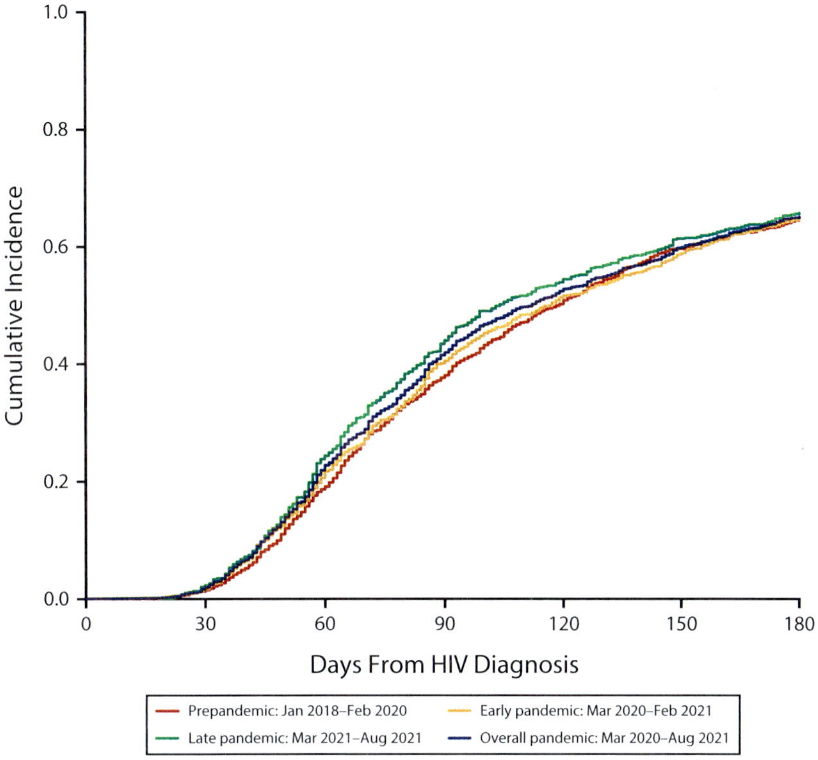

FIGURE 4— Cumulative Incidence Curves for Overall Initial HIV Viral Suppression by COVID-19 Pandemic Period: North Carolina, 2018–2022

Note. Initial HIV viral suppression = HIV RNA laboratory record less than 200 copies per milliliter of blood between 15 and 180 days after HIV diagnosis.

certain systematically marginalized groups, such as persons of color, adolescents, and gender minorities, appear to have been initially linked to care slightly faster during the pandemic, the same level of HIV care access was not maintained for stable linkage. Future research to probe mechanisms behind our descriptive findings may shed additional light on the observed variability in linkage and suppression.

We note that our study population only included persons whose new HIV diagnoses were reported by a provider or laboratory to the state's HIV surveillance system. Although reporting of all new HIV diagnoses and HIV RNA and CD4 measurements is required by law,[14] there is some possibility of reporting delays or underreporting, especially during the pandemic. In addition, although HIV RNA and CD4 measurements are standard components of HIV care initiation, and laboratory measures have been shown to be reliable proxies for HIV care,[34] there is the potential for misclassification of care linkage that could be differential across the prepandemic and pandemic periods.

It is also important to highlight that patients may not attend HIV care visits at regularly scheduled intervals, and some providers may prescribe ART upon HIV diagnosis, depending on patient needs and visit attendance. Persons with early ART initiation at diagnosis may not return for a follow-up visit until the recommended 4 to 8 weeks, leaving these persons vulnerable to being misclassified as not yet linked to care. To mitigate these potential issues common to surveillance-based analyses of HIV care engagement,[18] we included several linkage measures to capture both early and late laboratory tests over different follow-up lengths. We also acknowledge that some estimates were imprecise and that although the HIV epidemic in North Carolina is similar in many ways to the broader epidemic in the US Southeast, results may be less generalizable outside this region.

PUBLIC HEALTH IMPLICATIONS

The HIV care system in North Carolina appears to have been robust to COVID-19 pandemic impacts overall; however, statewide HIV care programs will need to build on past successes while further strengthening current efforts to meet 2025 EHE goals. Concerted efforts may be required to rectify pandemic-related harms, safeguard against future disruptions in widescale emergencies, and advance EHE efforts in gender minorities and persons of color who experienced adverse HIV care outcomes during the COVID-19 pandemic. AJPH

ABOUT THE AUTHORS

Courtney N. Maierhofer, Brian W. Pence, William C. Miller, and Kimberly A. Powers are with the Department of Epidemiology, Gillings School of Global Public Health, University of North Carolina at Chapel Hill. Abigail N. Turner is with the Division of Infectious Diseases, College of Medicine, and Division of Epidemiology, College of Public Health, The Ohio State University, Columbus. Erika Samoff, Victoria Mobley, and Jason Maxwell are with the North Carolina Department of Health and Human Services, Raleigh.

CORRESPONDENCE

Correspondence should be sent to Courtney N. Maierhofer, Department of Epidemiology, Gillings School of Global Public Health, University of North Carolina at Chapel Hill, Campus Box 7435, 135 Dauer Dr, Chapel Hill, NC 27599-7435 (e-mail: cmaierhofer@unc.edu). Reprints can be ordered at https://www.ajph.org by clicking the "Reprints" link.

Note. The findings and conclusions in this report are those of the authors and do not necessarily represent the official views of the North Carolina Department of Health and Human Services, Division of Public Health.

PUBLICATION INFORMATION

Full Citation: Maierhofer CN, Pence BW, Samoff E, et al. HIV care linkage and initial viral suppression among persons newly diagnosed with HIV in North Carolina before and after the start of the COVID-19 pandemic. *Am J Public Health*. 2025;115(9):1480–1489.

Acceptance Date: March 4, 2025.

DOI: https://doi.org/10.2105/AJPH.2025.308108

ORCID iDs:

Courtney N. Maierhofer https://orcid.org/0000-0003-3126-2022

Kimberly A. Powers https://orcid.org/0000-0001-7980-9846

CONTRIBUTORS

All authors contributed meaningfully to the completion of this article. C. N. Maierhofer and K. A. Powers led the conceptualization of this project. E. Samoff secured access to the data. C. N. Maierhofer, K. A. Powers, B. W. Pence, A. N. Turner, E. Samoff, V. Mobley, and W. C. Miller contributed to the design of the study. C. N. Maierhofer managed the data, conducted the data analysis, and drafted the article. K. A. Powers, B. W. Pence, A. N. Turner, E. Samoff, V. Mobley, J. Maxwell, and W. C. Miller assisted in interpretation of results and critically revised the article for important intellectual content. All authors take responsibility for and approve of the final version of this article.

ACKNOWLEDGMENTS

This work was supported by the National Institute of Nursing Research and the National Institute of Allergy and Infectious Diseases at the National Institutes of Health (NIH; R21 NR018805 to KAP and T32 AI070114 to CNM through BWP) and the University of North Carolina at Chapel Hill Center for AIDS Research, an NIH-funded program (P30 AI050410).

We thank Spencer Gee and Sara Levintow for their assistance with data storage, security, and management in support of these analyses.

Note. The content is solely the responsibility of the authors and does not necessarily represent the official views of the National Institutes of Health.

CONFLICTS OF INTEREST

C. N. Maierhofer is an employee at GSK but declares no nonfinancial competing interests.

HUMAN PARTICIPANT PROTECTION

The University of North Carolina at Chapel Hill institutional review board approved this study (21-0429).

REFERENCES

1. Hogg RS. Understanding the HIV care continuum. *Lancet HIV*. 2018;5(6):e269–e270. https://doi.org/10.1016/S2352-3018(18)30102-4
2. US Department of Health and Human Services. Ending the HIV Epidemic. 2019. Available at: https://www.hiv.gov/federal-response/ending-the-hiv-epidemic/overview. Accessed August 11, 2021.
3. Centers for Disease Control and Prevention. HIV Surveillance Report: Supplemental Report. Monitoring selected national HIV prevention and care objectives by using HIV surveillance data—United States and 6 dependent areas, 2021. 2023. Available at: https://www.cdc.gov/hiv/library/reports/hiv-surveillance/vol-28-no-4/index.html. Accessed July 17, 2023.
4. Bailey ZD, Krieger N, Agénor M, Graves J, Linos N, Bassett MT. Structural racism and health inequities in the USA: evidence and interventions. *Lancet*. 2017;389(10077):1453–1463. https://doi.org/10.1016/S0140-6736(17)30569-X
5. Lesko CR, Bengtson AM. HIV and COVID-19: Intersecting epidemics with many unknowns. *Am J Epidemiol*. 2021;190(1):10–16. https://doi.org/10.1093/aje/kwaa158
6. Kucharski AJ, Klepac P, Conlan AJK, et al. Effectiveness of isolation, testing, contact tracing, and physical distancing on reducing transmission of SARS-CoV-2 in different settings: a mathematical modelling study. *Lancet Infect Dis*. 2020;20(10):1151–1160. https://doi.org/10.1016/S1473-3099(20)30457-6
7. Budak JZ, Scott JD, Dhanireddy S, Wood BR. The impact of COVID-19 on HIV care provided via telemedicine—past, present, and future. *Curr HIV/AIDS Rep*. 2021;18(2):98–104. https://doi.org/10.1007/s11904-021-00543-4
8. Stephenson R, Walsh AR, Chavanduka TMD, et al. Widespread closure of HIV prevention and care services places youth at higher risk during the COVID-19 pandemic. *PLoS One*. 2021;16(9):e0249740. https://doi.org/10.1371/journal.pone.0249740
9. Dawson L, Kates J. Delivering HIV care prevention in the COVID era: a national survey of Ryan White providers. December 16, 2020. Available at: https://www.kff.org/report-section/delivering-hiv-care-prevention-in-the-covid-era-a-national-survey-of-ryan-white-providers-issue-brief. Accessed November 24, 2021.
10. Winwood JJ, Fitzgerald L, Gardiner B, Hannan K, Howard C, Mutch A. Exploring the social impacts of the COVID-19 pandemic on people living with HIV (PLHIV): a scoping review. *AIDS Behav*. 2021;25(12):4125–4140. https://doi.org/10.1007/s10461-021-03300-1
11. El-Nahal WG, Shen NM, Keruly JC, et al. Time between viral loads for people with HIV during the COVID-19 pandemic. *J Acquir Immune Defic Syndr*. 2022;91(1):109–116. https://doi.org/10.1097/QAI.0000000000003026
12. Santos G-M, Ackerman B, Rao A, et al. Economic, mental health, HIV prevention and HIV treatment impacts of COVID-19 and the COVID-19 response on a global sample of cisgender gay men and other men who have sex with men. *AIDS Behav*. 2021;25(2):311–321. https://doi.org/10.1007/s10461-020-02969-0
13. North Carolina Department of Health and Human Services. North Carolina Electronic Disease Surveillance System (NC EDSS). 2019. Available at: https://epi.dph.ncdhhs.gov/cd/about/ncedss.html. Accessed June 17, 2021.
14. North Carolina Department of Health and Human Services. HIV/AIDS reporting for healthcare providers. 2020. Available at: https://epi.dph.ncdhhs.gov/cd/hiv/providers/report.html. Accessed February 5, 2025.
15. Centers for Disease Control and Prevention. Monitoring selected national HIV prevention and care objectives by using HIV surveillance data—United States and 6 dependent areas, 2017. Vol 24; 2019. Available at: https://stacks.cdc.gov/view/cdc/160192. Accessed January 4, 2021.
16. Dombrowski JC, Kent JB, Buskin SE, Stekler JD, Golden MR. Population-based metrics for the timing of HIV diagnosis, engagement in HIV care, and virologic suppression. *AIDS*. 2012;26(1):77–86. https://doi.org/10.1097/QAD.0b013e32834dcee9
17. Crepaz N, Song R, Lyss S, Hall HI. Trends in time from HIV diagnosis to first viral suppression following revised US HIV treatment guidelines, 2012–2017. *J Acquir Immune Defic Syndr*. 2020;85(1):46–50. https://doi.org/10.1097/QAI.0000000000002398
18. Lesko CR, Sampson LA, Miller WC, et al. Measuring the HIV care continuum using public health

surveillance data in the United States. *J Acquir Immune Defic Syndr.* 2015;70(5):489–494. https://doi.org/10.1097/QAI.0000000000000788

19. US Department of Health and Human Services. *Guidelines for the Use of Antiretroviral Agents in Adults and Adolescents Living With HIV.* 2021. Available at: https://clinicalinfo.hiv.gov/sites/default/files/guidelines/documents/adult-adolescent-arv/guidelines-adult-adolescent-arv.pdf. Accessed June 14, 2021.
20. Thompson CN, Baumgartner J, Pichardo C, et al. COVID-19 outbreak—New York City, February 29–June 1, 2020. *MMWR Morb Mortal Wkly Rep.* 2020;69(46):1725–1729. https://doi.org/10.15585/mmwr.mm6946a2
21. Goldstein J, McKinley J. Manhattan woman is first confirmed coronavirus case in state. *New York Times.* March 1, 2020. Available at: https://www.nytimes.com/2020/03/01/nyregion/new-york-coronvirus-confirmed.html. Accessed January 28, 2025.
22. North Carolina Department of Health and Human Services. North Carolina identifies first case of COVID-19. March 3, 2020. Available at: https://www.ncdhhs.gov/news/press-releases/2020/03/03/north-carolina-identifies-first-case-covid-19. Accessed January 28, 2025.
23. State of North Carolina. COVID-19 orders & directives. 2022. Available at: https://www.nc.gov/covid-19/covid-19-orders-directives. Accessed February 25, 2022.
24. North Carolina Department of Health and Human Services. North Carolina Rural and Urban Counties. 2019. Available at: https://www.ncdhhs.gov/ruralurban-2019/open. Accessed July 15, 2023.
25. Lau B, Cole SR, Gange SJ. Competing risk regression models for epidemiologic data. *Am J Epidemiol.* 2009;170(2):244–256. https://doi.org/10.1093/aje/kwp107
26. Efron B. The efficiency of Cox's likelihood function for censored data. *J Am Stat Assoc.* 1977;72(359):557–565. https://doi.org/10.1080/01621459.1977.10480613
27. Poteat T, German D, Kerrigan D. Managing uncertainty: a grounded theory of stigma in transgender health care encounters. *Soc Sci Med.* 2013;84:22–29. https://doi.org/10.1016/j.socscimed.2013.02.019
28. *National HIV/AIDS Strategy Federal Implementation Plan, 2022–2025.* Washington, DC: The White House; 2022.
29. Freeman R, Gwadz MV, Silverman E, et al. Critical race theory as a tool for understanding poor engagement along the HIV care continuum among African American/Black and Hispanic persons living with HIV in the United States: a qualitative exploration. *Int J Equity Health.* 2017;16(1):54. https://doi.org/10.1186/s12939-017-0549-3
30. Magesh S, John D, Li WT, et al. Disparities in COVID-19 outcomes by race, ethnicity, and socioeconomic status. *JAMA Netw Open.* 2021;4(11):e2134147. https://doi.org/10.1001/jamanetworkopen.2021.34147
31. Lopez L, Hart LH, Katz MH. Racial and ethnic health disparities related to COVID-19. *JAMA.* 2021;325(8):719–720. https://doi.org/10.1001/jama.2020.26443
32. Zhou S, Long N, Moeser M, et al. Use of next-generation sequencing in a state-wide strategy of HIV-1 surveillance: impact of the SARS-COV-2 pandemic on HIV-1 diagnosis and transmission. *J Infect Dis.* 2023;228(12):1758–1765. https://doi.org/10.1093/infdis/jiad211
33. Magno L, da Silva LAV, Veras MA, Pereira-Santos M, Dourado I. Stigma and discrimination related to gender identity and vulnerability to HIV/AIDS among transgender women: a systematic review. *Cad Saude Publica.* 2019;35(4):e00112718. https://doi.org/10.1590/0102-311x00112718
34. Zetola NM, Bernstein K, Ahrens K, et al. Using surveillance data to monitor entry into care of newly diagnosed HIV-infected persons: San Francisco, 2006–2007. *BMC Public Health.* 2009;9(1):17. https://doi.org/10.1186/1471-2458-9-17

African Immigrants and the End of the HIV Epidemic in the United States: Actionable Recommendations to Enhance Equity

Gloria Aidoo-Frimpong, PhD, MPH, MA, Emmanuel Koku, PhD, Nipher Malika, PhD, Chioma Nnaji, MPH, and Roxanne Kerani, PhD

See also Okoro, p. 1357.

African immigrants in the United States are disproportionately affected by HIV yet remain overlooked in public health strategies such as the Ending the HIV Epidemic (EHE) initiative. Many reside in EHE-prioritized counties, but their categorization under the broad "Black/African American" label obscures their distinct pathways to HIV acquisition and barriers to care.

We explore how African immigrants can be more effectively prioritized in the EHE framework. We examine key challenges, including stigma, cultural and linguistic barriers, and structural inequities, that limit access to prevention and treatment services. Additionally, sociocultural factors, such as traditional health beliefs and immigration-related stressors, exacerbate these barriers.

We propose actionable strategies to address these gaps, including disaggregated data collection, culturally tailored interventions, and partnerships with African immigrant communities. By aligning EHE efforts with the unique needs of this population, public health strategies can better address disparities and advance equity in the fight to end the HIV epidemic. (*Am J Public Health*. 2025;115(9):1490–1499. https://doi.org/10.2105/AJPH.2025.308160)

AJPH September 2025, Vol. 115, No. 9

As the United States intensifies its efforts to end the HIV epidemic, it is crucial to ensure that all communities are equitably represented and adequately served. Despite significant progress, disparities persist in access to prevention and treatment resources.[1,2] One key group, African immigrants, individuals born in African countries who have relocated to and reside in the United States, remains largely overlooked. Although they are significantly present in US counties heavily affected by HIV, African immigrants are often subsumed under the broad category of Black/African American owing to US racial classification systems that aggregate data on different Black subgroups (e.g., African Americans, Afro-Caribbeans, and African immigrants) with varying histories, cultures, and health profiles.[3] Such aggregation overlooks critical historical background and cultural, linguistic, and socioepidemiological differences these groups embody.

African immigrants experience remarkably higher rates of HIV diagnosis, approximately 2 times higher than other US-born Black populations.[4] This disparity is even more startling among African-born Black women, who were reported to have an 85-fold higher HIV diagnosis rate than White women.[5] Moreover, HIV transmission among African immigrants occurs primarily through heterosexual contact, compared with the male-to-male contact predominant in the broader US population.[4] Thus, African immigrants may not benefit fully from US prevention efforts that prioritize interventions designed for populations at risk through male-to-male transmission and injection drug use.[6] In particular, messaging and interventions that broadly define their intended audience with such broad racial terms as "Black" or "people of color" often fail to resonate with African immigrants, who typically identify more strongly with their national, ethnic, or linguistic backgrounds.[7,8]

To end the HIV epidemic, public health efforts must move beyond homogenized approaches that obscure epidemiological differences and cultural identities among ethnoracial groups such as African immigrants.[9] Such efforts must recognize and address the unique sociocultural structural barriers they face as African immigrants in the US health care system and the interventions needed to address their specific challenges effectively. Consequently, we argue for prioritizing African immigrants in tailored interventions and programs to end the HIV epidemic. The article is divided into 3 sections. We first discuss the overlap between EHE hotspots with communities where African immigrants reside. Second, we discuss the 4 pillars of the EHE framework, focusing on barriers African immigrants experience in efforts for diagnosis, treatment, prevention, and response to HIV epidemics. We include strategies to address the barriers within each pillar. The final section concludes and reflects on the future agenda for ending the HIV epidemic and reducing HIV rates among African immigrant populations.

GEOGRAPHIC FOCUS

The Ending the HIV Epidemic (EHE) initiative in the US aims to reduce new HIV infections by 75% by 2025 and by 90% by 2030.[10] This federal effort concentrates on 57 jurisdictions, known as EHE counties and states, which are prioritized because of their high rates of HIV incidence.[10] Funding is allocated to these jurisdictions to develop and implement tailored EHE plans that address their specific epidemiological and social contexts. This localized approach ensures that interventions are culturally responsive and effectively meet the unique needs of each community. Many of these EHE jurisdictions overlap with regions that have substantial African immigrant populations.

As Table 1 shows, about half of African immigrants in the United States reside in these priority EHE regions. Between 60% and 80% of African immigrants residing in Arizona, California, Florida, Georgia, New York, Ohio, Texas, and Washington reside in EHE priority counties. For instance, 70% of African immigrants in Maryland reside in EHE priority counties, such as Prince George's, Montgomery, and Baltimore counties, reflecting significant overlap between HIV hotspots and immigrant communities (Table 2 provides county-level data). The geographic alignment of EHE counties with African immigrant communities reflects the disproportionate burden of HIV in communities of color.[11] However, current EHE plans lack targeted strategies for these populations. Hence, it is critically important that EHE plans respond to broader ethnoracial differences underlying HIV prevalence in priority EHE communities.

THE FRAMEWORK IN CONTEXT

The EHE framework provides a comprehensive roadmap to reduce HIV disparities through its 4 pillars: diagnose, treat, prevent, and respond.[10] Although these pillars aim to address gaps in the HIV continuum nationally, their implementation often fails to account for the unique challenges faced by African immigrant populations. Examining these pillars in the context of African immigrant HIV outcomes highlights critical service gaps and opportunities for more inclusive strategies.

Diagnose

In the first pillar of the EHE framework, which emphasizes early detection and testing, African immigrants face a significant and unique service gap: inadequate access to early HIV detection and testing services. African immigrants are disproportionately more likely to enter care later in the course of infection. In a comparative analysis of HIV-related outcomes among US-born and non–US-born Blacks (most of whom were African immigrants), a higher percentage of non–US-born Black males received a late-stage diagnosis, compared with non–US-born Black females (33.2% male vs 24.0% female), at the time of diagnosis.[12] Late testing and diagnosis often result in significant HIV-related morbidities, low CD4 counts (as low as an average of 285), and increased potential for onward HIV transmission.[4]

This gap is driven by multifaceted barriers, including language differences, cultural stigma, mistrust of health care systems, and limited awareness of HIV testing services.[8,13] Despite the EHE framework's goal of expanding access, African immigrants often encounter information about HIV testing only in English, limiting accessibility for those more comfortable in their native languages or dialects.[13,14] Additionally, concerns about confidentiality arise when interpretation services involve individuals from the local African immigrant community, deterring individuals from seeking testing because of fears of stigma and breach of privacy.[15]

African immigrants underuse the prevention methods of condoms, HIV testing, and preexposure prophylaxis (PrEP) despite their effectiveness.[16] A widespread lack of awareness regarding the availability and importance of these HIV prevention methods exacerbates this service gap, preventing many African immigrants from using early detection and intervention resources.[14]

TABLE 1— Distribution of African Immigrant Population in Ending the HIV Epidemic (EHE) Priority Counties and States: United States, 1987–2024

	National, No. (%)[a]	EHE Priority Counties and States, No. (%)[b]
Alabama	8 000 (0.4)	8 000 (NA)
Arkansas	3 900 (0.2)	3 900 (NA)
Arizona	31 500 (1.5)	24 200 (76.8)
California	152 000 (7.0)	112 100 (73.8)
Florida	51 900 (2.4)	33 300 (64.2)
Georgia	111 000 (5.1)	80 900 (72.9)
Illinois	65 200 (3.0)	37 500 (57.5)
Indiana	36 000 (1.7)	19 000 (52.8)
Kentucky	21 600 (1.0)	21 600 (NA)
Louisiana	6 500 (0.3)	1 200 (18.5)
Maryland	179 400 (8.3)	126 000 (70.2)
Massachusetts	98 300 (4.6)	20 000 (20.3)
Michigan	30 600 (1.4)	6 300 (20.6)
Mississippi	3 700 (0.2)	3 700 (NA)
Missouri	23 900 (1.1)	23 900 (NA)
Nevada	18 900 (0.9)	17 700 (88.4)
New Jersey	88 400 (4.1)	37 500 (42.4)
New York	169 200 (7.8)	113 600 (67.1)
North Carolina	60 000 (2.8)	18 100 (30.2)
Ohio	84 900 (3.9)	64 300 (75.7)
Oklahoma	12 200 (0.6)	12 200 (NA)
Pennsylvania	70 400 (3.3)	22 200 (31.5)
South Carolina	8 900 (0.4)	8 900 (NA)
Tennessee	28 700 (1.3)	6 200 (21.6)
Texas	260 300 (12.1)	167 400 (64.3)
Washington	66 400 (3.1)	42 300 (63.7)
Washington, DC	14 800 (0.7)	14 800 (NA)
Total population of African immigrants		
Non-EHE priority counties and states	451 700 (20.90)	NA
African immigrants in US	2 158 300 (100.0)	1 046 800 (48.5)

Note. NA = not applicable.
Source. Migration Policy Institute. Tabulation of data from the US Census Bureau's pooled 2018–2022 American Community Survey (available in Lorenzi J, Batalova J. Sub-Saharan African immigrants in the United States. Migration Policy Institute; May, 11, 2022. Available at: https://www.migrationpolicy.org/article/sub-saharan-african-immigrants-united-states-2019).
[a]Proportion of total African immigrant population in state.
[b]Proportion of African immigrant population in EHE counties (in each state).

Even when services are available, the stigma surrounding HIV in African immigrant communities negatively affects engagement with health care services.[1] It discourages HIV testing and hinders the adoption of effective prevention methods such as condom use and PrEP, exacerbating existing challenges in managing and ending the HIV epidemic. These stigmas are rooted in and shaped by cultural beliefs and expectations regarding sex and sexuality, which link HIV risk behaviors to immorality, shame, and violations of religious and cultural edicts.[17] These beliefs drive fears of casual transmission, rejection, social distance from others, and discrimination against those suspected of having or living with HIV.[1,17] As a result, community members tend to underestimate their risk or avoid testing to prevent societal judgment.[14]

TABLE 2— Number of African Immigrants in All Ending the HIV Epidemic (EHE) Counties and States: United States, 1987–2024

EHE Counties and States	No. (%)[a]
Alabama	8 000 (0.4)
Arizona	31 500 (1.5)
Maricopa County	24 200
Arkansas	3 900 (0.2)
California	152 000 (7)
Alameda County	17 000
Los Angeles County	43 500
Orange County	9 600
Riverside County	7 400
Sacramento County	8 200
San Bernardino County	7 100
San Diego County	16 000
San Francisco County	3 300
Florida	51 900 (2.4)
Broward County	5 100
Duval County	4 600
Hillsborough County	6 200
Miami-Dade County	5 500
Orange County	4 700
Palm Beach County	5 000
Pinellas County	2 200
Georgia	111 000 (5.1)
Cobb County	13 100
DeKalb County	27 700
Fulton County	13 700
Gwinnett County	26 400
Illinois	65 200 (3.0)
Cook County	37 500
Kentucky	21 600 (1.0)
Michigan	30 600 (1.4)
Wayne County	6 300
Mississippi	3 700 (0.2)
Missouri	23 900 (1.1)
Nevada	18 900 (0.9)
Clark County	16 700
New Jersey	88 400 (4.1)
Essex County	30 600
Hudson County	6 900
New York	169 200 (7.8)
Bronx County	54 000
Kings County	22 800
New York County	18 900
Queens County	17 900
Suffolk County	20 000

Continued

Such individual-level experiences are further compounded by institutional practices such as the now-repealed US HIV travel ban, which may still influence attitudes toward HIV testing because of lingering fears of discrimination or legal repercussions.[18] HIV stigma is compounded by a mistrust of health care providers, often linked to past negative experiences with health care systems or a general suspicion of Western medical practices, including HIV treatments,[8] resulting in a reluctance to engage in testing and care services.[19] Community and personal network stigma exacerbates these barriers, discouraging disclosure and adherence to care while increasing risky sexual behaviors.[17]

To address these gaps and ensure that African immigrants are engaged in the EHE initiative, several targeted strategies must be implemented through dedicated funding and strategic partnerships. Allocating targeted funding to community-based organizations that serve African immigrant populations can support the development of multilingual educational materials in languages such as Amharic, Somali, Swahili, French, and Arabic. Partnering with community-based organizations and local health departments to host culturally tailored testing and health-screening events can enhance accessibility and acceptance. Holding these events at trusted locations—such as cultural centers, churches, mosques, and community festivals—has proven effective, as demonstrated by the Clinics Without Walls initiative of Philadelphia, Pennsylvania.[8] Designing and disseminating culturally sensitive messaging that addresses HIV-related stigma and emphasizes the importance of testing should be done in collaboration with community leaders and influencers to ensure resonance

TABLE 2— Continued

EHE Counties and States	No. (%)[a]
Oklahoma	12 200 (0.6)
South Carolina	8 900 (0.4)
Texas	260 300 (12.1)
Bexar County	5 300
Dallas County	50 500
Harris County	65 400
Tarrant County	34 700
Travis County	11 500
Washington	66 400 (3.1)
King County	42 300
Washington, DC	14 800 (0.7)
Total population of African immigrants	
All US states	2 158 300
EHE counties and states	1 045 800

Source. Migration Policy Institute tabulation of data from the US Census Bureau's pooled 2018–2022 American Community Survey.
[a]Percentages in parenthesis represent the proportion of the total number of African immigrants (2 158 300) in each state.

and trust.[14] Furthermore, creating specific funding streams and technical support for these initiatives will help build sustainable, community-led responses that align with the EHE pillars, ultimately improving HIV testing and prevention outcomes among African immigrants.

Treat

The second pillar of the EHE framework emphasizes ensuring that individuals diagnosed with HIV receive timely treatment and remain consistently engaged in care. African immigrants, however, often face substantial delays to treatment, as evidenced by frequent diagnoses at advanced stages of HIV infection.[1] As a result of these delays, African immigrants are more likely to enter care late, with worsened disease progression and outcomes. An analysis of clinical characteristics of people with HIV in King County, Washington, indicated that Black African immigrants are more likely to enter care with an AIDS diagnosis (45%) compared with both US-born non-Blacks (25%) and US-born Blacks (35%).[20] These delays are shaped by the intersection of preimmigration experiences, such as trauma, disrupted health care access, and systemic inequities, as well as US-based barriers such as language, mistrust, and structural discrimination.[1]

As a critical determinant, migration status[21] and trajectories contribute to disparities in HIV outcomes. African immigrants carry the historical legacy of colonization, including systemic oppression and postcolonial traumas that have left enduring scars on their identities and socioeconomic realities.[22,23] Migration and resettlement introduce unique stressors (e.g., complexities in securing legal status, language barriers, economic and financial hardship, limited health insurance coverage, bias, discrimination, and difficulties navigating new health care systems)[21,24–26] that exacerbate health disparities and limit African immigrants' access to and engagement in HIV prevention services and care.

Once diagnosed, African immigrants encounter additional challenges in maintaining consistent engagement in HIV care because of insufficient culturally competent health care services and outreach. Even when services are available, health care providers may not possess the cultural competence or humility needed to understand and address the unique needs of African immigrants.[27] This gap in understanding can lead to suboptimal care and deter individuals from remaining engaged in treatment. Additionally, traditional HIV outreach often targets groups perceived as high risk, such as men who have sex with men, leaving African immigrants unaware of critical resources such as the AIDS Drug Assistance Program, which provides financial support for HIV treatment.[28]

Social determinants of health, such as housing instability, employment challenges, and social isolation, further complicate treatment access and adherence in this population.[29] There is evidence, however, that once linked to care, African immigrants tend to fare better in later stages of the HIV care continuum, with high levels of engagement and consequent viral suppression.[4] For example, comparative analysis of US HIV surveillance data revealed that a larger proportion of African-born Blacks had been retained in care (65% vs 61%) and achieved higher viral suppression (69% vs 58%) than their counterparts, US-born Blacks.[12] This evidence underscores the urgent need for tailored interventions to increase linkage and retention in care.

To address treatment and retention challenges and meet EHE goals, the initiative must prioritize culturally and linguistically competent care by training health care providers and equipping health care systems to understand the cultural backgrounds, traditional health practices, and communication preferences of African immigrant communities. Coled community and clinical training programs focusing on bidirectional learning, cultural humility, and systems-level change, such as the AI Health model, have demonstrated success. These programs have improved provider practices and organizational approaches to HIV care for African immigrants.[30] In addition, efforts should be supported by hiring staff who reflect the cultural and linguistic diversity of the populations they serve.[8] Additionally, the use of community health workers and patient navigators who share the cultural and linguistic backgrounds of African immigrants can significantly improve access and retention in care through culturally relevant messaging and programming.[8]

These navigators can guide patients through the complex health care system, help them understand their treatment options, schedule appointments, and connect them to essential support services in furtherance of treatment as prevention mandates. A few local initiatives, such as the Harambee! program in Seattle, Washington, demonstrate how employing culturally trained patient navigators can improve care retention.[14,31] Furthermore, advocating policy changes, such as expanding Medicaid eligibility to all immigrants regardless of legal status, would significantly reduce barriers to treatment and ensure equitable access to HIV care for all. By integrating these strategies, the EHE initiative can more effectively support African immigrants in accessing and remaining engaged in HIV treatment, ultimately improving health outcomes and advancing the goal of ending the HIV epidemic.

Prevent

The third pillar of the EHE framework emphasizes comprehensive prevention strategies, including PrEP and HIV self-testing. However, African immigrants face a critical gap in using these preventive measures, largely because of limited awareness and accessibility challenges caused by structural barriers.[16] Awareness of PrEP and HIV self-testing remains low among many African immigrants, often because prevention programs fail to engage this population effectively.[2] Even when individuals are informed about PrEP, structural barriers such as cost, transportation, and clinic hours that conflict with typical work schedules further restrict access.[32] Moreover, cultural and religious beliefs may discourage the use of PrEP, further limiting its uptake.[32]

To bridge these gaps, it is essential for the EHE initiative to require local health departments to prioritize targeted prevention campaigns in states and counties with large African immigrant populations. These campaigns should include education on HIV self-testing, highlighting its privacy and convenience as a nonclinical option for those hesitant to access traditional testing services. By mandating a focus on these communities, local health departments can allocate resources effectively and address the unique needs of African immigrants. Campaigns should be culturally tailored and delivered by trusted community figures and ethnic-based organizations embedded in African immigrant communities to ensure credibility and acceptance. Additionally, it is crucial to make PrEP and HIV self-testing services more accessible and affordable in clinics and health centers located in areas with high concentrations of African immigrants.

For example, implementing outreach programs, such as mobile clinics and health fairs that offer PrEP and HIV self-testing information and services near workplaces or cultural centers where African immigrants live, could address logistical barriers such as transportation and clinic hours.[8] Partnering with faith leaders for culturally specific prevention messaging can significantly improve engagement and uptake of these preventive methods.[31] By incorporating these strategies, the EHE initiative can enhance prevention efforts and ensure that African immigrants are fully engaged in the fight to end the HIV epidemic.

Respond

The fourth pillar of the EHE framework focuses on rapid and effective responses to HIV outbreaks. For African immigrants, outbreak response efforts are often limited by a lack of disaggregated data and insufficient community engagement.[9] In many jurisdictions, current data collection practices aggregate African immigrants under the broader Black/African American category, making it difficult to identify specific outbreak patterns and unique risk factors for this population and guide response efforts. As experiences from Ebola and COVID-19 outbreaks show,[33,34] limited resource allocation and engagement strategies that do not actively involve African immigrant communities reduce the reach and impact of outbreak interventions.[35] Without comprehensive support services tailored to this group, public health responses may miss critical opportunities to effectively control HIV transmission in African immigrant populations.

Additionally, African immigrant communities are often not sufficiently engaged in planning and implementing outbreak responses, resulting in strategies that may not be culturally appropriate or effectively communicated, as experiences with the recent COVID-19 outbreak demonstrated.[35] Although local and state health departments are required to include community engagement in their EHE plans and are instructed to include additional or new community representatives as needed,[36] if local jurisdictions do not routinely disaggregate their HIV surveillance data, they may not be aware of the degree to which HIV affects the local African immigrant population. Additionally, because African immigrant communities are often organized based on their country of origin, it may be challenging to identify the best representative or group to partner with in a local jurisdiction; a single representative or organization may not reflect the diversity of local African immigrant communities. As a result, resource allocation during outbreaks tends to be general rather than tailored to the specific needs of African immigrants, limiting the reach and effectiveness of comprehensive support services. Given the significant gaps in disaggregated HIV outbreak data for African immigrants, future surveillance efforts should prioritize this data collection.

As effective community-based outreach programs for COVID-19 and other emergencies have revealed,[37] engaging African immigrant communities in outbreak response planning and implementation ensures that strategies are culturally appropriate and effectively communicated. This engagement can be facilitated through partnerships with community organizations and leaders who have established trust in these communities.[35] For example, during the COVID-19 pandemic, a Seattle-based coalition partnered with African community leaders to implement culturally tailored vaccine drives,[38] achieving vaccination rates 15% higher than the city average, similar to what was observed in Philadelphia.[35] Providing comprehensive support services—including social determinants of health, such as housing and employment, which may be affected during outbreaks—can further support the resilience and well-being of African immigrant communities. Similar approaches can be adapted to ensure access to HIV testing, treatment, and preventive measures during outbreaks.

THE WAY FORWARD

To address these challenges and ensure the success of the EHE framework among African immigrants, 3 key priorities emerge: fostering community partnerships, securing dedicated funding, and advancing data disaggregation.

Community Partnerships

Community-based initiatives have proven effective in reaching African immigrants, but sustained partnerships are necessary to expand their reach and impact. This can be achieved through engaging trusted voices in African communities and allied affiliated networks of service providers and stakeholders, such as local health departments, academic and research institutions, and religious communities. Partnerships can be vital for capacity building and training community health workers and navigators in HIV prevention and treatment modalities. For example, the Tulumbe! Project[39] in Massachusetts successfully mobilized African immigrants to coidentify HIV-related priorities and codevelop culturally responsive strategies, demonstrating the effectiveness of community-driven engagement in HIV prevention. Such partnerships can foster stronger relationships among African immigrant service providers, ensuring delivery of culturally competent care and improving the uptake of HIV prevention and treatment services.

Securing Dedicated Funding

Historically, federal funding for research on HIV prevention and treatment among African immigrant populations has lagged behind research funding for other minority groups in the United States (Figure 1). This funding disparity is often linked to the misperception that African immigrants are a small population or are adequately represented in the broader Black/African American category. Although African immigrants indeed constitute a small fraction of the US population, they account for a greater share of new HIV diagnoses compared with other immigrant (i.e., non-US born) populations.[40] As observed earlier, diagnosis rates and projections to end-stage HIV infection are comparatively higher among African immigrants than other groups.[4]

Given that African immigrants constitute approximately 4% of new HIV diagnoses, National Institutes of Health and Centers for Disease Control and Prevention (CDC) funding allocations should reflect this burden, with a proportional increase in research funding directed to immigrant-specific interventions, especially those targeting pilot and full-scale projects on African immigrant health. Involvement of other

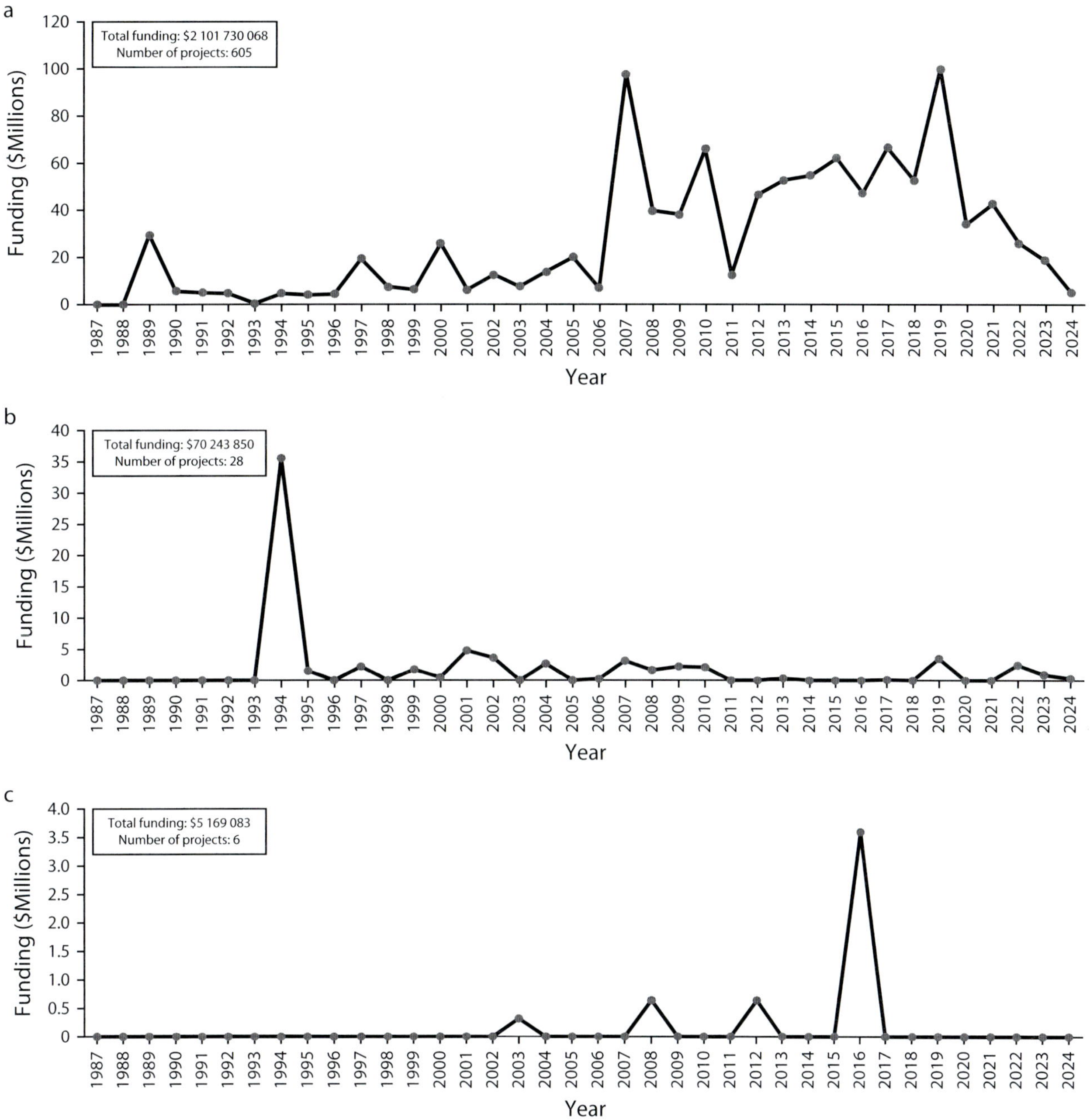

FIGURE 1— National Institutes of Health (NIH) Support for HIV Research Projects on (a) Latino, (b) Asian, and (c) African Immigrant Populations, by Year of Funding: United States, 1987–2024

Note. Only unique projects are included in the figure. Multiyear projects were collapsed into a single unit, with costs totaled across years of funding. Search criteria were as follows: Asian immigrants: ("Asian immigrant" OR "Asian-born" OR "Asian immigrants" OR "Asian-origin" OR "Asian- American" OR "Asian American" OR "Southeast Asian population" OR "Southeast Asian immigrant") AND HIV; Latino immigrants: ("Latino immigrant" OR "Latino immigrants" OR "Hispanic immigrant" OR "Hispanic immigrants" OR "Latino" OR "Hispanics" OR "Latinos" NOT "African" NOT "Black") AND HIV; African immigrants: ("African immigrant" OR "African-born" OR "African immigrants") AND HIV.
Source. National Institutes of Health RePORTER (https://reporter.nih.gov).

public, federal, and private funding agencies such as the National Science Foundation, the Health Resources and Services Administration, the Patient-Centered Outcomes Research Institute, the Robert Wood Johnson Foundation, and Gilead Sciences would advance efforts toward the elimination of ethnoracial health disparities. Among African immigrants in particular, such funding would be critical to scaling successful pilot projects such as

Tulumbe![39] and Harambee![14] and enable the development of targeted interventions that ensure that their unique needs are represented in public health efforts.

Data Disaggregation

US national data collection standards have often rendered African immigrants invisible in disease surveillance systems. Policymakers and funders must acknowledge the distinct identity of African immigrants and prioritize data disaggregation to reflect this diversity. The inclusion of "region of birth" variables in national surveys such as the National Health Interview Survey and the National Health and Nutrition Examination Survey is critical for tracking health trends among immigrant populations, and researchers must continue to disaggregate their findings by nativity or region of birth. The Office of Management and Budget released revised standards in March 2024, adopting a combined question approach for federal data on race and ethnicity. Although individuals can now identify as Black/African American and specify an ethnicity (e.g., Ghanaian, Nigerian), this represents only a minimum standard.

More detailed data collection is needed to fully capture the diversity and unique health needs of African immigrant communities. A feasible approach to disaggregated HIV data collection could involve modifying existing CDC HIV surveillance forms to include "country of birth" as a required field, alongside similar adaptations in electronic medical record systems already being implemented in local health departments in some states (e.g., New York, Washington, Massachusetts, and Georgia). In tandem with national efforts, the CDC and the US Department of Health and Human Services could also encourage medical providers in local jurisdictions to collect and record country of birth information in their medical charts and records to ensure that such data are available for larger HIV surveillance systems.

CONCLUSIONS

Ending the HIV epidemic requires strategies that address the unique challenges faced by African immigrants, including stigma, systematic barriers to care, and aggregation of HIV surveillance data that overlooks their unique needs. To achieve the national goal of ending the HIV epidemic, public health systems must act decisively to address disparities faced by African immigrants through community partnerships, equitable funding, and more inclusive data collection standards. By integrating these recommendations, the EHE framework can set a precedent for equitable health strategies that serve all communities. By recognizing African immigrants as integral to the broader public health strategy, we can make significant strides toward ending the HIV epidemic in a way that is inclusive, equitable, and impactful. AJPH

ABOUT THE AUTHORS

Gloria Aidoo-Frimpong is with the Department of Epidemiology and Environmental Health, School of Public Health and Health Professions, University at Buffalo, State University of New York, Buffalo. Emmanuel Koku is with the Department of Sociology, Drexel University, Philadelphia, PA. Nipher Malika is with the RAND Corporation, Santa Monica, CA. Chioma Nnaji is with the Multicultural AIDS Coalition, Boston, MA. Roxanne Kerani is with the Department of Medicine, Division of Allergy & Infectious Diseases, University of Washington, Seattle, and Public Health–Seattle & King County, Seattle.

CORRESPONDENCE

Correspondence should be sent to Gloria Aidoo-Frimpong, PhD, MPH, MA, School of Public Health and Health Professions, University at Buffalo, 193 Farber Hall, Buffalo, NY 14214 (e-mail: gloriaai@buffalo.edu). Reprints can be ordered at http://www.ajph.org by clicking the "Reprints" link.

PUBLICATION INFORMATION

Full Citation: Aidoo-Frimpong G, Koku E, Malika N, Nnaji C, Kerani R. African immigrants and the end of the HIV epidemic in the United States: actionable recommendations to enhance equity. *Am J Public Health*. 2025;115(9):1490–1499.

Acceptance Date: April 12, 2025.

DOI: https://doi.org/10.2105/AJPH.2025.308160

ORCID iDs:

Gloria Aidoo-Frimpong https://orcid.org/0000-0002-4658-2953

Nipher Malika https://orcid.org/0000-0001-5887-5481

Chioma Nnaji https://orcid.org/0000-0001-8512-7913

CONTRIBUTORS

G. Aidoo-Frimpong led the conceptualization and drafting of the article. E. Koku, N. Malika, C. Nnaji, and R. Kerani contributed to the conceptual development, provided critical revisions for intellectual content, and approved the final version.

CONFLICTS OF INTEREST

The authors have no conflicts of interest to declare.

HUMAN PARTICIPANT PROTECTION

This study did not involve human participants, and therefore institutional review board approval was not required.

REFERENCES

1. Nnaji C, O Ojikutu B. Intersecting stigmas: Being Black African, immigrant, and living with HIV in the United States. *Am J Public Health*. 2022; 112(suppl 4):S367–S370. https://doi.org/10.2105/ajph.2022.306734
2. Aidoo-Frimpong G, Agbemenu K, Adzrago D, Akyirem S, Boateng S, Nelson LE. The promise of pre-exposure prophylaxis—examining awareness, knowledge, and willingness to use different modalities among US-based African immigrants. *J Immigr Minor Health*. 2023;25(6):1331–1338. https://doi.org/10.1007/s10903-023-01515-z
3. Tamir C, Anderson M. One-in-ten Black people living in the US are immigrants. January 20, 2022. Available at: https://www.pewresearch.org/race-ethnicity/2022/01/20/one-in-ten-black-people-living-in-the-u-s-are-immigrants. Accessed June 1, 2025.
4. Kerani RP, Lugg A, Berzins B, et al. Post-migration HIV acquisition among African immigrants in the US. *J Immigr Minor Health*. 2022;24(6):1459–1468. https://doi.org/10.1007/s10903-022-01356-2
5. Demeke HB, Johnson AS, Wu B, Moonesinghe R, Dean HD. Unequal declines in absolute and relative disparities in HIV diagnoses among Black women, United States, 2008 to 2016. *Am J Public*

Health. 2018;108(suppl 4):S299–S303. https://doi.org/10.2105/ajph.2018.304641

6. Connor JJ, Lund SM, Ciesinski A, Finsaas M, Bichanga T, Robinson BBE. The East African HIV prevention model: perspectives from HIV-positive male immigrants living in the USA. *Cogent Med*. 2016;3(1):1175402. https://doi.org/10.1080/2331205X.2016.1175402
7. Commodore-Mensah Y, Turkson-Ocran RA, Nmezi NA, et al. Commentary: Engaging African immigrants in research experiences and lessons from the field. *Ethn Dis*. 2019;29(4):617–622. https://doi.org/10.18865/ed.29.4.617
8. Aidoo-Frimpong G, Agbemenu K, Orom H. A review of cultural influences on risk for HIV and culturally-responsive risk mitigation strategies among African immigrants in the US. *J Immigr Minor Health*. 2021;23(6):1280–1292. https://doi.org/10.1007/s10903-020-01138-8
9. Koku EF, Rajab-Gyagenda WM, Korto MD, et al. HIV/AIDS among African immigrants in the US: the need for disaggregating HIV surveillance data by country of birth. *J Health Care Poor Underserved*. 2016;27(3):1316–1329. https://doi.org/10.1353/hpu.2016.0128
10. Centers for Disease Control and Prevention. Ending the HIV epidemic in the US (EHE). Available at: https://www.cdc.gov/ehe/?CDC_AAref_Val=https://www.cdc.gov/endhiv/about-ehe/index.html. Accessed June 1, 2025.
11. Centers for Disease Control and Prevention. HV surveillance supplemental report: estimated HIV incidence and prevalence in the United States, 2018–2022. 2024. May 21, 2024. Available at: https://stacks.cdc.gov/view/cdc/156513. Accessed June 1, 2025.
12. Demeke HB, Johnson AS, Zhu H, Gant Z, Duffus WA, Dean HD. HIV infection-related care outcomes among US-born and non–US-born Blacks with diagnosed HIV in 40 US areas: the National HIV Surveillance System, 2016. *Int J Environ Res Public Health*. 2018;15(11):2404. https://doi.org/10.3390/ijerph15112404
13. Hassan SA, Mohamed F, Sheikh N, et al. "They wait until the disease has taking over you and the doctors cannot do anything about it": qualitative insights from Harambee! 2.0. *Int J Environ Res Public Health*. 2021;18(23):12706. https://doi.org/10.3390/ijerph182312706
14. Daniel NA, Hassan SA, Mohamed F, et al. Harambee! 2.0: the impact of HIV-related and intersectional stigmas on HIV testing behaviors among African immigrant communities in Seattle, Washington. *AIDS Behav*. 2021;26(suppl 1): 149–164. https://doi.org/10.1007/s10461-021-03396-5
15. Koku E. Pathways to care: HIV testing among African born persons in the USA. Evidence from the National Health Interview Survey, 2000–2010. *Sociological Imagination*. 2023;59(1):1–22.
16. Aidoo-Frimpong G, Orom H, Agbemenu K, Collins RL, Morse GD, Nelson LE. Exploring awareness, perceptions, and willingness to use HIV pre exposure prophylaxis: a qualitative study of Ghanaian immigrants in the United States. *AIDS Patient Care STDS*. 2022;36(1):8–16. https://doi.org/10.1089/apc.2021.0156
17. Koku EF. Social networks and stigma: the experiences of African immigrants living with HIV in the United States. *SSM Qual Res Health*. 2024;6:100493. https://doi.org/10.1016/j.ssmqr.2024.100493
18. Kerani RP, Kwakwa HA. Scaring undocumented immigrants is detrimental to public health. *Am J Public Health*. 2018;108(9):1165–1166. https://doi.org/10.2105/ajph.2018.304596
19. Nipher M, Lisa R, Qais A, Carlos AC, Susanne M. Medical mistrust on prostate cancer screening: a mixed method study among African Americans, Caribbean immigrants and African immigrants. *Med Res Arch*. 2024;12(8):10.18103/mra.v12i8.5727. https://doi.org/10.18103/mra.v12i8.5727
20. Page LC, Goldbaum G, Kent JB, Buskin SE. Access to regular HIV care and disease progression among Black African immigrants. *J Natl Med Assoc*. 2009;101(12):1230–1236. https://doi.org/10.1016/s0027-9684(15)31134-2
21. Castañeda H, Holmes SM, Madrigal DS, Young ME, Beyeler N, Quesada J. Immigration as a social determinant of health. *Annu Rev Public Health*. 2015;36:375–392. https://doi.org/10.1146/annurev-publhealth-032013-182419
22. Bogart LM, Takada S, Cunningham WE. Medical mistrust, discrimination, and the domestic HIV epidemic. In: Ojikutu BO, Stone VE, eds. *HIV in US Communities of Color*. Cham, Switzerland: Springer International Publishing; 2021:207–231.
23. Herschthal E. Slavery, health, and healing now: the state of the field. *J Hist Med Allied Sci*. 2022;77(1):1–23. https://doi.org/10.1093/jhmas/jrab042
24. Hassan S, Mohamed F, Patel R, Kerani R. When culture and preventative care collide. *Public Health Post*. March 23, 2022. Available at: https://publichealthpost.org/health-equity/culture-preventative-care-collide. Accessed June 1, 2025.
25. Ross J, Akiyama MJ, Slawek D, et al. Undocumented African immigrants' experiences of HIV testing and linkage to care. *AIDS Patient Care STDS*. 2019;33(7):336–341. https://doi.org/10.1089/apc.2019.0036
26. Ojikutu BO, Nnaji C, Sithole-Berk J, et al. African born women living with HIV in the United States: unmet needs and opportunities for intervention. *AIDS Care*. 2018;30(12):1542–1550. https://doi.org/10.1080/09540121.2018.1497767
27. Roberts DA, Abera S, Basualdo G, et al. Barriers to accessing preventive health care among African-born individuals in King County, Washington: a qualitative study involving key informants. *PLoS ONE*. 2021;16(5):e0250800. https://doi.org/10.1371/journal.pone.0250800
28. Health Resources and Services Administration. Part B: AIDS Drug Assistance Program (ADAP). December 2024. Available at: https://ryanwhite.hrsa.gov/about/parts-and-initiatives/part-b-adap. Accessed November 27, 2024.
29. Omenka OI, Watson DP, Hendrie HC. Understanding the healthcare experiences and needs of African immigrants in the United States: a scoping review. *BMC Public Health*. 2020;20(1): 27–27. https://doi.org/10.1186/s12889-019-8127-9
30. Nnaji C, Adigwe A, Patel RC, Day PG, Escobar MF. A community-based, multidisciplinary training program to improve HIV services for US-based African immigrants: lessons learned over 5 years of implementation. *BMC Med Educ*. In press.
31. Roberts DA, Kerani R, Tsegaselassie S, et al. Harambee!: a pilot mixed methods study of integrated residential HIV testing among African-born individuals in the Seattle area. *PLoS One*. 2019;14(5):e0216502. https://doi.org/10.1371/journal.pone.0216502
32. Aidoo-Frimpong G, Collins RL, Agbemenu K, Orom H, Morse GD, Nelson LE. Barriers to HIV pre-exposure prophylaxis uptake and ways to mitigate them: perspectives of Ghanaian immigrants in the United States. *AIDS Educ Prev*. 2022;34(3):209–225. https://doi.org/10.1521/aeap.2022.34.3.209
33. Whembolua G-LS, Conserve DF, Tshiswaka DI. Socio-cultural factors influencing the Ebola virus disease-related stigma among African immigrants in the United States. *Irikirendo: Journal of African Migration*. 2017(9):114–136. Available at: https://africamigration.com/issue/dec2017/Whembolua_Conserve_Tshiswaka_issue_9.pdf. Accessed June 1, 2025.
34. Johansen I, Selim M, Hoffman SJ, Dawson-Hahn E, Yu K. Pivoting from influenza to COVID-19 vaccinations: how a Minnesota vaccination program reduced barriers for refugee, immigrant, and migrant communities accessing vaccines during the COVID-19 pandemic. *J Public Health Manag Pract*. 2024;30(5):701–709. https://doi.org/10.1097/phh.0000000000001931
35. Koku EF, Johnson-Yengbeh N, Muhr A. Addressing COVID-19 vaccine hesitancy and uptake among African immigrants: lessons from a community-based outreach program. *J Racial Ethn Health Disparities*. 2025;12(2):1124–1138. https://doi.org/10.1007/s40615-024-01947-9
36. Centers for Disease Control and Prevention. Ending the HIV epidemic in the US jurisdictions and plans. March 12, 2024. Available at: https://www.cdc.gov/ehe/php/jurisdictions-plans/index.html. Accessed November 27, 2024.
37. Suva C, Liu J, Sigurdson E, Torio JE, Benson OG. A case study of community-based, cross-sectoral crisis response to the COVID-19 pandemic: serving racialized immigrant communities. *Glob Soc Welf*. 2022;9(3):193–202. https://doi.org/10.1007/s40609-022-00223-0
38. Abdi N, Ebengho S, Mohamed N, et al. Early pandemic access to COVID-19 testing in the Somali community in King County, Washington, USA: a mixed-methods evaluation. *J Racial Ethn Health Disparities*. 2023;10(6):2930–2943. https://doi.org/10.1007/s40615-022-01470-9
39. Nnaji C, Anyango L, Bova C, et al. The Tulumbe! partnership: a case study in developing a community-led research agenda to address HIV among African immigrants in the United States. *Front Public Health*. 2024;12:1406397. https://doi.org/10.3389/fpubh.2024.1406397
40. Kerani RP, Satcher Johnson A, Buskin SE, et al. The epidemiology of HIV among people born outside the United States, 2010–2017. *Public Health Rep*. 2020;135(5):611–620. https://doi.org/10.1177/0033354920942623

Critical Reflections From the Black Women First Initiative

Linda S. Sprague Martinez, PhD, Judith C. Scott, PhD, LICSW, Melanie Rocco, MSW, MPH, Masill Miranda, MSW, Cynthia Tucker, DrPH, and Angela Wangari Walter, PhD, MPH, MSW

In 2020, the Health Resources and Services Administration launched the first initiative focused on Black women in nearly 40 years of the HIV epidemic: the Black Women First initiative. A critical step toward advancing racial equity, the initiative addressed the health and social needs of diverse Black women in HIV care and treatment.

In this essay, we posit that the disproportionate burden of HIV/AIDS experienced by Black women is rooted in racism, not race. Using critical reflexivity and the Public Health Critical Race praxis, we critically discuss the Black Women First initiative's framing and components, the factors contributing to successes and challenges, opportunities to deepen efforts, and recommendations to focus on dismantling racism in future efforts addressing care and treatment for Black women with HIV. We reflect on how racism was challenged through the involvement of Black women with lived experiences and racial justice organizations, although racism was not a focus of the initiative.

Advancing the health of Black women with HIV needs a comprehensive and critical approach that addresses racism by changing intervention funding, service delivery, and the measurement of success. (*Am J Public Health*. 2025;115(9):1500–1507. https://doi.org/10.2105/AJPH.2025.308138)

AJPH September 2025, Vol. 115, No. 9

Black women are disproportionately impacted by HIV. They represent nearly 14% of the female population in the United States[1] and 54% of women newly diagnosed with HIV.[2,3] When the HIV/AIDS epidemic first emerged in the United States during the 1980s, rates of HIV diagnoses were highest among White gay men in large metropolitan areas, and by the 1990s, pronounced racial inequities, which persist today, emerged.[4] In the mid-1980s, the White gay community began receiving HIV education and information about how to stay healthy; however, tailored information for communities of color and focused outreach were lacking.[4,5] Messaging related to HIV/AIDS risk and transmission was characterized by stereotypes, othering, and stigmatized behaviors,[5] focusing on Haitians, heroin users, homosexuals, and hemophiliacs; thus, many in the Black community believed it was not a threat.[5] By 1993, the dearth of public health intervention efforts, combined with racialized policies discussed in the following sections, contributed to HIV/AIDS inequities among Black women.[5–7] These inequities are unnecessary, avoidable, and unjust.

The Ryan White HIV/AIDS Program (RWHAP) has made important contributions to addressing racial and gender inequity over the years and continues to invest in initiatives to reach and provide medical and social services to populations most affected by the HIV/AIDS epidemic.[8,9] Building on the experience of previous initiatives for women of color, the Health Resources and Services Administration (HRSA) addressed a critical need by launching the first initiative in nearly 40 years of the HIV epidemic focused on Black women. The Improving Care and Treatment Coordination: Focusing on Black Women With HIV initiative, also known as the Black Women First initiative (BWF), was funded by the Department of Health and Human Services Office of the Assistant Secretary for Health Minority HIV/AIDS Fund, and the HIV/AIDS Bureau RWHAP Program Part F: Special Projects of National Significance.[10] The BWF initiative includes 12 sites and an Evaluation and Technical Assistance Provider (ETAP), designed specifically to center the priorities and needs of diverse Black women and provide a critical step toward advancing racial equity.

We reflect from our perspectives as members of the initiative on the implementation of the BWF and propose recommendations for research, policy, and practice to improve care and treatment of Black women with HIV. We posit that the inequities experienced by Black women with HIV are not the result of Blackness because racial inequity is rooted in racism,[11,12] and, as such, efforts to address racial inequity call for antiracism.[4,13] We provide background discussion on racism as a driver of the disproportionate burden of HIV and poorer outcomes among Black women, and antiracism as an approach to intervention. Then, drawing on critical reflexivity, we examine the BWF initiative by (1) critically discussing the framing of the initiative and its components, (2) reflecting on the initiative's successes and challenges, and (3) identifying recommendations for future efforts to improve care and treatment of Black women with HIV.[14]

RACE AND RACISM

The notion of race is rooted in an ideology of White supremacy that ties value, expertise, and power to Whiteness. In the colonies, race was rarely used to categorize and stratify humans before the 1600s. The term, "race," in its current conceptualization, emerged during the Enlightenment and was used by Europeans to justify the colonization and enslavement of populations across the Americas.[15] In the United States, laws were established and instituted to systematically strip Africans of their rights, and unlike other enslaved populations, Africans lost the opportunity to obtain freedom and were eventually classified as property.[15] Black women, specifically, faced horrific conditions; they were held in bondage, beaten, sexually exploited, and bred.[16,17] Laws in the mid-1600s that ensured slave status was inherited further fueled the breeding of Black women.[16,17] These new conceptualizations of race and racial hierarchy were used by intellectuals and religious leaders, among others, to justify the institution of slavery.[15] The construction of race was deeply tied to the economics of slavery.

The racial stratification of US society, in which Whiteness and maleness were superior, created the conditions in which Black women remain systematically oppressed.[18] White supremacy remains the dominant ideology in the United States and is embedded in and reinforced by institutions across sectors. The dominant ideology of White supremacy, coupled with patriarchy, creates a culture in which Blackness and womanhood are unfairly disadvantaged, stigmatized, and demeaned. Within this context, Black women are objectified and their value is negated, giving way to multiple forms of racialized oppression, including commodification, exploitation, sexual violence, mutilation, and murder, as well as social stereotypes and marginalization that have spurred generational poverty.[19] Examples of commodification include how Black women's bodies continue to be hypersexualized in popular culture for financial gain.[20] Exploitation, meanwhile, can be seen in how Black women continue to be marginalized and exploited in the labor market.[20] Moreover, Black women experience both health care[21] and state-sponsored violence (e.g., police violence, maternal health neglect),[18,22] which have been justified through cultural tropes (i.e., mammy, welfare queen, jezebel, and sapphire),[20] and are reinforced through economic and social policies such as the Personal Responsibility and Work Opportunity Reconciliation Act.

RACISM AND HIV DISPARITIES AMONG BLACK WOMEN

Racial inequity in the HIV epidemic is not explained by race. Rather, racial inequities are rooted in the racism experienced while living in a racially stratified society. Racism has been defined as a system of advantage based on race.[23] It is a multilevel construct that operates at the societal, institutional, interpersonal, and individual (internalized) levels.[24] At the societal level, racism is described as structural. Structural racism focuses on the interconnectedness between and across institutions. Institutional racism, meanwhile, describes the ways in which racism is embedded in political, economic, and legal institutions and, thus, becomes embedded in policies and practices.[24,25] Structural and institutional racism create the conditions for both interpersonal racism and internalized racism.[14]

For Black women, structural and institutional racism fuel racial inequities in HIV/AIDS outcomes and treatment.[19] Macrosocial factors, including historical context, economic order, legal codes, and ideology, together work to create a socially stratified and segregated society in which Black women are exposed to harmful conditions and deprived of resources.[19] Black women are overrepresented in poverty because of policies such as redlining, and are more likely to live in segregated neighborhoods with relatively higher rates of HIV.[19,26] They are also more likely to experience barriers to HIV treatment associated with transportation, employment, and housing, as well as limited access to high-quality care as the result of resource deprivation in communities of color.[19] Furthermore, historical medical exploitation and Black women's experiences of being denied care, dismissed, or ignored by their providers[19] have resulted in medical mistrust, which may inhibit treatment seeking, affect interpersonal aspects of care, and impact the uptake of preexposure prophylaxis among Black women.[27]

Early HIV transmission messaging was not tailored for Black women and was highly stigmatized; thus, transmission was believed to be the result of engaging in "risky behaviors," deemed immoral. Therefore, many in the Black community believed it was not a threat.[5] This messaging was reinforced by social and cultural institutions that have been characterized as protective for Black women's health. For example, the Black church has long been viewed as the social and religious center of the Black community, encouraging resistance, fostering hope, championing justice, and preserving tradition.[28] Early in the HIV epidemic, before collective efforts such as the National Week of Prayer for the Healing of AIDS, the church, influenced by values shaped by dominant cultural narratives, was silent.[29]

The core values of the Black church include love, inclusiveness, justice, freedom, and equality.[28] According to Douglas and Hopson, unpacking the values of the Black church is complex because, in addition to its core values, it also promulgates a set of contingent values that vary by denomination and the sociodemographics of a given church population. Indeed, the Black church is not a monolith, and its contingent values reflect the Black experience in our broader racialized society; thus, its core and contingent values are in some cases diametrically opposed.[28] For example, the church's rejection of homosexuality and its support of the patriarchal hierarchy contradict the core values of inclusiveness and equality.[28] A lack of acceptance by the church can drive men to hide their orientation and contribute to Black women's risk for and acquisition of HIV.[28]

The national dialogue framing HIV/AIDS as "immoral" at the beginning of the epidemic, as the result of stigmatized behavior, likely contributed to the church's silence and the association of HIV/AIDS with racialized tropes.[29] The Black church's lack of action in the early years of the epidemic fueled stigma and exacerbated the gap in HIV-related resources for the Black community and left the community with a false sense of security with respect to HIV exposure.[28,29]

ANTIRACISM AS A STRATEGY TO ADDRESS HIV INEQUITIES

Racial inequity is the result of racism, and efforts to improve outcomes for Black women with HIV and to advance racial equity require a focus on unraveling the structures and social interpretations that uphold racism. Kendi defines antiracism as "actively opposing and dismantling the policies, practices, and structures of oppression that uphold racism."[30(p106)] Jones elevates the antiracism strategy that involves naming racism, interrogating how racism operates, and then organizing and strategizing the health intervention. Similarly, in the context of improving HIV outcomes for Black women and ending the HIV epidemic, Bowleg et al. stress the importance of confronting racism and intentionally strategizing ways to dismantle it.[31]

Drawing on antiracism and critical scholarship more broadly, Ford and Airhihenbuwa put forward a framework for public health researchers to advance antiracism, Public Health Critical Race praxis (PHCR).[32] PHCR, seen in Table 1, involves 4 areas of focus and 10 underlying principles.

This framework illustrates how antiracism involves an active approach that includes naming race and racism, having a shared understanding of how it operates and influences public health practice, and the study of public health problems, as well as the need for ongoing critical reflection and intentionality. Using this framework, we critically reflect on the BWF initiative and how, although racism was not an initiative focus, it addressed racism to improve the care and treatment coordination for Black women with HIV.

CRITICAL REFLECTIONS ON THE BLACK WOMEN FIRST INITIATIVE

The BWF initiative included 12 community-based organizations and clinics that were funded to implement evidence-based bundled interventions that address socio-cultural health determinants, expand the delivery and utilization of comprehensive HIV care and treatment services, support continuous engagement in care, and improve health outcomes for Black women with HIV in a culturally responsive manner.[33] Racism was not mentioned in the funding announcement, and, as a result, the initiative did not focus on racism and racialization. A goal stated in the funding announcement was to address the sociocultural health determinants that contributed to limited access to care

TABLE 1— Public Health Critical Race Praxis Focus Areas

Focus Area	Description	Embedded Principles
Race consciousness	Understanding racialization, recognizing racism, and attending to how it operates in different contexts	Race consciousness, the primacy of racialization, race as a social construct, the ordinariness of racism, and structural determinism
Knowledge production	Understanding how knowledge production is shaped by structural racism and how racialization impacts projects	Race consciousness, the social construction of knowledge, critical approaches needed, and voice
Conceptualization and measurement	Having context-specific constructs and measures that can account for differences across population, place, and time	Race consciousness, race as a social construct, and intersectionality
Action	Engaging in action to disrupt racism and the systems that sustain it	Race consciousness, disciplinary self-critique, intersectionality, and voice

Source. Ford and Airhihenbuwa.[32]

and treatment of Black women with HIV with consideration of race and gender.[10]

MOVING TOWARD RACE CONSCIOUSNESS

Despite the absence of racism in the funding notice, some of the organizations' proposals discussed racism because those organizations had an explicit focus on addressing racism. Furthermore, at the start of the initiative, racism was consistently discussed in early site planning and implementation meetings. Following the first virtual multisite convening in December 2020, we listened to attendee feedback and recognized the need for active discussions about racism. This led to a 2-part racial equity planning session in August 2021. Part 1 focused on racialization, racism, racial capitalism, and the ways White supremacy operates at the organizational level as well as strategies for organizational change. In part 2, organizations worked on a racial equity planning template.

After the convening, ETAP coaches, who advised organizations on implementation, were asked to follow up with implementation staff during monthly meetings to support continued racial equity planning. Annual visits to organizations continued to explore progress on racial equity planning. Racial equity planning was not built into proposals or required as part of funding, and not all of the 12 BWF organizations had the capacity to plan and implement additional racial equity strategies.

In April 2023, a follow-up session reflecting on racial equity planning was held to engage BWF site staff in an assessment of their racial equity planning process, their progress, and the barriers they encountered. Reflections were shared across sites, and common themes that emerged were discussed. Themes centered on the challenges and facilitators of racial equity planning. Organizational leadership buy-in for racial equity planning was described as a major challenge. Racial equity planning facilitators described by participants included elevating community participation and stakeholder engagement and having an explicit racial equity focus and an organizational strategy focused on advancing racial equity.

KNOWLEDGE PRODUCTION AND ACTION

The centering of Black women's ideas and input and their meaningful involvement in intervention design, adaptation, implementation, and evaluation in the initiative is progress toward challenging racism. This occurred through trainings; community and client advisory boards,[34] which were critical for making cultural adaptations to the original evidence-based and evidence-informed interventions for Black women with HIV at the initiative and organizational levels; and arts-based approaches. Direct staff training, which included in-person workshops, was also used to increase race consciousness and awareness of how power operates in organizations. For example, we hosted cultural humility workshops, which included objectives focused on (1) illustrating the relationship of one's identity to social power, (2) describing how power enacted through structural racism contributes to HIV health disparities, (3) identifying the ways power is enacted to empower or disempower clients in the health care setting, and (4) exploring culturally humble practices to challenge power imbalances. Workshops were facilitated by Black women with similar lived experiences, who engaged participants in interactive reflective activities as well as peer-to-peer and case-based learning.

In addition, the ETAP and its BWF advisory board, which was compensated, developed a leadership development program for Black women with HIV to further support their meaningful involvement in the initiative and beyond. The program was led by Black women with HIV for Black women with HIV and focused on promoting strategies for their meaningful involvement, elevating Black women's lived experience, and addressing topics including racial and gender inequity. We facilitated power-sharing between local partners and initiative staff to redesign interventions and reshape their approaches to working with Black women. At some organizations, adaptations focused on acknowledging and coping with the impacts of racism.

Black women with HIV from advisory boards and across organizations also participated in multisite convenings, which leveraged their expertise to inform design, implementation, and evaluation. For example, 4 women from across the organizations were panelists at the 2023 convening. These efforts facilitated co-learning across organizations and increased the integration of Black women's voices in intervention implementation and adaptation. However, there were also missed opportunities to continue meaningful engagement of the BWF advisory board throughout the implementation of bundled interventions and tailoring of site programs. Advisory board members shared wanting a clearer, more involved role beyond the Leadership Development Program and throughout the initiative, to allow them to bring more of their lived experience to design and implementation.

Storytelling and participatory arts–based methods, which can foster meaningful involvement and inclusivity, were embraced within the BWF initiative to advance change.[35] We actively sought ways to integrate storytelling into BWF programs, such as creating safe spaces and healing circles where women could share their narratives and preserving their overlooked or unheard stories and experiences. Through participatory arts–based methods such as photovoice, films, theater, visual arts, and music,[36,37] we witnessed the emergence of a powerful medium for self-expression and community building.[38] The participatory nature of these artistic endeavors encouraged collaborative storytelling, inviting Black women to co-create narratives that resonated with their lived realities.[35] This approach validated lived experiences and also empowered Black women to take ownership of their stories, fostering a sense of agency and pride. They provided alternative means of expression, catering to diverse learning styles and preferences, ensuring that every woman had a voice regardless of their background or communication abilities.[35] For example, one site partnered with The Medea Project to incorporate storytelling through theater to illustrate the relationships between structural oppression and the lived experience of formerly incarcerated Black women with HIV.

Storytelling is an important element of antiracism practice[32]; it facilitates inclusion and challenges the dominant narrative rooted in White supremacy, which situates expertise and knowledge production in the context of Whiteness.[39] By incorporating narratives and personal experiences, the program created a more engaging and relatable environment. In addition, arts-based efforts, storytelling, and Black women's meaningful involvement seen across the initiative were a form of resistance in that they celebrated and centered Black women's expertise. This approach and the active participation of Black women contributed to more comprehensive and relevant interventions that addressed the unique needs and aspirations of Black women with HIV and more sustained health care engagement.

CONCEPTUALIZATION AND MEASUREMENT

During the initiative, a shared conceptualization of racism was not developed. In addition, how racism operates across geographic contexts and the relationship between interlocking systems of oppression and implementation were not examined. Perceptions of discrimination based on race and the impacts of racism, as well as intersectionality, were explored qualitatively in the context of implementation. In addition, qualitative interviews were added at the end of the intervention period to explore perceptions of racism and its impact on implementation.

LESSONS LEARNED

Throughout the initiative, Black women's health and quality of life were prioritized, and their expertise was integrated to inform intervention design, implementation, and evaluation. It was Black women's voices that moved the initiative toward a focus on racism. Racism was not viewed as a peripheral issue by implementation staff or client advisory board members. Instead, it was considered a fundamental factor that impedes any attempts at intervention because racialized policies and initiatives such as redlining, Jim Crow laws, discriminatory criminal sentencing, the War on Drugs, and child welfare policies shape communities and, in turn, how systems operate. Improving treatment for Black women with HIV requires plans for addressing racism[13,31,40] because racism is embedded in all organizations and shapes practice, including service delivery.[41]

While an important conversation about racism and racial equity was started as a part of this initiative, racial equity planning was challenging, and more time, resources, and focused attention needed to be invested. We did not coalesce around a shared understanding of racism, its impact on our work, and ways to address it. For example, during our convening debrief, implementation teams described the difficulty of having leadership who were not interested in organizational change and did not consider racial equity a priority. It was also noted that being a predominantly Black organization is not enough and that intentional racial equity planning is needed in all organizations.

Although we discussed racism as it relates to knowledge production, it was not adequately examined, addressed, or evaluated by the initiative. Implementation staff, partners, and research team members came to spaces with varying understandings of racism that often reflected their journeys and the microcosms of their individual and contextual environments (e.g., organizations, communities, society). Starting the conversation by naming racism, reflecting on racialization, and developing a shared language about racism allows for effective and ongoing conversations and the ability to move from meaningful discussion to actions with measurable impact.[13] This process entails a fundamental respect for persons, understanding of the systemic structural scaffolding of racism (e.g., pillars of White supremacy, social construction of race),[42] understanding of organizational culture (e.g., how organizational members come to learn about the expectations of the organization and how they behave),[43] and a process for managing ideological differences.

While language may evolve over time, training and education toward a shared understanding of racism, particularly when working with multiple groups, allows for greater knowledge and awareness, responsiveness, transparency, skill, and capacity building, as well as the opportunity for individual and collective learning, unlearning, and relearning. Through ongoing collective training, individuals and organizations can establish goals, objectives, and accountability benchmarks to address racism and move toward racial justice. As this was not included in the original funding notice and expectations for the initiative, we identify this as an important lesson learned for the BWF initiative. This is critical if we are to end the HIV epidemic.

The literature emphasizes that conceptual models that fail to explicitly identify racism perpetuate racism and, in turn, further proliferate health inequity.[13,31] Racism underlies barriers to high-quality health care, including HIV treatment.[31] Acknowledging the role of racialized policy in perpetuating inequity was a missed opportunity in the context of the intervention and evaluation framework.

FUTURE DIRECTIONS

There is an increased recognition of the role of racism in shaping the distribution of disease, health outcomes, and mortality. Continued investment in this area is paramount. We echo the work of Bowleg, Bailey, Ford, Jones, and the many other scholars who are calling on our fields to center racism and to engage in critical public health practice to effectively improve health and reform policies and programs that stand in the way of addressing racial inequity.[11–13,31,32] In the following sections, we provide a set of recommendations for funders, researchers, and practitioners to consider in advancing this work.

- Funders, especially those in the private sector, can lead by acknowledging racism as the root cause of inequities and providing a clear definition of what racism is and how it operates at different levels, and funding initiatives focused on dismantling racism embedded in policies to reshape practice and address the priorities of Black women.[11] Funders can also require the use of frameworks informed by critical and antiracism scholarship[13,32] and set expectations for measurement that captures racism, thus creating conditions that hold grantees accountable for supporting efforts to dismantle racism and advance racial equity. We have seen some progress in this area with research and prevention programs funded by the National Institutes of Health[44] and the Centers for Disease Control and Prevention.[45]
- Institutions and organizations can examine the ways in which practices, procedures, and policies reinforce oppressive structures and identify opportunities for change. Intervention needs to go beyond service delivery to focus on organizational practices, procedures, and policies such as hiring practices to ensure staff reflect the population; opportunities for professional development and growth and salary equity; and training for all staff,

administrative leaders, and medical providers on implicit bias and the ways it shapes organizational practice.[13] Meaningfully involving Black women with HIV in the redesign of organizational practices, procedures, and policies, as well as service delivery, can ensure priorities are aligned.

- Research and evaluation efforts should be designed in collaboration with Black women with HIV and should include systems to monitor and measure racism at multiple levels. The meaningful involvement of Black women in decision-making can allow researchers and partners to engage in critical reflection to identify how disciplinary norms are racialized and promulgate bias. However, it is also important that community members serving in leadership roles and on boards are compensated for their expertise and labor so as not to replicate societal extractive practices. These are elements funders can encourage and champion through proposal requirements.
- Through community partnerships, organizations can provide wraparound services when they are not provided on site. This approach leverages each partner's strength and increases capacity and access to resources for the community being served.[46] We found that partnership increased the participation of Black women with HIV. Their participation across all aspects of the work led to meaningful adaptations and increased engagement within the bundled set of care services. They informed planning and implementation at sites through participation in advisory boards and feedback groups.

CONCLUSION

Although the intention of the initiative was not to address racism, racism was challenged during the initiative through the meaningful involvement of Black women with HIV. We learned that focusing on a racialized population is not enough to end the HIV epidemic; it is just 1 piece of the puzzle. Addressing racism and advancing the health of Black women with HIV will take a comprehensive and critical approach, including changing the way we fund interventions, deliver them, and measure success. This will be no easy feat in the coming years. Racial inequities are the result of racism, and it is long overdue that we address it. AJPH

ABOUT THE AUTHORS

Linda S. Sprague Martinez and Melanie Rocco are with the Health Disparities Institute, University of Connecticut School of Medicine, UConn Health, Hartford, CT. Judith C. Scott is with the Boston University School of Social Work, Boston, MA. Masill Miranda is with AIDS United in Washington, DC. Cynthia Tucker is with the AIDS Foundation Chicago in Chicago, IL. Angela Wangari Walter is with the Department of Public Health, Zuckerberg College of Health Sciences, University of Massachusetts, Lowell.

CORRESPONDENCE

Correspondence should be sent to Linda Sprague Martinez, Health Disparities Institute, University of Connecticut School of Medicine, UConn Health, 241 Main St, 5th Floor, Hartford, CT 06106 (e-mail: spraguemartinez@uchc.edu). Reprints can be ordered at https://ajph.org by clicking the "Reprints" link.

PUBLICATION INFORMATION

Full Citation: Sprague Martinez LS, Scott JC, Rocco M, Miranda M, Tucker C, Walter AW. Critical reflections from the Black Women First initiative. *Am J Public Health*. 2025;115(9):1500–1507.

Acceptance Date: March 24, 2025.

DOI: https://doi.org/10.2105/AJPH.2025.308138

ORCID iDs:

Linda S. Sprague Martinez https://orcid.org/0000-0002-5070-7640

Judith C. Scott https://orcid.org/0000-0002-1561-9354

Melanie Rocco https://orcid.org/0009-0003-4787-731X

Masill Miranda https://orcid.org/0009-0007-0376-0450

Cynthia Tucker https://orcid.org/0000-0003-0645-5308

Angela Wangari Walter https://orcid.org/0000-0003-0098-6802

CONTRIBUTORS

L. Sprague Martinez contributed to conceptualization and writing the original draft. J. C. Scott, M. Rocco, M. Miranda, C. Tucker, and A. Wangari Walter contributed to conceptualization, writing, review, and editing.

ACKNOWLEDGMENTS

This study is funded by the Health Resources and Services Administration (HRSA) of the US Department of Health and Human Services (HHS) grant U90HA39727.

The authors would like to thank the 12 demonstration sites as well as the many participants who engaged with and informed the initiative. In addition, we would like to thank Cecilia Flores-Rodriguez, PhD, for her efforts to inform racial equity action planning across sites. Finally, we thank Serena Rajabiun, PhD, MPH, who reviewed the many iterations of this essay over the past 18 months.

Note. The contents are those of the authors and do not necessarily represent the official views of nor an endorsement by HRSA/HHS, or the US government.

CONFLICTS OF INTEREST

The authors declare that they have no competing interests, commercial associations, or sources of support that might pose a conflict of interest.

HUMAN PARTICIPANT PROTECTION

Ethics approvals were obtained from the University of Massachusetts, Lowell, and the Boston University Charles River Campus institutional review boards, protocol numbers 20-147 and 5832X.

REFERENCES

1. Annual estimates of the resident population by sex, race, and Hispanic origin for the United States: April 1, 2020 to July 1, 2022 (NC-EST2022-SR11H). Washington, DC: US Census Bureau; 2023.
2. Centers for Disease Control and Prevention. *HIV Surveillance Report*. US Department of Health and Human Services. Available at: https://stacks.cdc.gov/view/cdc/149071. Accessed May 24, 2024.
3. Hassan KS, Coon DW. The provider's role in retaining Black women with HIV in care: a scoping review. *J Int Assoc Provid AIDS Care*. 2024;23:23259582231224232. https://doi.org/10.1177/23259582231224
4. Harrison SE, Muessig K, Poteat T, et al. Addressing racism's role in the US HIV epidemic: qualitative findings from three Ending the HIV Epidemic prevention projects. *J Acquir Immune*

Defic Syndr. 2022;90(suppl 1):S46–S55. https://doi.org/10.1097/QAI.0000000000002965

5. Scott A. Erased by respectability: the intersections of AIDS, race, and gender in Black America. *Women, Gender, and Families of Color.* 2022;10(1): 71–99. https://doi.org/10.5406/23260947.10.1.04
6. Hutchinson J. AIDS and racism in America. *J Natl Med Assoc.* 1992;84(2):119–124.
7. Schneider CL. Racism, drug policy, and AIDS. *Polit Sci Q.* 1998;113(3):427–446. https://doi.org/10.2307/2658075
8. Cheever LW, Rich J, Adashi EY. The Ryan White HIV/AIDS Program: thirty years of addressing health disparities. *J Health Care Poor Underserved.* 2024;35(2):726–730. https://doi.org/10.1353/hpu.2024.a928642
9. Goyal R, Hotchkiss J, Gilman B, et al. The health equity implications of the HRSA Ryan White HIV/AIDS Program. *AIDS.* 2024;38(7):1025–1032. https://doi.org/10.1097/QAD.0000000000003836
10. Improving care and treatment coordination: focusing on Black women with HIV. Rockville, MD: Health Resources and Services Administration; 2020.
11. Bailey ZD, Feldman JM, Bassett MT. How structural racism works—racist policies as a root cause of US racial health inequities. *N Engl J Med.* 2021; 384(8):768–773. https://doi.org/10.1056/NEJMms2025396
12. Jones CP. Invited commentary: "Race," racism, and the practice of epidemiology. *Am J Epidemiol.* 2001;154(4):299–304, discussion 305–306. https://doi.org/10.1093/aje/154.4.299
13. Jones CP. Toward the science and practice of anti-racism: launching a national campaign against racism. *Ethn Dis.* 2018;28(suppl 1): 231–234. https://doi.org/10.18865/ed.28.S1.231
14. Wendel ML, Garney WR, Castle BF, Ingram CM. Critical reflexivity of communities on their experience to improve population health. *Am J Public Health.* 2018;108(7):896–901. https://doi.org/10.2105/AJPH.2018.304404
15. Smedley A. "Race" and the construction of human identity. *Am Anthropol.* 1998;100(3):690–702.
16. Jennings T. "Us colored women had to go through a plenty": sexual exploitation of African-American slave women. *Journal of Women's History.* 1990;1(3):45–74. https://doi.org/10.1353/jowh.2010.0050
17. Cooper I. Commodification of the Black body, sexual objectification and social hierarchies during slavery. *Earlham Historical Journal.* 2015;7(2):21–41.
18. Laster Pirtle WN. Racial capitalism: a fundamental cause of novel coronavirus (COVID-19) pandemic inequities in the United States. *Health Educ Behav.* 2020;47(4):504–508. https://doi.org/10.1177/1090198120922942
19. Prather C, Fuller TR, Jeffries WL, et al. Racism, African American women, and their sexual and reproductive health: a review of historical and contemporary evidence and implications for health equity. *Health Equity.* 2018;2(1):249–259. https://doi.org/10.1089/heq.2017.0045
20. Rousseau N. Understanding commodification. In: Rousseau N, ed. *Black Woman's Burden: Commodifying Black Reproduction.* New York, NY: Palgrave Macmillan US; 2009:173–176.
21. Campbell C. Medical violence, obstetric racism, and the limits of informed consent for Black women. *Mich J Race L.* 2021;26:47.
22. Sprague Martinez L, Scott JC, Rocco M, et al. Policies enacted during COVID-19 came with unintended health benefits: why go back? *BMC Health Serv Res.* 2023;23(1):496–498. https://doi.org/10.1186/s12913-023-09448-x
23. Wellman DT. *Portraits of White Racism.* 2nd ed. Cambridge, England: Cambridge University Press; 1993.
24. Bailey ZD, Krieger N, Agénor M, Graves J, Linos N, Bassett MT. Structural racism and health inequities in the USA: evidence and interventions. *Lancet.* 2017;389(10077):1453–1463. https://doi.org/10.1016/S0140-6736(17)30569-X
25. Jones CP. Levels of racism: a theoretic framework and a gardener's tale. *Am J Public Health.* 2000;90(8): 1212–1215. https://doi.org/10.2105/ajph.90.8.1212
26. Brawner BM, Kerr J, Castle BF, et al. A systematic review of neighborhood-level influences on HIV vulnerability. *AIDS Behav.* 2022;26(3):874–934. https://doi.org/10.1007/s10461-021-03448-w
27. Tekeste M, Hull S, Dovidio JF, et al. Differences in medical mistrust between Black and White women: implications for patient–provider communication about PrEP. *AIDS Behav.* 2019;23(7): 1737–1748. https://doi.org/10.1007/s10461-018-2283-2
28. Douglas KB, Hopson RE. Understanding the Black church: the dynamics of change. *The Journal of Religious Thought.* 2001;56(2/1):95–113.
29. Otchere A. *"Our Church Lights the Way": The Black Church Response to HIV/AIDS in Connecticut, 1981–2005.* Dissertation. Yale University; April 3, 2023. Available at: https://hshm.yale.edu/sites/default/files/files/Otchere%2C%20Amma%20-%20Final%20Project.pdf. Accessed June 7, 2025.
30. Kendi IX. *How to Be an Antiracist.* New York, NY: One World, Random House; 2023.
31. Bowleg L, Malekzadeh AN, Mbaba M, Boone CA. Ending the HIV epidemic for all, not just some: structural racism as a fundamental but overlooked social-structural determinant of the US HIV epidemic. *Curr Opin HIV AIDS.* 2022;17(2): 40–45. https://doi.org/10.1097/COH.0000000000000724
32. Ford CL, Airhihenbuwa CO. The public health critical race methodology: praxis for antiracism research. *Soc Sci Med.* 2010;71(8):1390–1398. https://doi.org/10.1016/j.socscimed.2010.07.030
33. Rajabiun S, Heath C, Walter AW, et al. The Black Women First initiative: using implementation science to examine bundled interventions to improve care and treatment coordination for Black women with HIV. *BMC Health Serv Res.* 2023;23(1):551. https://doi.org/10.1186/s12913-023-09446-z
34. Rocco M, Downes A, Tucker C, et al. Using advisory boards to enhance and implement interventions for Black women. 2022. Available at: https://targethiv.org/sites/default/files/media/documents/2023-03/BWF_CABs_HIV_Care_Brief.pdf. Accessed June 7, 2025.
35. Etmanski C, Kyte A, Cassidy M, Bade N. Three examples of engagement through photovoice. *Engaged Scholar Journal.* 2022,8(1).20–36. https://doi.org/10.15402/esj.v8i2.70754
36. Rocco M, Meshesha M, Scott J, et al. Using participatory art approaches to promote health and empower client voice: examples from the Black Women First initiative. 2023. Available at: https://targethiv.org/sites/default/files/media/documents/2023-03/BWF_ParticipatoryArts_IssueBrief.pdf. Accessed June 7, 2025.
37. Martinez LS, Scott JC, Rocco M, Walter AW, Rajabiun S. How is COVID-19 impacting you? A community-based photovoice workshop. *Am J Public Health.* 2022;112(11):1541–1542. https://doi.org/10.2105/AJPH.2022.307054
38. Strand M, Albany Y, Buthelezi MNL, et al. Snow. Reflecting on arts-based participatory research: considerations for more equitable transdisciplinary collaborations. *Ecology and Society.* 2024. 29(4):29. https://doi.org/10.5751/ES-15563-290429
39. Petteway RJ. On epidemiology as racial-capitalist (re) colonization and epistemic violence. *Crit Public Health.* 2023;33(1):5–12. https://doi.org/10.1080/09581596.2022.2107486
40. El-Bassel N. Why addressing racism against Black women in health care is key to ending the US HIV epidemic. *The Conversation.* December 6, 2021. Available at: https://theconversation.com/why-addressing-racism-against-black-women-in-health-care-is-key-to-ending-the-us-hiv-epidemic-172842. Accessed May 24, 2024.
41. Ray V. A theory of racialized organizations. *Am Sociol Rev.* 2019;84(1):26–53. https://doi.org/10.1177/0003122418822335
42. Tourse R, Hamilton-Mason J, Wewiorski NJ. *Systemic Racism in the United States.* Cham, Switzerland: Springer International. 2018.
43. Schein EH. *Organization Culture and Leadership.* 4th ed. San Francisco, CA: Jossey-Bass; 2010.
44. National Institutes of Health. Ending structural racism. 2023. Available at: https://www.nih.gov/ending-structural-racism. Accessed January 31, 2024.
45. Centers for Disease Control and Prevention. CDC's efforts to address racism as a fundamental driver of health disparities. 2023. Available at: https://www.cdc.gov/minorityhealth/racism-disparities/cdc-efforts.html. Accessed January 31, 2024.
46. Farhang L, Morales X. Building community power to achieve health and racial equity: principles to guide transformative partnerships with local communities. *NAM Perspect.* 2022;2022. https://doi.org/10.31478/202206d

Primary Prevention of Drug Overdoses in Rural Low-Resource and Tribal Communities: A Cluster Randomized Trial

Kelli A. Komro, PhD, MPH, Melvin D. Livingston, PhD, Juli R. Skinner, MSW, LMSW, Bethany J. Livingston, BS, Terrence K. Kominsky, PhD, Ashna Jagtiani, MBBS, MPH, Caroline M. Barry, PhD, MPH, Alexander C. Wagenaar, PhD, Hannah L. F. Cooper, ScD, Megan Harmon, BA, Emily Ivanich, MSPH, Hannah LaBounty, LCSW, Ashley N. Gassaway, MSW, and Sierra L. Talavera-Brown, BS

See also Adolescent Mental Health, pp. 1377–1453.

Objectives. To determine the Connect intervention's effectiveness in reducing substance use among rural and tribal adolescents in northeastern Oklahoma.

Methods. We conducted a 2-arm cluster randomized trial from 2021 to 2024, with 10 high schools per condition.

Results. At baseline, 919 students were enrolled (mean age = 15 years), and the majority were American Indian or White. Alcohol-use days during the past 30 days was reduced by 18% per survey wave in the intervention compared with the control condition (rate ratio [RR] = 0.82; 95% confidence interval [CI] = 0.72, 0.93; t = −3.02; *P* = .003), binge drinking was reduced by 26% (RR = 0.74; 95% CI = 0.64, 0.86; t = −3.90; *P* < .001), cannabis use was reduced by 11% (RR = 0.89; 95% CI = 0.80, 1.00; t = −2.03; *P* = .04), and prescription opioid misuse was reduced by 40% (RR = 0.60; 95% CI = 0.43, 0.85; t = −2.86; *P* = .004). Model-predicted means revealed the control condition followed the expected developmental trajectory of increased substance use and the intervention condition showed a flat or decreasing use pattern.

Conclusions. The Connect intervention prevented the typical escalation of substance use during adolescence.

Trial Registration. ClinicalTrials.gov NCT04839978. Registered on April 9, 2021. Version 10, April 30, 2025. (*Am J Public Health*. 2025;115(9):1508–1517. https://doi.org/10.2105/AJPH.2025.308205)

AJPH September 2025, Vol. 115, No. 9

Rural White and American Indian/Alaska Native (AI/AN) populations face disproportionate substance use harms.[1] Historical and structural inequities, including colonization, forced assimilation, and systemic racism, contributed to lasting disparities among AI/AN populations.[2,3] These challenges are compounded by factors shared with rural White populations, such as economic instability, poverty, limited health care access, and isolation.[4] By 2022, during the fourth wave of the US overdose crisis, AI/ANs aged 15 to 34 years had the highest overdose death rates of all racial/ethnic groups.[5]

Decades of prevention research have identified effective strategies,[6] yet rates of alcohol-, cannabis-, and opioid-related harms among youths and young adults continue at high levels,[7] disparities widen,[8] and tragic consequences prevail.[9,10] These patterns indicate an urgent need for prevention strategies addressing inequities and providing culturally relevant, sustainable solutions for rural and AI/AN communities.

The current trial was funded by the National Institute on Drug Abuse through the Preventing Opioid Use Disorder in Older Adolescents and

Young Adults Initiative, part of the National Institutes of Health's Helping to End Addiction Long-Term Initiative.[11] Designed collaboratively between academic prevention scientists and members of Cherokee Nation Behavioral Health, a department within the Cherokee Nation health system,[12] the trial was implemented in rural, multiracial communities within tribal reservation boundaries. The objective of this trial was to determine whether the Connect intervention (a combined school and family drug use preventive intervention) is effective at reducing substance use among rural and tribal adolescents in northeastern Oklahoma.

METHODS

A 2-arm, cluster randomized controlled trial tested the effectiveness of a combined school and family drug use preventive intervention, compared with a delayed-intervention control (schools offered the treatment following the trial) in rural communities in northeastern Oklahoma.[13] The target population was older adolescents (10th-grade students at baseline; mean age = 15.5 years) in high schools in low-resource, sparsely populated rural towns. Eligible high schools were located within counties overlapping the tribal reservation, with town populations under 3000 and class sizes of 30 to 100 students. We excluded schools within metropolitan or micropolitan cores or with existing community drug prevention coalitions. All 10th-grade students (ages 15–17 years) enrolled in fall 2021 who could understand English were eligible.[13]

Figure A (available as a supplement to the online version of this article at http://www.ajph.org) displays the CONSORT flowchart for the study. Of 28 schools that met the study inclusion criteria, 22 were invited to a recruitment meeting based on geographic dispersion, and 20 agreed to participate in the study and to be randomized to intervention (n = 10) or delayed-intervention control (n = 10) conditions. Among the 20 high schools, nearly 70% of students were eligible for free or reduced price lunch and nearly 50% of students were American Indian. Community populations ranged from 386 to 2888 (mean = 1103), each with only 1 high school.

To ensure balance across study conditions and valid inference, we used constrained randomization to allocate communities to either the intervention or control. Full details of the constrained randomization process are described elsewhere.[13] Briefly, we enumerated all possible randomization schemes and then restricted them to those that met a priori balance constraints on school and community factors. We selected the final randomization scheme from the restricted schemes by sampling a single scheme from the pool of possible schemes with equal probability.

Parent or guardian consent and student assent were obtained following randomization. In fall 2021, a baseline survey was conducted with the 10th grade cohort in all 20 study high schools (n = 919; response rate = 87%). We conducted 5 follow-up surveys of the study cohort approximately every 6 months over 3 years (response rates: spring 2022, 89%; fall 2022, 88%; spring 2023, 85%; fall 2023, 83%; spring 2024, 83%). Response rates did not differ by study condition. The school and family interventions began in spring 2022 and continued through spring 2024. For 3 years, an annual $750 incentive was provided to each study school to help offset administrative burdens. Students were provided a $5 cash incentive for each survey completed.

Intervention

Intervention framework. Interventions were guided by previous research,[14–18] culturally responsive and promising intervention practices with Indigenous communities,[12,19] socio-ecological and risk and protective frameworks,[20] and an Indigenous relational worldview perspective.[21,22] They aimed to influence and reinforce interrelationships between contextual (e.g., family, school, community) and intra- and interlevel (i.e., mind, body, spirit) factors promoting health and well-being.

Connect Brief Intervention. Connect Brief Intervention (CBI) with motivational interviewing (MI) was adapted from our previously designed and tested CBI[17] and an effective brief intervention for school-based health centers.[23,24] Adaptations facilitated digital delivery despite extensive pandemic-related school disruptions and maximized reach to in-person as well as remote students. We implemented CBI using the Computerized Intervention Authoring System platform[25,26] and administered it in schools.

All students in the intervention condition were eligible to participate in CBI once per semester for 4 semesters. A Connect coach from the youth services branch of Cherokee Nation Behavioral Health facilitated CBI delivery to students. Remote students were sent an e-mail invitation with instructions via their school e-mail address. Students in school were individually invited by the Connect coach or school counselor to participate in the 15-minute-maximum CBI in a private location during school periods determined by the school. CBI used an animated narrator that assessed risk, delivered information, and initiated MI. For low-risk students, MI affirmed drug-free decisions and set personal goals. For students assessed at moderate-to-high risk (at least monthly use of alcohol or cannabis or misuse of opioids during the past 6 months), MI encouraged students to avoid risky situations and drug use. Moderate-to-high-risk students also received follow-up MI sessions with the Connect coach at school or over Zoom to reassess risk and promote change.

Among all eligible students, 87%, 83%, 87%, and 87% completed CBI each semester during 10th-grade spring, 11th-grade fall, 11th-grade spring, and 12th-grade fall, respectively. Because of hiring challenges during the early part of the COVID-19 pandemic, no Connect coach was available during the 10th-grade spring semester for follow-up sessions with moderate-to-high-risk students. During both 11th-grade semesters and the 12th-grade fall semester, follow-up sessions were completed among 82% (n = 49), 56% (n = 30), and 78% (n = 40) of eligible students per semester, respectively. All students flagged for follow-up during 11th and 12th grade were invited for a second follow-up during 12th-grade spring semester, with 62% (n = 69) completed. Details on CBI design and implementation are provided in Appendix A (available as a supplement to the online version of this article at https://www.ajph.org). We offered schools 2 options for teacher training on youth mental health support; however, because of demands on teacher time, we were only able to conduct a brief training in 4 of the 10 schools.

Connect Kits for Family Action. We developed and implemented a multiyear home-based intervention as a low-cost feasible prevention tool for rural communities, addressing challenges due to geographic dispersion, limited infrastructure and human resources, and COVID-19 pandemic-related barriers.[27] Although we retained core principles of environmental prevention and adult proficiency to promote healthy youth behaviors, we modified our community organizing intervention[14,16] to (1) focus on families and (2) minimize person-to-person contact. Our resultant Connect Kits for Family Action (CKFA) included 9 kits mailed to parents and guardians over 3 years (10th–12th grade). On average, 3% of kits per mailing were undeliverable.

Yearly themes provided the overall framework for developmentally tailored information, cues to action, interactive activities, and resources. The first-year kits, themed "Connection Matters to Teens," encouraged family mealtimes and spending time together. The second-year kits, themed "Safe Places Matter to Teens," provided guidance and resources for safe alcohol and medication storage and disposal, mental health promotion, and ensuring safe celebrations. The third-year kits, themed "Community Matters to Teens," included media literacy and advocacy skill development, with special information on youth exposure to local medical marijuana dispensary advertisements, as well as skill development and resources for future planning, goal setting, and healthy transition to adulthood. Details on kit contents, cultural tailoring, and implementation are described in Appendix B (available as a supplement to the online version of this article at https://www.ajph.org).

Outcome Measures

Prespecified trial primary outcome measures, drawn from standard items from the Monitoring the Future study,[28] included frequency (number of days) during the past 30 days of any (1) alcohol use, (2) binge drinking (defined as having at least 4 [among young women and those not disclosing gender] or 5 [among young men] standard alcoholic drinks within a couple of hours), (3) cannabis (marijuana) use, and (4) prescription opioid misuse (defined as "without a doctor's prescription or differently than how a doctor or medical provider told you to use it").

Secondary outcome measures included depression and anxiety. Depression was measured with the Patient Health Questionnaire 8-item depression scale (PHQ-8), established as a valid measure of current depression in the general population.[29] We measured anxiety with the Generalized Anxiety Disorder 7-item scale (GAD-7), found to have acceptable specificity and sensitivity and to differentiate between mild and moderate generalized anxiety disorder among adolescents.[30] The risk and protective measures collected included normative estimates, social normative beliefs, perceived access to drugs, social support, self-efficacy, and perceptions of getting in trouble for use. For scales without existing scoring metrics, we used mean scoring. There were no changes to the primary outcome measures. After baseline data collection, but prior to the collection of follow-up waves, we changed social support from a single scale to separate scales for each relationship (parent, friend, teacher, and community) following psychometric analysis. A detailed description of survey measures, reliability and validity was described previously.[18,31]

Statistical Analysis

After describing baseline characteristics, we estimated generalized linear

AJPH September 2025, Vol. 115, No. 9

mixed models assessing the effects of the preventive intervention on substance use behaviors and related outcomes among the cohort present at baseline (n = 919). The fixed effects portion of the model is:

$$(1)\quad g(y_{1\text{-}5}) = \beta_0 + \beta_1\ \text{TimeL} + \beta_2\ \text{IntG} + \beta_3\ \text{TimeL} * \text{IntG} + \beta_4 y_0 + \beta_{5\text{-}12} X_i + \beta_{13\text{-}21} Z_s$$

where $g()$ represents the link function for outcome y at follow-up times 1 to 5, TimeL is modeled as a continuous linear variable representing the survey wave (wave is the time point at which surveys were administered), IntG is an indicator for treatment condition, y_0 is the baseline value of the corresponding outcome, X_i is a series of individual-level baseline covariates, and Z_s is the series of school-level covariates used in the constrained randomization. X_i is included to increase precision and includes race, gender, age, and food insecurity. The parameter of primary interest is β_3, the difference in slope between the intervention and control conditions. For Poisson models, this coefficient is exponentiated to provide a rate ratio interpreted as the relative change per survey wave between the intervention and control conditions. Our models account for both school-level clustering and repeated measures within students over time by estimating a random intercept for school, and allow within-student residuals to correlate over time following an AR(1) covariance structure. We estimated all models using PROC GLIMMIX in SAS version 9.4 (SAS Institute, Cary, NC). Poisson mixed effects models were estimated for count outcomes, and linear mixed models were estimated for scale outcomes. All models used the containment method for approximating the denominator degrees of freedom. As a sensitivity analysis, we reran all models treating survey wave as categorical. To facilitate interpretation, we estimated model-predicted outcomes by wave and study condition, and they are presented alongside tests of the difference in slope by study condition.

Missing data in our models arises from 2 processes. First, baseline measures may be missing because of item nonresponse during the baseline survey. Second, wave-level missingness may occur through attrition or absence during a specific survey wave. Missingness due to item nonresponse is minimal, ranging from 2% to 4% across our primary outcome models, and is considered ignorable. Missingness due to attrition is handled via maximum likelihood, assuming missingness at random conditional on the measured outcomes.[32]

RESULTS

Of 919 enrolled students at baseline, 465 (88% of eligible sample) were in the intervention and 454 (85%) in the control condition. There were no statistically significant differences in response rates or loss to follow-up by study condition. Among the 465 students in the intervention condition, 289 (62%) completed all survey waves, 50 (11%) were middle censored (i.e., missed at least 1 wave and returned at a subsequent wave), and 126 (27%) were right censored (i.e., lost to follow-up). Of the 454 students in the control condition, 274 (60%) completed all waves, 47 (10%) were middle censored, and 133 (29%) were right censored (Figure A). Reasons for attrition included any absence or long-term absence, parent or student refusal, special education, disabled, moved, graduated, or dropped out.

Table 1 and Table A (available as a supplement to the online version of this article at https://www.ajph.org) show baseline characteristics for the overall cohort and by intervention condition.

Trial Outcomes

The intervention effectively prevented the well-established typical escalation during adolescence of all 4 primary outcomes, including past 30-day frequency of alcohol use, binge drinking, cannabis use, and prescription opioid misuse. The number of alcohol-use days during the past 30 days was reduced by 18% per survey wave among students in the intervention compared with control condition (rate ratio [RR] = 0.82; 95% confidence interval [CI] = 0.72, 0.93; $t = -3.02$; $P = .003$). Similarly, binge drinking was reduced 26% per survey wave (RR = 0.74; 95% CI = 0.64, 0.86; $t = -3.90$; $P < .001$), cannabis use was reduced 11% per wave (RR = 0.89; 95% CI = 0.80, 1.00; $t = -2.03$; $P = .04$), and prescription opioid misuse was reduced 40% per wave (RR = 0.60; 95% CI = 0.43, 0.85; $t = -2.86$; $P = .004$).

In Figures 1 through 3, we present model-predicted means by survey wave and study condition for the primary outcomes. For each outcome, the control condition followed the long-standing expected developmental trajectory of increased substance use. Among students in the intervention condition, substance use trajectories showed a flat or decreasing use pattern over the study period. For number of alcohol-use days during the past 30 days, the control condition reported a 20% increase per wave (RR = 1.20; 95% CI = 1.09, 1.32), whereas no increase was observed in the intervention condition (RR = 0.98; 95% CI = 0.90, 1.08;

TABLE 1— Student Baseline Characteristics Overall and by Study Condition: Northeastern Oklahoma, Fall 2021

Characteristic	Overall, Mean ±SD or No. (%) (n = 919)	Control, Mean ±SD or No. (%) (n = 454)	Intervention, Mean ±SD or No. (%) (n = 465)
Demographics			
Age, y	15.5 ±0.7	15.6 ±0.7	15.5 ±0.6
Gender			
Female	444 (48.5)	214 (47.5)	230 (49.5)
Male	437 (47.7)	222 (49.2)	215 (46.2)
Decline to answer	35 (3.8)	15 (3.3)	20 (4.3)
Race			
American Indian only	266 (29.2)	136 (30.3)	130 (28.2)
White only	323 (35.5)	149 (33.2)	174 (37.7)
American Indian and White	205 (22.5)	103 (22.9)	102 (22.1)
Other	116 (12.7)	61 (13.6)	55 (11.9)
Receive free or reduced price lunch			
Yes	673 (74.0)	344 (76.8)	329 (71.2)
No	86 (9.5)	35 (7.8)	51 (11.0)
Don't know	151 (16.6)	69 (15.4)	82 (17.8)
Food insecurity			
A lot	35 (3.8)	20 (4.4)	15 (3.2)
Sometimes	123 (13.5)	68 (15.1)	55 (11.9)
Never	756 (82.7)	363 (80.5)	393 (84.9)
Substance use in the past 30 days			
Alcohol use	166 (18.2)	92 (20.4)	74 (16.1)
No. of alcohol use days	0.5 ±1.9	0.6 ±2.1	0.5 ±1.8
Binge drinking	95 (10.5)	52 (11.6)	43 (9.3)
No. of binge drinking days	0.4 ±1.8	0.5 ±2.0	0.3 ±1.5
Cannabis use	136 (15.1)	68 (15.3)	68 (14.8)
No. of cannabis use days	1.7 ±5.9	1.8 ±6.1	1.5 ±5.8
Rx opioid misuse	38 (4.3)	17 (3.9)	21 (4.6)
No. of Rx opioid misuse days	0.2 ±1.7	0.2 ±2.2	0.2 ±1.0
Related Outcomes			
Depression (PHQ-8)	7.5 ±6.0	7.7 ±6.1	7.2 ±5.9
Anxiety (GAD-7)	6.6 ±5.7	7.0 ±5.8	6.3 ±5.6

Note. GAD-7 = Generalized Anxiety Disorder 7-item scale; PHQ-8 = Patient Health Questionnaire 8-item depression scale; Rx = prescription.

Figure 1). For frequency of binge drinking, there was a 31% increase per wave in the control condition (RR = 1.31; 95% CI = 1.18, 1.47), whereas no increase was observed in the intervention condition (RR = 0.97; 95% CI = 0.88, 1.08; Figure B [available as a supplement to the online version of this article at https://www.ajph.org]). For frequency of cannabis use, there was a 10% increase per wave in the control condition (RR = 1.10; 95% CI = 1.02, 1.19), whereas no increase was observed in the intervention condition (RR = 0.98; 95% CI = 0.90, 1.06; Figure 2). For frequency of prescription opioid misuse, the control condition started follow-up with lower prescription opioid misuse than the intervention condition. Thereafter, the control condition increased use by 33% each wave (RR = 1.33; 95% CI = 1.01, 1.75), whereas the intervention condition decreased use by 20% per wave (RR = 0.80; 95% CI = 0.65, 1.00; Figure 3).

Results for secondary outcomes of anxiety, depression, and 13 other measures are presented in Table B

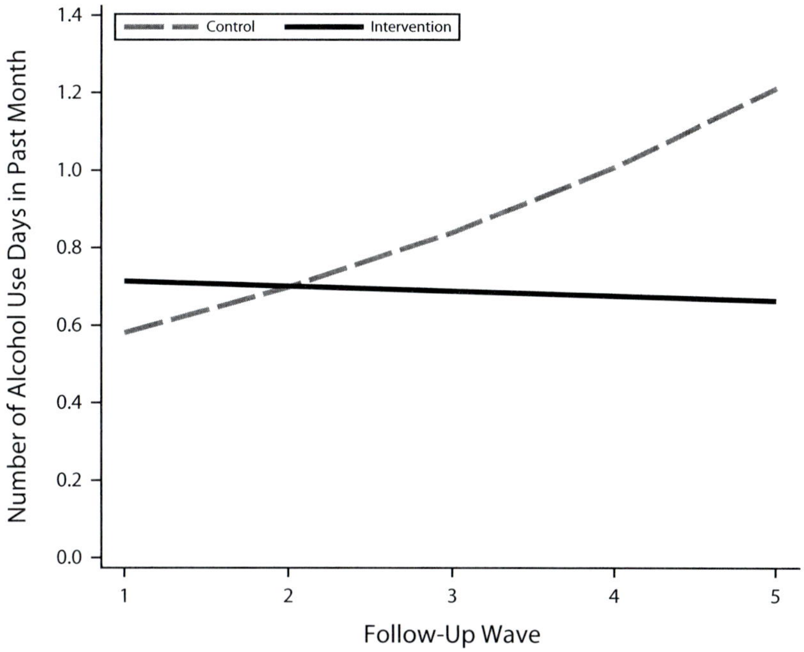

No. of Days, Control	0.58	0.70	0.84	1.01	1.21
No. of Days, Intervention	0.71	0.70	0.69	0.68	0.66

FIGURE 1— Alcohol Use by Study Condition and Follow-Up Wave at Ages 16 to 18 Years: Northeastern Oklahoma, 2021–2024

Note. Figure presents model-predicted means by wave and study condition. Summary statistics for the slope by study condition (study condition by time) from the generalized linear mixed model: rate ratio = 0.82; 95% confidence interval = 0.72, 0.93; t = −3.02; *P* = .003.

(available as a supplement to the online version of this article at https://www.ajph.org). Although effects were in the protective direction, no statistically significant effects by study condition were found on anxiety (b = −0.17; 95% CI = −0.36, 0.02; t = −1.76; *P* = .08) or depression (b = −0.08; 95% CI = −0.27, 0.11; t = −0.76; *P* = 0.44). Among the other 13 secondary outcomes, 2 statistically significant differences in trajectories were observed between conditions, with reductions among the intervention condition in normative estimates of peer substance use (b = −0.05; 95% CI = −0.08, −0.01; t = −2.70; *P* = .007) and perceived access to prescription opioids (b = −0.03; 95% CI = −0.06, −0.002; t = −2.11; *P* = .04).

Sensitivity analyses treating time categorically showed similar results, with 1 notable exception. The pattern of effects for cannabis use was appreciably nonlinear, with stronger mean differences at the last wave of follow-up. With the increased number of parameters and subsequent loss of precision, the corresponding tests were no longer statistically significant ($F_{4,3447}$ = 2.06; *P* = .08).

DISCUSSION

The combined school and family intervention, CBI with MI and CKFA, significantly reduced the expected escalation of substance use during late adolescence (ages 16–18 years). Frequency of use during the past month of alcohol, binge drinking, and prescription opioid misuse increased among the control condition, but not in the intervention condition. We observed fewer days of past-month cannabis use in the intervention group relative to the control group. However, this finding should be interpreted with caution as the results were no longer statistically significant in models allowing for nonlinear trajectories.

To contextualize the observed reductions in frequency of use, prior research suggests that even modest decreases in substance use can have meaningful effects. For example, reducing alcohol use by 1 day per month has been linked to lower odds of high-risk sexual behaviors.[33] Similarly, a reduction of 1 binge drinking episode per month has been associated with slight but significant increases in grade point average among adolescents in a dose–respondent manner.[34] Reducing

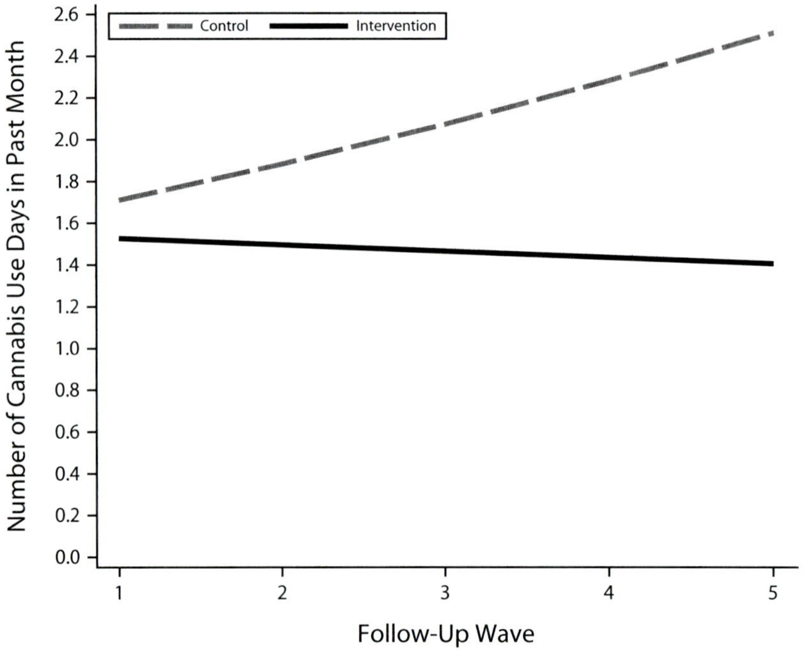

No. of Days, Control	1.71	1.88	2.07	2.28	2.51
No. of Days, Intervention	1.53	1.50	1.46	1.44	1.41

FIGURE 2— Cannabis Use by Study Condition and Follow-Up Wave at Ages 16 to 18 Years: Northeastern Oklahoma, 2021–2024

Note. Figure presents model-predicted means by wave and study condition. Summary statistics for the slope by study condition (study condition by time) from the generalized linear mixed model: rate ratio = 0.89; 95% confidence interval = 0.80, 1.00; t = −2.03; *P* = .04.

cannabis use by 1 day per month has been associated with decreased odds of suicidal ideation and behavior.[35] Although these translations required assumptions due to differences in reporting and study design, they show that even small linear reductions in adolescent substance use can yield meaningful clinical and functional benefits.

All prespecified primary trial outcomes with prespecified analytic models showed statistically significant and substantively important preventive effects. Analyses of 15 other potentially relevant secondary measures showed few significant effects; only 2 were significantly different between study conditions: reductions in normative estimates of substance use and perceptions of access to prescription opioids, both important risk factors for use addressed by the intervention. Many of these other measures conceptually might be considered possible mechanisms for observed intervention effects. Perhaps the primary effects were achieved by inducing a small change in each of these 15 measures, individually not detectable (i.e., not significant) because the trial was not designed or powered for such analyses. Perhaps there are other unmeasured factors that better account for the observed effects on the primary outcomes. The exact psychological, social, and environmental mechanisms of the significant intervention effects remain a topic for further research, requiring trials with larger numbers of communities.

Despite rapid adaptations necessitated by the COVID-19 pandemic and its aftermath, including reduced staff, the intervention effectively suspended the expected escalation in substance use during high school. These results are consistent with our first collaborative trial, which involved in-person delivery of CBI by Connect coaches along with community organizing, both substantially more resource-intensive than the current adapted intervention.[15,16] The magnitude of Connect intervention effects is equivalent to or greater than those reported for other brief interventions and family interventions.[36,37]

Strengths and Limitations

The trial has notable strengths. We successfully embraced a strong collaboration between academic researchers and practitioners at Cherokee Nation

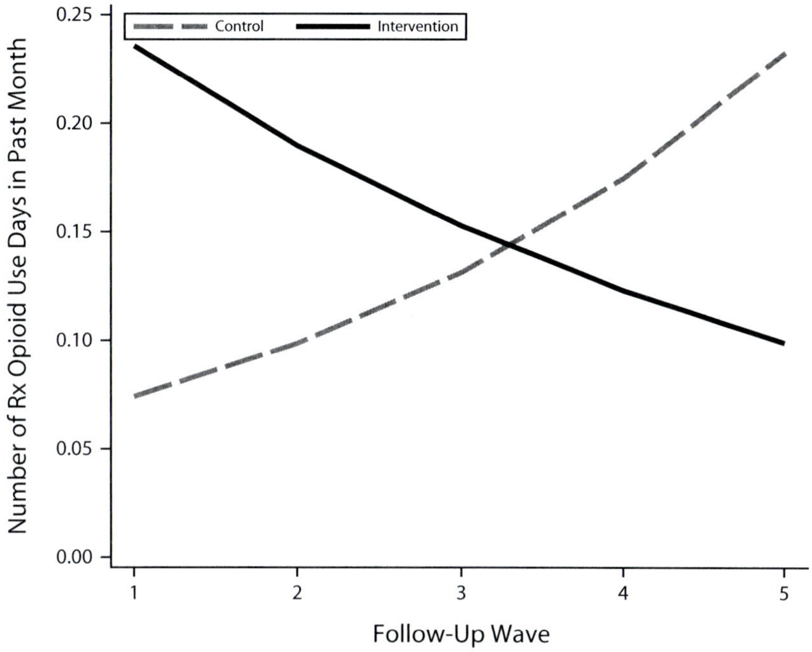

No. of Days, Control	0.07	0.10	0.13	0.17	0.23
No. of Days, Intervention	0.24	0.19	0.15	0.12	0.10

FIGURE 3— Prescription Opioid Misuse by Study Condition and Follow-up Wave at Ages 16 to 18 Years: Northeastern Oklahoma, 2021–2024

Note. Figure presents model-predicted means by wave and study condition. Summary statistics for the slope by study condition (study condition by time) from the generalized linear mixed model: rate ratio = 0.60; 95% confidence interval = 0.43, 0.85; t = −2.86; *P* = .004.

Behavioral Health. We successfully implemented a rigorous cluster randomized trial design in real-world settings during and after the COVID-19 pandemic, using constrained randomization that optimized baseline equivalence, and sustained a youth cohort over 3 years. We recruited and retained 20 small rural high schools during challenging times, ensuring sufficient power to detect meaningful intervention effects.

Study limitations include a slow start and ramp-up of the intervention because of COVID-19–related hiring challenges that necessitated rapid adaptation of the planned intervention. Despite this limitation, we benefited from the expertise and diversity of our team to redesign the intervention and rapidly advance to implementation.

A second important limitation is the 28% loss to follow-up over 3 years. However, we observed no differential attrition by study condition, and our estimates are conditioned on prior outcomes. Given that prior substance use is one of the strongest predictors of current substance use among adolescents, our missingness at random assumption is likely to hold, resulting in minimal bias. Third, although our constrained randomization produced conditions that were similar across most outcomes, some differences in key outcomes were observed at baseline (i.e., binge drinking). Although some variation is to be expected even under randomization, these differences are accounted for by our a priori control of baseline outcome values.

Fourth, with 20 sites, the trial was not powered sufficiently to reliably assess specific mechanisms of intervention effect or differential effects. Fifth, although the control school students received identical attention and activities associated with the surveys, they did not receive a sham or alternative intervention at the same time the treatment schools were treated. Sixth, although the intervention focused on individual- and family-level determinants of drug use with primary prevention delivered by a tribal health system in partnership with rural school districts, comprehensive approaches also require more thoroughly addressing system and structural factors affecting drug use. Finally, the trial was conducted in small, remote rural communities within the boundaries of tribal nations.

Although we believe the intervention is appropriate for many diverse communities, results are best generalized to similar communities.

Public Health Implications

The low cost and efficient intervention package, comprising CBI and CKFA, collaboratively designed with a team from Cherokee Nation Behavioral Health and academic researchers, was effective at preventing the escalation of substance use among older adolescents, a particularly vulnerable age for the development of substance use disorders.[38] The preventive effects are equivalent to or greater than those seen with other effective practices.[36,37] The results highlight the importance and feasibility of primary prevention in addressing the overdose epidemic.[39] AJPH

ABOUT THE AUTHORS

At the time of the study, Kelli A. Komro, Melvin D. Livingston, Bethany J. Livingston, Ashna Jagtiani, Caroline M. Barry, Alexander C. Wagenaar, Hannah L. F. Cooper, Emily Ivanich, and Sierra L. Talavera-Brown were with the Rollins School of Public Health, Emory University, Atlanta, GA. Juli R. Skinner, Terrence K. Kominsky, Hannah LaBounty, and Ashley N. Gassaway were with Cherokee Nation Behavioral Health, Cherokee Nation Health, Tahlequah, OK. Megan Harmon was with Neighbors Building Neighborhoods, Muskogee, OK.

CORRESPONDENCE

Correspondence should be sent to Kelli A. Komro, MPH, PhD (e-mail: kkomro@emory.edu). Reprints can be ordered at https://www.ajph.org by clicking the "Reprints" link.

PUBLICATION INFORMATION

Full Citation: Komro KA, Livingston MD, Skinner JR, et al. Primary prevention of drug overdoses in rural low-resource and Tribal communities: a cluster randomized trial. *Am J Public Health*. 2025;115(9):1508–1517.

Acceptance Date: May 20, 2025.

DOI: https://doi.org/10.2105/AJPH.2025.308205

ORCID iD:

Kelli A. Komro https://orcid.org/0000-0002-7893-9558

CONTRIBUTORS

K. A. Komro, M. L. Livingston, J. R. Skinner, T. K. Kominsky, A. C. Wagenaar, and H. L. F. Cooper conceptualized the study and acquired funding. K. A. Komro, J. R. Skinner, B. J. Livingston, E. Ivanich, H. LaBounty, A. N. Gassaway, S. L. Talavera-Brown, and C. M. Barry developed the intervention. T. K. Kominsky and M. Harmon collected data. M. L. Livingston and A. Jagtiani analyzed data. K. A. Komro, M. L. Livingston, and A. Jagtiani wrote the first draft of the article. All authors revised the article and read and approved the final version.

ACKNOWLEDGMENTS

We acknowledge the contributions of Eugena Atkinson, connect coach for brief intervention; Brittany Beasley, prevention coordinator; Kim Lynch, director of Neighbors Building Neighborhoods Nonprofit Resource Center; Lisa Merlo, PhD (University of Florida) connect brief intervention and motivational interviewing consultant; Dallas Pettigrew, MSW (University of Oklahoma), intervention consultant; and Brianna Reynolds, connect brief intervention. We appreciate the collegiality and generosity of Steven Ondersma, PhD (Michigan State University), for sharing his expertise and open-source Computerized Intervention Authoring System (cias.app) and Jan Gryczynski, PhD (Friends Research Institute) for sharing his CIAS-based brief intervention and manual, which enabled rapid intervention adaptation in response to challenges posed by the COVID-19 pandemic. Most importantly, we sincerely thank the students, parents/caregivers, and high school counselors, principals, and superintendents for their trust and participation in this trial.

Research reported in this publication was supported by the National Institute on Drug Abuse of the National Institutes of Health (NIH) through the NIH HEAL Initiative under award numbers UG3DA050234 and UH3DA050234 to Emory University (principal investigators [PIs], K. A. Komro and M. D. Livingston), with subaward to Cherokee Nation (PI, J. Skinner; T. Kominsky, 2019–2023), as well as training grant 5T32DA050552. The funder did not influence the specific research question, data analysis, or results reporting. As part of the NIH UG3/UHS mechanism, the funder assigned a National Institute on Drug Abuse co-investigator to the project, Kathy Etz, PhD, and she participated in monthly meetings through January 2023.

Note. The contents are solely the responsibility of the authors and do not necessarily represent the views of the NIH, NIH HEAL Initiative, Emory University, or the Cherokee Nation.

CONFLICTS OF INTEREST

The authors have no conflicts of interest to disclose.

HUMAN PARTICIPANT PROTECTION

The study protocol was approved by the Cherokee Nation Institutional Review Board (IRB; USA Federal-Wide Assurance #0000047). Emory University and Cherokee Nation signed a Reliance Agreement that designated Cherokee Nation as the organization providing IRB review. The Cherokee Nation IRB reviewed and approved this manuscript for publication. A model consent form is available on request.

REFERENCES

1. Committee on Rising Midlife Mortality Rates and Socioeconomic Disparities, Committee on National Statistics, Committee on Population, Division of Behavioral and Social Sciences and Education, National Academies of Sciences, Engineering, and Medicine. *High and Rising Mortality Rates Among Working-Age Adults.* Harris KM, Majmundar M, Becker T, eds. Washington, DC: National Academies Press; 2021.
2. Blue Bird Jernigan V, D'Amico EJ, Duran B, Buchwald D. Multilevel and community-level interventions with Native Americans: challenges and opportunities. *Prev Sci.* 2020;21(suppl 1): 65–73. https://doi.org/10.1007/s11121-018-0916-3
3. Wendt DC, Hartmann WE, Allen J, et al. Substance use research with Indigenous communities: exploring and extending foundational principles of community psychology. *Am J Community Psychol.* 2019;64(1–2):146–158. https://doi.org/10.1002/ajcp.12363
4. Thomas N, van de Ven K, Mulrooney KJD. The impact of rurality on opioid-related harms: a systematic review of qualitative research. *Int J Drug Policy.* 2020;85:102607. https://doi.org/10.1016/j.drugpo.2019.11.015
5. Friedman JR, Nguemeni Tiako MJ, Hansen H. Understanding and addressing widening racial inequalities in drug overdose. *Am J Psychiatry.* 2024;181(5):381–390. https://doi.org/10.1176/appi.ajp.20230917
6. National Academies of Sciences, Engineering, and Medicine, Division of Behavioral and Social Sciences and Education, Board on Children, Youth, and Families, Committee on Fostering Healthy Mental, Emotional, and Behavioral Development Among Children and Youth. *Fostering Healthy Mental, Emotional, and Behavioral Development in Children and Youth: A National Agenda.* Washington, DC: National Academies Press; 2020.
7. Office of Disease Prevention and Health Promotion, US Dept of Health and Human Services. Reduce the proportion of adolescents who used drugs in the past month—SU-05. Available at: https://health.gov/healthypeople/objectives-and-data/browse-objectives/drug-and-alcohol-use/reduce-proportion-adolescents-who-used-drugs-past-month-su-05. Accessed April 2, 2024.
8. Friedman J, Godvin M, Shover CL, Gone JP, Hansen H, Schriger DL. Trends in drug overdose deaths among US adolescents, January 2010 to June 2021. *JAMA.* 2022;327(14):1398–1400. https://doi.org/10.1001/jama.2022.2847
9. Friedman J, Hadland SE. The overdose crisis among US adolescents. *N Engl J Med.* 2024;390(2):97–100. https://doi.org/10.1056/NEJMp2312084
10. Woolf SH, Wolf ER, Rivara FP. The new crisis of increasing all-cause mortality in US children and adolescents. *JAMA.* 2023;329(12):975–976. https://doi.org/10.1001/jama.2023.3517
11. Ridenour TA, Saavedra LM, Fernandes CSF, Cance JD, Graham PW, Oudekerk BA. Introduction to helping to end addiction long-term prevention cooperative: overview and strategies.

Prev Sci. 2023;24(suppl 1):1–7. https://doi.org/10.1007/s11121-023-01503-7

12. Komro KA, D'Amico EJ, Dickerson DL, et al. Culturally responsive opioid and other drug prevention for American Indian/Alaska Native people: a comparison of reservation- and urban-based approaches. *Prev Sci.* 2023;24(suppl 1):88–98. https://doi.org/10.1007/s11121-022-01396-y
13. Komro KA, Kominsky TK, Skinner JR, et al. Study protocol for a cluster randomized trial of a school, family, and community intervention for preventing drug misuse among older adolescents in the Cherokee Nation. *Trials.* 2022;23(1):175. https://doi.org/10.1186/s13063-022-06096-0
14. Wagenaar AC, Livingston MD, Pettigrew DW, Kominsky TK, Komro KA. Communities mobilizing for change on alcohol (CMCA): secondary analyses of a randomized controlled trial showing effects of community organizing on alcohol acquisition by youth in the Cherokee nation. *Addiction.* 2018;113(4):647–655. https://doi.org/10.1111/add.14113
15. Livingston MD, Komro KA, Wagenaar AC, Kominsky TK, Pettigrew DW, Garrett BA. Effects of alcohol interventions on other drug use in the Cherokee Nation. *Am J Public Health.* 2018;108(2):259–261. https://doi.org/10.2105/AJPH.2017.304188
16. Komro KA, Livingston MD, Wagenaar AC, Cherokee Nation Prevention Trial Team, et al. Multilevel prevention trial of alcohol use among American Indian and white high school students in the Cherokee Nation. *Am J Public Health.* 2017;107(3):453–459. https://doi.org/10.2105/AJPH.2016.303603
17. Garrett BA, Komro KA, Merlo LJ, et al. CONNECT: implementation of a school-based alcohol screening and brief intervention for youth in the Cherokee Nation. *J Sch Health.* 2019;89(11):874–882. https://doi.org/10.1111/josh.12830
18. Livingston MD, Barry CM, Jagtiani A, et al. Theory, measurement, and psychometric properties of risk and protective factors for drug misuse among adolescents living on or near the Cherokee Nation Reservation. *Advers Resil Sci.* 2023;4(4):401–413. https://doi.org/10.1007/s42844-023-00112-1
19. Whitesell NR, Mousseau A, Parker M, Rasmus S, Allen J. Promising practices for promoting health equity through rigorous intervention science with Indigenous communities. *Prev Sci.* 2020;21(suppl 1):5–12. https://doi.org/10.1007/s11121-018-0954-x
20. Hawkins JD, Catalano RF, Miller JY. Risk and protective factors for alcohol and other drug problems in adolescence and early adulthood: implications for substance abuse prevention. *Psychol Bull.* 1992;112(1):64–105. https://doi.org/10.1037/0033-2909.112.1.64
21. Blackstock C. Revisiting the breath of life theory. *Br J Soc Work.* 2019;49(4):854–859. https://doi.org/10.1093/bjsw/bcz047
22. Cross TL. Through Indigenous eyes: rethinking theory and practice. Presented at: SNAICC National Conference, National Indian Child Welfare Association; September 20, 2007; Adelaide, Australia. Available at: https://www.snaicc.org.au/wp-content/uploads/2015/12/02242.pdf. Accessed July 20, 2025.
23. Gryczynski J, Mitchell SG, Schwartz RP, et al. Computer- vs. nurse practitioner-delivered brief intervention for adolescent marijuana, alcohol, and sex risk behaviors in school-based health centers. *Drug Alcohol Depend.* 2021;218:108423. https://doi.org/10.1016/j.drugalcdep.2020.108423
24. Gryczynski J, Mitchell SG, Gonzales A, et al. A randomized trial of computerized vs. in-person brief intervention for illicit drug use in primary care: outcomes through 12 months. *J Subst Abuse Treat.* 2015;50:3–10. https://doi.org/10.1016/j.jsat.2014.09.002
25. Ondersma SJ, Svikis DS, Thacker LR, Beatty JR, Lockhart N. Computer-delivered screening and brief intervention (e-SBI) for postpartum drug use: a randomized trial. *J Subst Abuse Treat.* 2014;46(1):52–59. https://doi.org/10.1016/j.jsat.2013.07.013
26. Ondersma SJ, Svikis DS, Schuster CR. Computer-based brief intervention a randomized trial with postpartum women. *Am J Prev Med.* 2007;32(3):231–238. https://doi.org/10.1016/j.amepre.2006.11.003
27. van Zyl C, Badenhorst M, Hanekom S, Heine M. Unravelling "low-resource settings": a systematic scoping review with qualitative content analysis. *BMJ Glob Health.* 2021;6(6):e005190. https://doi.org/10.1136/bmjgh-2021-005190
28. Miech RA, Johnston LD, O'Malley PM, Bachman JG, Schulenberg JE, Patrick ME. Monitoring the Future: National Survey Results on Drug Use, 1975–2020: Secondary School Students. Institute for Social Research, The University of Michigan; 2021. https://monitoringthefuture.org/wp-content/uploads/2022/08/mtf-vol1_2020.pdf. Accessed June 23, 2025.
29. Kroenke K, Strine TW, Spitzer RL, Williams JBW, Berry JT, Mokdad AH. The PHQ-8 as a measure of current depression in the general population. *J Affect Disord.* 2009;114(1-3):163–173. https://doi.org/10.1016/j.jad.2008.06.026
30. Mossman SA, Luft MJ, Schroeder HK, et al. The Generalized Anxiety Disorder 7-item scale in adolescents with generalized anxiety disorder: signal detection and validation. *Ann Clin Psychiatry.* 2017;29(4):227–234A.
31. Ridenour TA, Cruden G, Yang Y, et al. Methodological strategies for prospective harmonization of studies: application to 10 distinct outcomes studies of preventive interventions targeting opioid misuse. *Prev Sci.* 2023;24(suppl 1):16–29. https://doi.org/10.1007/s11121-022-01412-1
32. Allison PD, Statistical Horizons. Handling missing data by maximum likelihood. Available at: https://statisticalhorizons.com/wp-content/uploads/MissingDataByML.pdf. Accessed March 18, 2021.
33. Muchimba M, Haberstick BC, Corley RP, McQueen MB. Frequency of alcohol use in adolescence as a marker for subsequent sexual risk behavior in adulthood. *J Adolesc Health.* 2013;53(2):215–221. https://doi.org/10.1016/j.jadohealth.2013.02.005
34. Hjarnaa L, Møller SP, Curtis AB, et al. Alcohol intake and academic performance and dropout in high school: a prospective cohort study in 65,233 adolescents. *J Adolesc Health.* 2023;73(6):1083–1092. https://doi.org/10.1016/j.jadohealth.2023.07.008
35. Hinckley JD, Mikulich-Gilbertson SK, He JP, et al. Cannabis use is associated with depression severity and suicidality in the National Comorbidity Survey-Adolescent Supplement. *JAACAP Open.* 2023;1(1):24–35. https://doi.org/10.1016/j.jaacop.2023.02.002
36. The Community Guide. Substance use: family-based interventions to prevent substance use among youth. September 14, 2023. Available at: https://www.thecommunityguide.org/findings/substance-use-family-based-interventions-to-prevent-substance-use-among-youth.html. Accessed July 8, 2024.
37. The Community Guide. Alcohol Excessive Consumption: Electronic Screening and Brief Interventions (e-SBI). April 27, 2023. Available at: https://www.thecommunityguide.org/findings/alcohol-excessive-consumption-electronic-screening-and-brief-interventions-e-sbi.html. Accessed July 8, 2024.
38. Volkow ND, Han B, Einstein EB, Compton WM. Prevalence of substance use disorders by time since first substance use among young people in the US. *JAMA Pediatr.* 2021;175(6):640–643. https://doi.org/10.1001/jamapediatrics.2020.6981
39. Adams E, Komro K, Bonar E. A renewed outlook on substance use prevention. The Medical Care Blog. February 3, 2023. Available at: https://www.themedicalcareblog.com/substance-use-prevention. Accessed March 20, 2024.

Excess Mortality and Containment Performance During the COVID-19 Pandemic: Evidence From 34 Countries

Chieh Cheng, MS, Hsiao-Yu Wu, MS, Shu-Chen Kuo, PhD, Brandon Fan, Ya-Ting Hsu, MS, Yi-Kai Chen, BS, Byron Fan, BS, Yung-An Jang, MS, Chih-Fan Hung, BS, Wei-Ming Jiang, MS, Hung-Yi Chiou, PhD, Wei J. Chen, MD, ScD, and Hsiao-Hui Tsou, PhD

Objectives. To expand COVID-19 containment indicators to evaluate the relationship between excess mortality and government response.

Methods. We developed a longitudinal study analyzing excess mortality, COVID-19 containment, and structural conditions in 34 countries between 2020 and 2022.

Results. The average excess mortality ratios of the 34 countries were 1.09, 1.14, and 1.11 in 2020, 2021, and 2022, respectively. Thirteen countries experienced continuous annual rises, while only 2 had consistent annual declines. Top-performing countries significantly reduced excess deaths by 5.7% (b = −0.06; 95% CI [confidence interval] = −0.10, −0.01; P = .02) in 2020 and 12.9% (b = −0.13; 95% CI = −0.17, −0.08; P < .001) in 2021, compared to bottom performers. Middle-performing countries saw reductions of 6.7% (b = −0.07; 95% CI = −0.11, −0.02; P = .01) and 10.6% (b = −0.11; 95% CI = −0.15, −0.06; P < .001). These findings suggest that better containment is associated with fewer excess deaths, even after accounting for preexisting structural differences.

Conclusions. The COVID-19 containment indicators' precision emphasizes the association between better containment and lower excess mortality during early and postvaccine development periods.

Public Health Implications. Our findings urge governments to utilize new metrics that balance flexibility and strictness for pandemic strategies, informing future policy interventions. (*Am J Public Health*. 2025;115(9):1518–1528. https://doi.org/10.2105/AJPH.2025.308136)

AJPH September 2025, Vol. 115, No. 9

Excess mortality stands as a widely accepted and more comprehensive index evaluating the impact of the COVID-19 pandemic.[1] Defined as the difference between the number of people who die in a given period and the baseline death number of recent years,[2] excess mortality captures both direct and indirect mortality effects of COVID-19, including factors such as health care utilization,[3,4] chronic disease exacerbation,[5] and psychological distress.[6] Furthermore, it overcomes differences in reporting and testing between countries,[1] enhancing comparability between countries. Moreover, excess mortality is less affected by the misclassification of deaths, facilitating comparisons of before and after COVID-19 within the same country.[1] Previous research on excess mortality has included calculations of total excess mortality[7–9] and the investigation of potentially associated structural conditions, which are underlying factors that shape the quality and outcomes for health services received by various groups of people.[5,10–12] Research has shown that excess mortality is associated with structural conditions such as the health care system,[13–16] chronic diseases,[5,12,17] and socioeconomic determinants of health.[18,19]

The different governments' responses are correlated with varying levels of excess mortality. Responses that effectively contain the spread of COVID-19 variants do not necessarily ensure a decrease in excess mortality.[5,12,13,20] The effectiveness of the containment measures in reducing excess mortality depends on several factors, including the timing of implementation, health care system capacities, and population vulnerability. For instance, delayed interventions may fail to curb highly infectious periods, and limited health care resources could exhaust treatment capabilities, especially in countries with greater proportions of high-risk demographics. There have been various criteria, such as the Oxford COVID-19 Government Response Tracker,[21] developed to evaluate containment performance, that have inconsistent findings on their relationship with excess deaths.[22–25] Notably, the Oxford Tracker has developed several indices for government response, containment and health, stringency, and economics—each using a distinct subset of 16 available indicators (details in Table A, available as a supplement to the online version of this article at https://ajph.org). Tsou et al.[21] developed a comprehensive evaluation of COVID-19 containment performance indicators in 2022, evaluating government interventions based on COVID-19 case numbers, hygiene education, physical and mental health, and socioeconomic impact to gain insight into the effectiveness of government response.

In this study, we aimed to expand the use of indicators to clarify the relationship between excess mortality and COVID-19 containment performance. This was a global, longitudinal study covering 34 countries through the Alpha, Delta, and Omicron waves, spanning 2020 to 2022. Acknowledging the influence of structural conditions on the relationship between government response and excess mortality, this study incorporates health care, vaccination, diabetes and cardiovascular disease death rates, percentage of the population aged 65 years and older, pandemic severity, and gross national income per capita for model adjustment through literature review. This study provides a more comprehensive perspective on the impact of government containment measures during the COVID-19 pandemic and provides policymakers with valuable insights into the direct and indirect effects of pandemic policies.

METHODS

The analysis focused on data from 2020 to 2022. Figure 1 illustrates the inclusion and exclusion criteria used to select countries for the study. Initially, we considered 117 countries with weekly or monthly mortality data from the Economist Intelligence Unit (EIU) as candidates (n = 117).[22] We excluded 83 countries because of a lack of complete death count data or because they were missing a comprehensive assessment of COVID-19 containment performance.[21] Ultimately, 34 countries emerged as eligible for the subsequent analysis (n = 34).

Data Collection

We used the 2020–2022 data collected for each country to investigate the

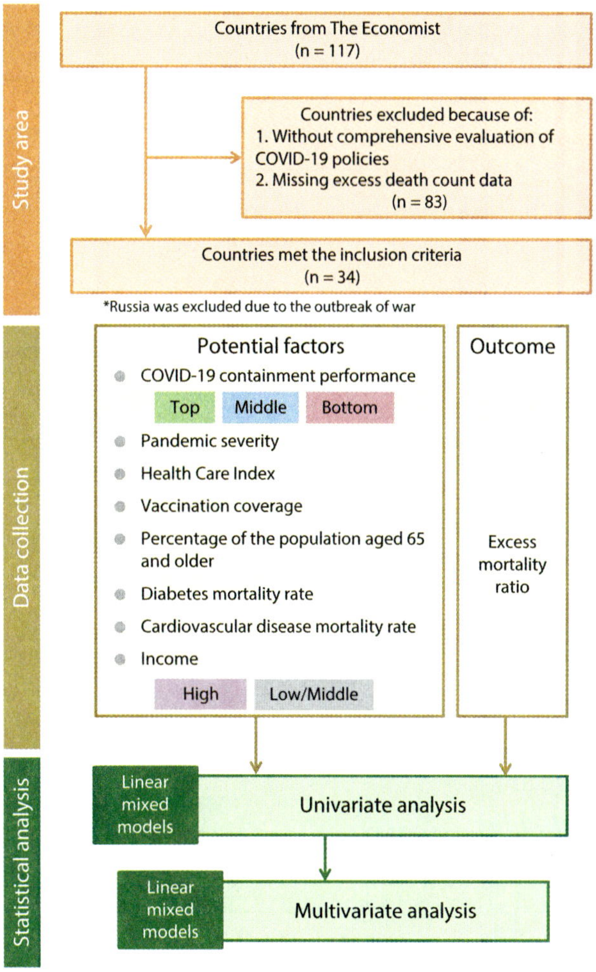

FIGURE 1— Flowchart of Studies Analyzing the Relationship Between Excess Mortality and Containment Performance

Note. The orange shade represents the country selection criteria; the yellow shade indicates data collection (including COVID-19 containment performance and a high-income country binary indicator, where both were categorical variables, while others were continuous variables); and the green shade signifies the statistical analysis phase.

association between excess mortality and potential risk factors or protective factors. These factors included COVID-19 containment performance scores, pandemic severity, health care system ranking, the percentage of the population aged 65 years and older, diabetes and cardiovascular disease death rates, COVID-19 vaccination coverage, and income (Figure 1).

Excess Mortality

The outcome variable was the excess mortality ratio. Tracking COVID-19 excess deaths across countries from the EIU provides observed mortality data (particularly monthly deaths for 117 countries) and estimates of expected mortality.[22] We normalized excess mortality per 100 000 people for consistent comparison. We analyzed the excess mortality ratio by dividing the number of observed deaths by the number of expected deaths to provide a more accurate basis for comparisons and effectively address nuances in demographic differences[23] (excess mortality rate using subtraction can be found in Section A, available as a supplement to the online version of this article at https://ajph.org). The complete data for each country, along with the underlying code, can be downloaded from the GitHub repository of the EIU (https://github.com/TheEconomist/covid-19-excess-deaths-tracker). The EIU has employed statistical models to establish the baseline expected number of deaths in each region for 2020, 2021, and 2022 (Table B, available as a supplement to the online version of this article at https://ajph.org).

COVID-19 Containment Performance

The COVID-19 containment performance score proposed by Tsou et al.[21] served as an evaluative tool for assessing the effectiveness of COVID-19 containment. The containment performance score is composed of 10 indicators: lockdown efficiency, health system policies, health literacy, vaccine coverage of the population, 1-month cases per capita, infection growth rate, fatality rate, gross domestic product loss, unemployment rate, and insomnia (Table C and Figure A, available as supplements to the online version of this article at https://ajph.org). The indicators were then standardized, 0 to 100, to score relative containment performance for each country. Each country's containment performance score was a simple monthly average of the standardized scores of 10 indicators of equal weight from March 2020 to November 2021. According to the rankings of countries' average containment performance scores, the 34 countries were divided into 3 roughly equal-sized groups: top (1st–12th), middle (13th–23rd), and bottom (24th–34th; Table D, available as a supplement to the online version of this article at https://ajph.org). A higher score reflects superior containment performance.

Pandemic Severity

We used the annual cumulative COVID-19 cases to represent a time-varying evaluation of pandemic severity. The annual cumulative COVID-19 cases during 2020 to 2022 were calculated by daily COVID-19 cases from Our World in Data[24] at the country level to fully inform the time effects of the pandemic's impact across geographically distinct regions.

Health Care Index

The Health Care Index is the ranking of health care systems from *CEOWORLD Magazine*.[25] The index assesses 5 key health variables across 89 countries: health care infrastructure, competency of health care professionals, costs, availability of quality medicines, and government readiness. The ranking provides a comprehensive evaluation of the overall effectiveness and performance of health care systems worldwide.

COVID-19 Vaccination Coverage

We calculated COVID-19 vaccination coverage by using fully vaccinated people per 100 from Our World in Data.[24] We defined fully vaccinated people as the total number of individuals who received all doses prescribed by the initial vaccination protocol, divided by the total population of the country. We collected monthly data from 2020 to 2022 for correlation analysis with other variables to provide a comprehensive understanding of the vaccination landscape over time.

Diabetes and Cardiovascular Disease

The Global Burden of Disease Results Tool provided data on global all-cause deaths and disability-adjusted life years for the year 2019, along with trends since 1990.[26] For this study, we collected data on diabetes death rates and cardiovascular disease death rates from the year 2019 for correlation analysis with other variables.

Percentage of Population Aged 65 Years and Older

The data source of the percentage of those aged 65 years and older in each country in 2022 was Our World in Data.[24] This was one of the control variables, which was incorporated as a consideration toward age-related effects, particularly regarding the vulnerability of the elderly aged 65 years and older within our model.

High-Income Country Binary Indicator

The high-income country binary indicator was derived from The World Bank,[27] which classifies economies into 4 income groups: low, lower-middle, upper-middle, and high based on the gross national income per capita, representing the sum of incomes earned by residents in the economy divided by its population. We established a binary measure that distinguished high-income countries from low- and middle-income countries.

Statistical Analysis

Regression analysis evaluated the relationship between the outcome variables and 1 or more predictors, as illustrated in Figure 1. Potential predictors ($P < .2$) were identified through univariate analysis (Table F, available as a supplement to the online version of this article at https://ajph.org) and subsequently integrated into a multivariate regression model.[28] We used linear mixed models to explore the relationship between the excess mortality ratio and several variables, including COVID-19 containment performance, the health care index, COVID-19 vaccination coverage, the diabetes mortality rate, historical cardiovascular disease death rates, percentage of the population aged 65 years and older, pandemic severity, and the high-income country binary indicator.

Let Y_{ijk} denote the excess mortality ratio in year j and month k in the ith country. Each year, excess mortality accumulates anew. The model structure can be expressed as follows:

$$(1)\quad Y_{ijk} = \beta_0 + b_{i0} + \beta_1 X_{ijk} + \beta_2\, year_{ij} + \beta_3 X_{ijk} \times year_{ij} + \epsilon_{ijk},$$

where X_{ijk} denotes the predictor variables for year j and month k for the ith country. X_{ijk} could be COVID-19 containment performance, health care index, COVID-19 vaccination coverage, diabetes mortality rate, historic cardiovascular disease death rates, percentage of the population aged 65 years and older, pandemic severity, or high-income country binary indicator. The $year_{ij}$ was a categorical variable, which represented the observation year for the ith country. The $X_{ijk} \times year_{ij}$ was the interaction terms of the variables X_{ijk} and $year_{ij}$. If the 2-way interaction was significant, lower-order interaction terms must be retained. If the 2-way interaction was not significant, it was excluded from the model. The coefficient β_0 is an intercept term with a fixed effect, and coefficient b_{i0} is an intercept term with a random effect, representing the difference between the average intercept and intercept of the ith country. The standardized coefficients $\beta 1$, $\beta 2$, and $\beta 3$ are fixed effects. The coefficient ε_{ijk} is the error term, which is the error for the ith country in year j and month k. We assumed that the errors for country i follow a multivariate normal distribution.

To evaluate the models' performance in capturing the observed data, we included goodness-of-fit statistics. Additional details about the model can be found in the supplementary materials (Section B, available as a supplement to the online version of this article at https://ajph.org).

RESULTS

Figure 2 and Table B show the excess mortality in each year. In 2021 and 2022, the highlighted bars indicate that there were more excess deaths in that year than in the previous year. For example, the bars in Germany in 2021 and 2022 are highlighted, indicating that excess deaths in Germany increased yearly. Approximately one third of the countries ($n = 13$) experienced a consecutive increase in excess mortality, peaking in 2022. Approximately one third of the countries' ($n = 13$) maximum peak was in 2021 (Table E, available as a supplement to the online version of this article at https://ajph.org). In Mexico, excess mortality eventually decreased, with Mexico maintaining similar levels in 2020 and 2021, before a decline in 2022. Other countries, including Austria, Portugal, and the Netherlands, maintained relatively stable excess mortality ratios throughout the 3-year period. In some countries, such as New Zealand, Japan, Taiwan, Denmark, and Australia, the total number of excess deaths remained lower than in other countries, despite the excess mortality ratio increasing over the 3-year period. The annual number of deaths in these countries was lower than 1.05 (5% relative increase).

The excess mortality ratio and government response varied globally. Figure 3 shows a comprehensive

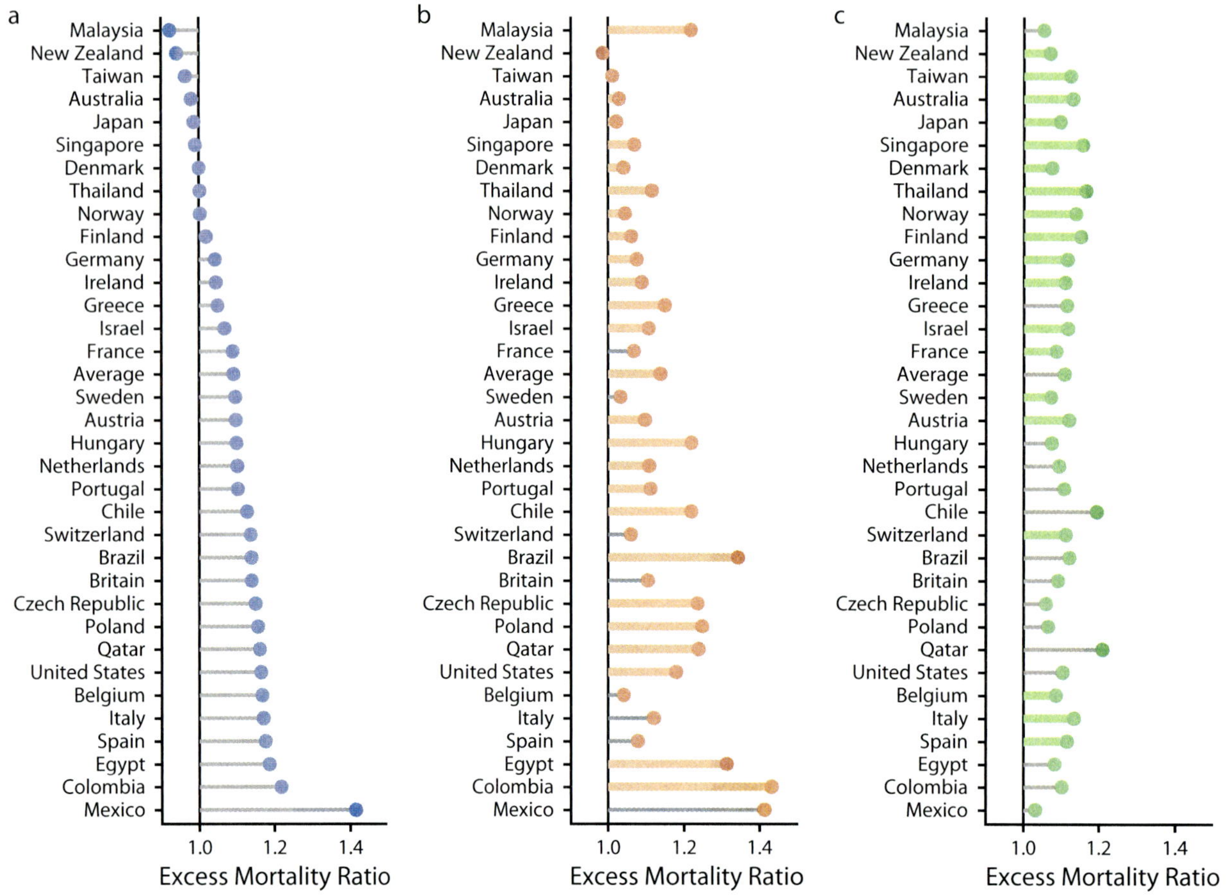

FIGURE 2— **Excess Mortality in Each Country in (a) 2020, (b) 2021, and (c) 2022**

Note. Highlighted color lines (orange, green) indicate that the excess mortality was greater than that in the previous year.

comparison of the mortality and containment performance—an index of COVID-19 control measures (as defined in the Methods section)—over the 3 years from 2020 to 2022. The ranking plots for each group are in Figure B (available as a supplement to the online version of this article at https://ajph.org). The countries were ranked by the excess mortality ratio, with those exhibiting lower mortality ratio placed higher in the ranking. In 2020 and 2021, we observed that the excess mortality ratio ranged from negative to more than 1.4 (40% relative increase). Countries with superior and middle containment performance tended to exhibit lower mortality ratios and higher rankings, whereas countries with poorer containment performance were predominantly associated with higher mortality ratios and lower rankings. However, we observed a reversal in ranking in the third year. The rankings of countries with bottom containment performance, such as the Czech Republic, Poland, and Mexico, surged sharply as mortality decreased. Conversely, the rankings of countries with top containment performance, such as Australia, Norway, and Finland, plunged as mortality increased. Moreover, in 2022, excess mortality showed a relatively small difference. Twenty-nine countries (including the containment performance top, middle, and bottom groups) had excess mortality within 1.1 (10% relative increase). Therefore, some countries' rankings declined even though their excess mortality ratios did not increase significantly. This bump chart (Figure 3) suggests a relationship between excess mortality and containment performance.

We conducted the univariate analysis for all predictors (Table F). All variables with *P* values smaller than 0.2 were included in the multivariate analysis. We also estimated the effect of COVID-19 containment performance on excess mortality by using the univariate analysis (Table G, available as a supplement to the online version of this article at https://ajph.org). The impact of the

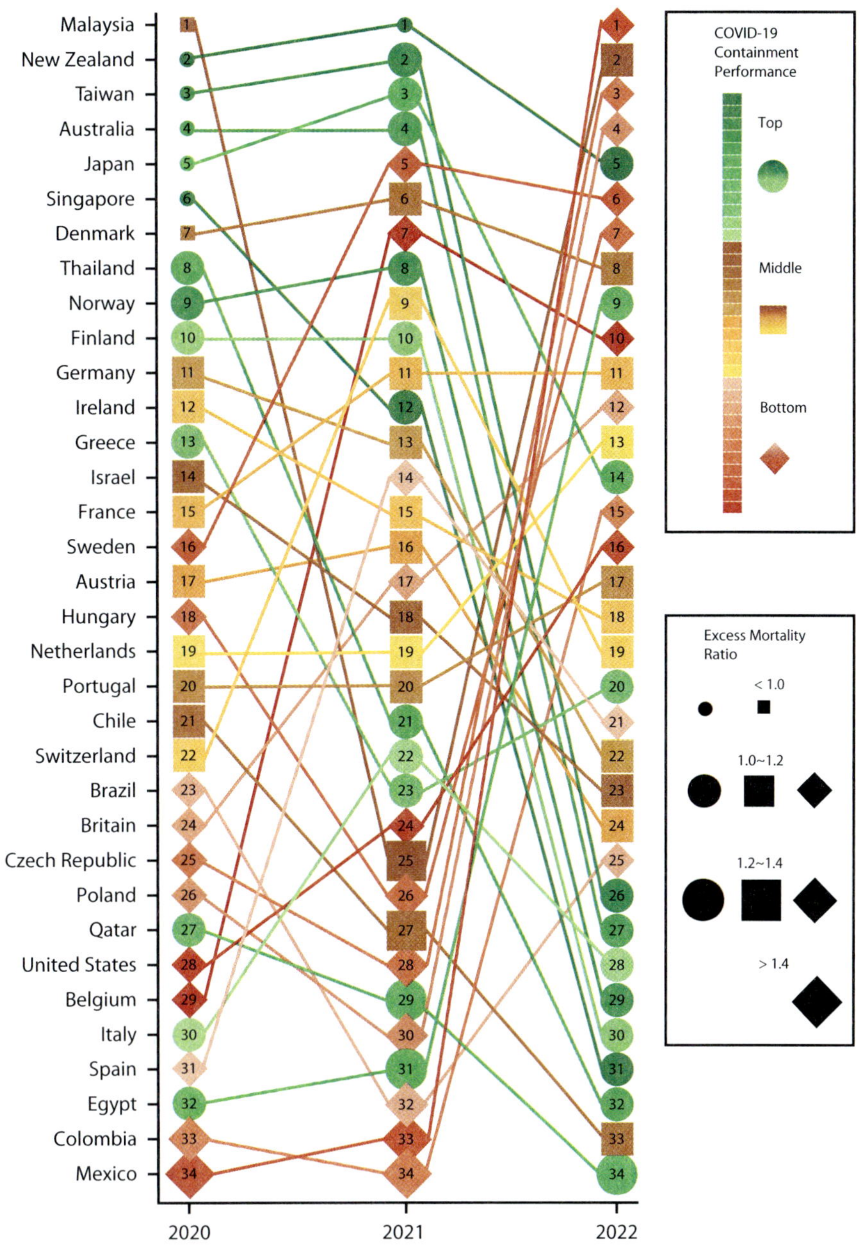

FIGURE 3— The Excess Mortality Ratio Ranking in 2020–2022

Note. The ranking was ordered according to the excess mortality ratio, with better rankings for countries with lower excess mortality ratios. The figure legend shows the groupings of the country's COVID-19 containment performance. The ranking of COVID-19 containment performance is represented by the color coding of the legend, with the first place dark green on the far top and the last place dark red on the far bottom. The size of the symbols in the figure legend indicates the excess mortality ratio.

COVID-19 containment performance on excess mortality was formally estimated using a multivariate linear mixed model. Figure 4 shows the association between excess mortality ratio and our indicators. For countries with top containment performance compared with bottom performance, excess deaths were reduced by 5.7% (P = .02) and 12.9% (P < .001) in 2020 and 2021, respectively. For countries with middle containment performance compared with bottom performance, excess deaths were reduced by 6.7% (P = .01) and 10.6% (P < .001) in 2020 and 2021, respectively. However, for countries with top containment performance compared with middle performance, there was no significant reduction. In 2022, no significant difference was observed among the 3 containment performance a

Group	b (SE)	P
Performance group, top vs bottom	−0.057 (0.023)	.02
Performance group, top vs middle	0.009 (0.022)	.68
Performance group, middle vs bottom	−0.067 (0.024)	.01
Health care index	−0.002 (0.001)	.13
% aged ≥ 65 y	0.001 (0.003)	.79
Diabetes mortality rate	0.001 (0.001)	.18
Cardiovascular disease mortality rate	−0.0002 (0.0001)	.05
High income vs low/middle income	0.020 (0.033)	.56

b

Group	b (SE)	P
Performance group, top vs bottom	−0.129 (0.024)	< .001
Performance group, top vs middle	−0.023 (0.023)	.32
Performance group, middle vs bottom	−0.106 (0.024)	< .001
Health care index	−0.004 (0.001)	< .001
% aged ≥ 65 y	−0.008 (0.003)	.03
Diabetes mortality rate	0.004 (0.001)	< .001
Cardiovascular disease mortality rate	−0.0001 (0.0001)	.69
High income vs low/middle income	−0.073 (0.033)	.04

c

Group	b (SE)	P
Performance group, top vs bottom	0.027 (0.024)	.27
Performance group, top vs middle	0.045 (0.023)	.05
Performance group, middle vs bottom	−0.018 (0.026)	.5
Health care index	−0.001 (0.001)	.27
% aged ≥ 65 y	−0.006 (0.003)	.07
Diabetes mortality rate	0.0003 (0.0008)	.69
Cardiovascular disease mortality rate	−0.0001 (0.0001)	.4
High income vs low/middle income	0.033 (0.034)	.34

d

Group	b (SE)	P
Pandemic severity	< 0.0001 (0)	< .001
Vaccination coverage	−0.0003 (0.0001)	.05

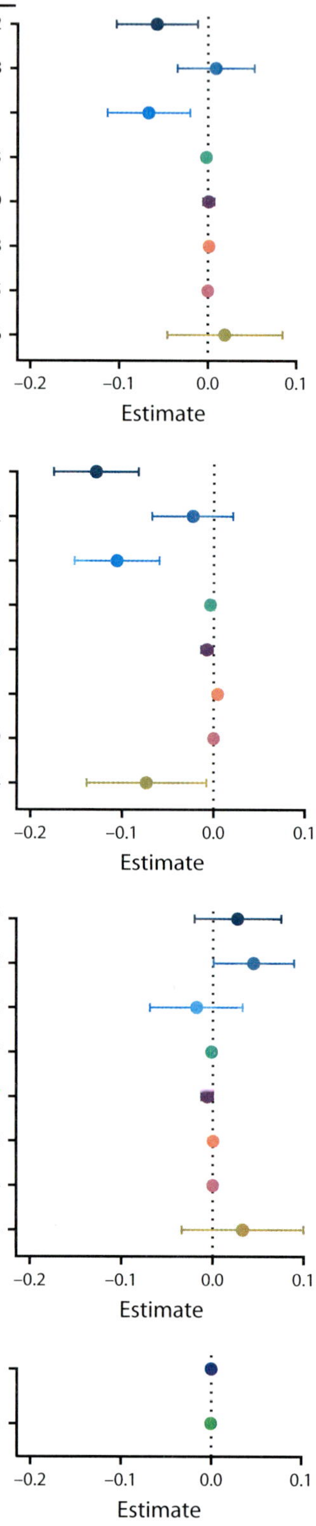

FIGURE 4— Association Between Excess Mortality Ratio and COVID-19 Containment Performance After Adjusting for Other Variables for (a) 2020, (b) 2021, (c) 2022, and (d) Pandemic Severity and Vaccination Coverage: 2020–2022

Note. Pandemic severity and vaccination coverage show no interaction with the variable representing the year.

groups. Although some variables were not statistically significant, the model indicates that higher health care index scores were associated with reductions in excess mortality. An increasing trend in diabetes-related death ratios was significantly associated with higher excess mortality, suggesting that chronic disease prevalence may exacerbate pandemic-related mortality. No statistically significant or consistent associations were observed between cardiovascular mortality, high-income country status, and the percentage of those aged 65 years and older with excess mortality during the 2020–2022 study period. Although the variable did not reach statistical significance, the excess mortality decreased as vaccination coverage increased. The pandemic severity, included as a time-varying covariate in the model, indicates a relationship between increasing COVID-19 infections and the excess mortality ratio.

DISCUSSION

Our research revealed that after adjusting for structural conditions—including pandemic severity, the percentage of the population aged 65 years and older, health care, vaccination ratios, diabetes, cardiovascular disease death ratios, and income—our findings on excess mortality ratios remained largely unchanged, indicating that these factors had minimal impact on the observed associations. In 2020 and 2021, the excess mortality ratios for the top and middle containment performance groups were significantly lower than those for the bottom containment performance group. The excess mortality ratio of the top containment performance group compared with that of the middle containment performance group was also reduced, although not significantly. The analysis revealed a diminished divergence in excess mortality across containment performance groups in 2022 compared with previous years. This convergence likely reflects the unique epidemiological context, especially Omicron's rapid global spread because of its high transmissibility. This herd immunity from Omicron's widespread infections may have lessened the observable impact of containment approaches on excess mortality, contributing to reduced disparities. Further research is needed to disentangle the roles of Omicron's characteristics, preexisting immunity, and ongoing public health measures in shaping mortality patterns. This finding suggests that the indicator accurately reflects better government containment, potentially leading to reduced excess mortality both in the early, prevaccine stages and the middle, postvaccine phases of the COVID-19 pandemic.

In an investigation of 34 countries, New Zealand exhibited the lowest total excess mortality. New Zealand has long focused on health care equity and subsidies for disadvantaged groups.[29] Early in the pandemic, New Zealand implemented an elimination strategy that included border closures and lockdowns.[30] Besides this strategy,[31] the decrease in deaths from respiratory viral infections[32,33] and external causes[34] contributed to the negative excess mortality reported in 2020. By Omicron's dominance in 2022, New Zealand already had more than 90% vaccination coverage, booster shots were administered, and there was a superior free rapid antigen testing strategy.[29] New Zealand's robust public health infrastructure and high vaccination coverage, supported by immunity brought by Omicron's high transmissibility with lower severity, facilitated effective COVID-19 management under a mitigation strategy. Thus, despite shifting strategies, New Zealand successfully managed to control transmission.

Mexico recorded the highest excess mortality ratio in 2020 and the second highest in 2021, primarily because of COVID-19. The conversion of hospitals to COVID-19 care facilities and fear of seeking medical assistance may have further increased mortality.[35] In addition, high rates of underlying conditions, such as hypertension, obesity, and diabetes, likely contributed to the elevated mortality figures.[36]

This study demonstrated that indicators show a decrease in excess mortality corresponding to containment performance during the first 2 years. While the pandemic lifestyle was sustained for a limited period, individuals eventually reverted to prepandemic norms. The study noted that excess mortality rose after restrictions were lifted in some countries with good containment performance, consistent with previous findings.[37,38] Several factors may have influenced this outcome. First, transitioning from an elimination strategy to a mitigation strategy before achieving sufficient vaccine coverage caused a rebound in deaths.[39–41] Second, disruptions in health care services, missed routine care, and delayed procedures likely impacted individuals with chronic conditions. While the direct impact of missed health checks on mortality may be limited,[42] these disruptions, coupled with delays in essential procedures, could have contributed to adverse outcomes.[43,44] Finally, the previous strict policies protected the lives of vulnerable individuals, such as the elderly. As a consequence, when the restrictions were lifted, countries with high aging populations experienced an increase in deaths, as observed in Finland and

Norway.[45] Therefore, in some countries with previously stronger containment performance, the lifting of restrictions in 2022, coupled with factors such as vaccine coverage, inconsistent availability of essential medical services, and population vulnerability, likely contributed to excess mortality.[38]

Our research found that robust health care systems were linked to decreased excess mortality, consistent with previous studies.[46] We suggest allocating more resources during epidemics to avoid shortages of medical personnel, interruptions in medical education, and deterioration in professional well-being.[47–49] In addition, there is a relationship between diabetes and an increase in excess mortality, aligning with previous findings.[50,51] High-income countries experienced higher excess mortality ratios in 2020, likely because of early virus spread and international mobility, but showed statistically significant reductions in excess mortality in 2021, possibly reflecting improved health care access and rapid vaccination rollout.[52,53] In addition, our research indicates that there was a negative correlation between vaccine coverage and excess mortality ratios. This finding is similar to the results of previous studies.[54] Therefore, high vaccine coverage was associated with a decrease in excess mortality ratios. We found that there was no significant interaction between vaccination coverage and years. A plausible reason is that vaccine coverage showed a rapid increase during 2021. During 2022, the growth in vaccine coverage rate in each country began to slow. This phenomenon may shed light on the importance of booster doses of the COVID-19 vaccine.[55,56]

A striking finding of our analysis is the apparent paradox of regions that experienced increases in excess mortality later in the pandemic also demonstrated the best overall outcomes. This suggests that strict early interventions, even if relaxed later, were crucial. Aggressive early containment suppressed initial viral circulation, buying time for vaccines and treatments. Although these regions eventually saw increased mortality as the pandemic evolved, the delayed and potentially less severe impact, because of prioritized early suppression, contributed to their lower overall excess mortality.

In the first 2 years of the pandemic, as countries navigated the emerging crisis, the elimination strategy proved effective. This containment performance indicator was instrumental in assessing how excess mortality was impacted when governments adopted elimination strategies. These early indicators showed that robust health policies and targeted lockdowns correlated with lower excess mortality. In the postpandemic phase, with widespread vaccine coverage, booster programs, and the lifting of lockdowns, a "new normal" emerged. Moving forward, a new indicator is needed to evaluate the efficacy of ongoing mitigation strategies and preparedness to address potential future epidemics.

Limitations

This study has several limitations. First, COVID-19 excess mortality data varied across research units, affecting study precision. Second, the grouping was based on containment performance data from 2020 and 2021, which is potentially not entirely reflective of countries' responses to COVID-19 in 2022. Third, this analysis encompassed only 34 countries, which requires cautious generalization of findings. Fourth, different testing capabilities may have had a potential impact on the data used in our model. Using cases per capita can be biased, as limited testing and high positivity rates can mask true infection numbers. Restricted testing may falsely suggest lower case numbers. This could underestimate the true COVID-19 burden and influence our results. Future research could explore alternative metrics less sensitive to testing variations or incorporate testing data to adjust for this potential bias. Finally, heterogeneous vaccination uptake across demographic groups, especially by age, may have influenced the analysis results. Although we analyzed overall vaccination rates, we acknowledge that these aggregate figures may not accurately reflect the distribution of vaccine coverage within populations. For example, high overall vaccination rates may mask low coverage among vulnerable elderly, increasing their risk of severe outcomes. Our analysis, lacking age-stratified vaccination data, cannot directly address this issue.

Public Health Implications

Our findings highlight the need for new metrics to assess long-term public health strategies after the acute pandemic phase, recognizing their evolving nature. We envision a new index encompassing the "One Health" approach, integrating our existing analysis of government COVID-19 response with veterinary and environmental health to address disease control and resilience. Assessing human–animal interactions, animal disease, and ecosystem health will improve emerging infectious disease prediction, prevention, and response—safeguarding overall health. AJPH

ABOUT THE AUTHORS

Chieh Cheng, Hsiao-Yu Wu, Ya-Ting Hsu, Yi-Kai Chen, Yung-An Jang, Chih-Fan Hung, and Wei-Ming Jiang were with the Institute of Population Health Sciences, National Health Research Institutes, Zhunan, Miaoli County, Taiwan, at the time of this study. Shu-Chen Kuo is with the National Institute of Infectious Diseases and Vaccinology, National Health Research Institutes, Zhunan. Brandon Fan is with the Richard Montgomery High School, Rockville, MD. Byron Fan is with the Department of Applied Mathematics, Brown University, Providence, RI. Hung-Yi Chiou and Hsiao-Hui Tsou are with the Institute of Population Health Sciences, National Health Research Institutes, Zhunan. Wei J. Chen is with the Center for Neuropsychiatric Research, National Health Research Institutes, Zhunan.

CORRESPONDENCE

Correspondence should be sent to Hsiao-Hui Tsou, Institute of Population Health Sciences, National Health Research Institutes, 35 Keyan Rd, Zhunan, Miaoli County 350, Taiwan (e-mail: tsouhh@nhri.edu.tw). Reprints can be ordered at https://www.ajph.org by clicking the "Reprints" link.

PUBLICATION INFORMATION

Full Citation: Cheng C, Wu H-Y, Kuo S-C, et al. Excess mortality and containment performance during the COVID-19 pandemic: evidence from 34 countries. *Am J Public Health*. 2025;115(9): 1518–1528.

Acceptance Date: March 23, 2025.

DOI: https://doi.org/10.2105/AJPH.2025.308136

ORCID iDs:

Chieh Cheng https://orcid.org/0009-0003-2359-1720

Hsiao-Yu Wu https://orcid.org/0000-0003-0904-0351

Shu-Chen Kuo https://orcid.org/0000-0002-6940-6450

Brandon Fan https://orcid.org/0009-0005-1581-241X

Yi-Kai Chen https://orcid.org/0009-0004-1851-9406

Byron Fan https://orcid.org/0000-0002-8373-715X

Yung-An Jang https://orcid.org/0009-0003-6744-0975

Wei-Ming Jiang https://orcid.org/0000-0002-2882-5392

Hsiao-Hui Tsou https://orcid.org/0000-0001-6773-4111

CONTRIBUTORS

C. Cheng, H.Y. Wu, Y.T. Hsu, Y.K. Chen, C.F. Hung, and H.H. Tsou contributed to the acquisition, analysis, or interpretation of data. C. Cheng, H.Y. Wu, Br. Fan, Y.T. Hsu, Y.K. Chen, By. Fan, and H.H. Tsou contributed to the drafting of the article. C. Cheng, H.Y. Wu, Y.T. Hsu, and C.F. Hung conducted the statistical analysis. S.C. Kuo and H.H. Tsou contributed to the concept and design of the study. S.C. Kuo, H.Y. Chiou, W.J. Chen, and H.H. Tsou obtained funding. S.C. Kuo, Br. Fan, and By. Fan contributed to the interpretation of data. Y.K. Chen, H.Y. Chiou, W.J. Chen, and H.H. Tsou provided administrative, technical, or material support. Y.A. Jang, W.M. Jiang, W.J. Chen, and H.H. Tsou conducted a critical review of the article for important intellectual content. C. Cheng and H.H. Tsou had full access to all data in the study and take responsibility for the integrity of the data and the accuracy of the data analysis.

ACKNOWLEDGMENTS

This work was supported by grants (PH-113-GP-02, PH-113-GP-12) from the National Health Research Institutes, a nonprofit foundation dedicated to medical research and improved health care in Taiwan.

The authors thank MengLi Lu, MS and Yu-Chun Lu, MS, from the National Health Research Institutes, Taiwan, for their valuable comments and support.

Note. The funders had no role in the design and conduct of the study; collection, management, analysis, and interpretation of the data; preparation, review, or approval of the article; and decision to submit the article for publication.

CONFLICTS OF INTEREST

All authors declare no conflicts of interest, including employment, consultancies, stock ownership, honoraria, paid expert testimony, patent applications, and travel grants.

HUMAN PARTICIPANT PROTECTION

The institutional review board of the National Health Research Institutes approved this study (EC1101202-E).

REFERENCES

1. Beaney T, Clarke JM, Jain V, et al. Excess mortality: the gold standard in measuring the impact of COVID-19 worldwide? *J R Soc Med*. 2020;113(9): 329–334. https://doi.org/10.1177/0141076820956802
2. Checchi F, Roberts L. Interpreting and using mortality data in humanitarian emergencies. Humanitarian Practice Network. 2005. Available at: https://odihpn.org/wp-content/uploads/2005/09/networkpaper052.pdf. Accessed January 11, 2024.
3. Ahmed T, Roberton T, Vergeer P, et al. Healthcare utilization and maternal and child mortality during the COVID-19 pandemic in 18 low- and middle-income countries: an interrupted time-series analysis with mathematical modeling of administrative data. *PLoS Med*. 2022;19(8):e1004070. https://doi.org/10.1371/journal.pmed.1004070
4. Arsenault C, Gage A, Kim MK, et al. COVID-19 and resilience of healthcare systems in ten countries. *Nat Med*. 2022;28(6):1314–1324. https://doi.org/10.1038/s41591-022-01750-1
5. Woolf SH, Chapman DA, Sabo RT, Weinberger DM, Hill L. Excess deaths from COVID-19 and other causes, March–April 2020. *JAMA*. 2020;324(5): 510–513. https://doi.org/10.1001/jama.2020.11787
6. Petterson S, Westfall JM, Miller BF. Projected deaths of despair from COVID-19. Well Being Trust. 2020. Available at: https://digitalcommons.providence.org/publications/3054. Accessed January 12, 2024.
7. Wang H, Paulson KR, Pease SA, et al. Estimating excess mortality due to the COVID-19 pandemic: a systematic analysis of COVID-19-related mortality, 2020–21. *Lancet*. 2022;399(10334):1513–1536. https://doi.org/10.1016/S0140-6736(21)02796-3
8. Rovetta A. Annual excess crude mortality in Europe during the COVID-19 pandemic: a longitudinal joinpoint regression analysis of historical trends from 2000 to 2021. *COVID*. 2022;2(12): 1778–1786. https://doi.org/10.3390/covid2120128
9. Msemburi W, Karlinsky A, Knutson V, Aleshin-Guendel S, Chatterji S, Wakefield J. The WHO estimates of excess mortality associated with the COVID-19 pandemic. *Nature*. 2023;613(7942): 130–137. https://doi.org/10.1038/s41586-022-05522-2
10. Zhu D, Ozaki A, Virani SS. Disease-specific excess mortality during the COVID-19 pandemic: an analysis of weekly US death data for 2020. *Am J Public Health*. 2021;111(8):1518–1522. https://doi.org/10.2105/AJPH.2021.306315
11. Demetriou CA, Achilleos S, Quattrocchi A, et al. Impact of the COVID-19 pandemic on total, sex- and age-specific all-cause mortality in 20 countries worldwide during 2020: results from the C-MOR project. *Int J Epidemiol*. 2023; 52(3):664–676. https://doi.org/10.1093/ije/dyac170
12. Lee WE, Woo Park S, Weinberger DM, et al. Direct and indirect mortality impacts of the COVID-19 pandemic in the United States, March 1, 2020 to January 1, 2022. *eLife*. 2023;12:e77562. https://doi.org/10.7554/eLife.77562
13. Kondilis E, Tarantilis F, Benos A. Essential public healthcare services utilization and excess non-COVID-19 mortality in Greece. *Public Health*. 2021;198:85–88. https://doi.org/10.1016/j.puhe.2021.06.025
14. Stokes AC, Lundberg DJ, Bor J, Elo IT, Hempstead K, Preston SH. Association of health care factors with excess deaths not assigned to COVID-19 in the US. *JAMA Netw Open*. 2021;4(9):e2125287. https://doi.org/10.1001/jamanetworkopen.2021.25287
15. Kapitsinis N. The underlying factors of excess mortality in 2020: a cross-country analysis of pre-pandemic healthcare conditions and strategies to cope with Covid-19. *BMC Health Serv Res*. 2021;21(1):1197. https://doi.org/10.1186/s12913-021-07169-7
16. Buja A, Paganini M, Fusinato R, et al. Health and healthcare variables associated with Italy's excess mortality during the first wave of the COVID-19 pandemic: an ecological study. *Health Policy*. 2022;126(4):294–301. https://doi.org/10.1016/j.healthpol.2022.03.002
17. Favaro E, Saugo C, Sandu B, et al. Estimation of excess deaths in Turin from COVID-19 and other causes, October to November 2020. *Eur J Public Health*. 2021;31(suppl 3):ckab164.554. https://doi.org/10.1093/eurpub/ckab164.554
18. Parkes B, Stafoggia M, Fecht D, et al. Community factors and excess mortality in the COVID-19 pandemic in England, Italy and Sweden. *Eur J*

Public Health. 2023;33(4):695–703. https://doi.org/10.1093/eurpub/ckad075

19. Wang W, Gurgone A, Martínez H, et al. COVID-19 mortality and economic losses: the role of policies and structural conditions. *J Risk Financ Manag.* 2022;15(8):354. https://doi.org/10.3390/jrfm15080354
20. Agrawal V, Cantor J, Sood N, Whaley C. The impact of COVID-19 shelter-in-place policy responses on excess mortality. *Health Econ.* 2023;32(11):2499–2515. https://doi.org/10.1002/hec.4737
21. Tsou HH, Kuo SC, Lin YH, et al. A comprehensive evaluation of COVID-19 policies and outcomes in 50 countries and territories. *Sci Rep.* 2022;12(1):8802. https://doi.org/10.1038/s41598-022-12853-7
22. Tracking COVID-19 excess deaths across countries. *The Economist.* October 20, 2021. Available at: https://www.economist.com/graphic-detail/coronavirus-excess-deaths-tracker. Accessed December 25, 2023.
23. Paglino E, Stokes AC. Excess mortality as a tool to monitor the evolution of health emergencies: choices, challenges, and future directions. *Am J Public Health.* 2024;114(6):583–586. https://doi.org/10.2105/AJPH.2024.307661
24. Mathieu E, Ritchie H, Rodés-Guirao L, et al. COVID-19 pandemic. Our World in Data. March 2020. Available at: https://ourworldindata.org/coronavirus. Accessed February 9, 2023.
25. Dimitropoulou A. Revealed: countries with the best health care systems, 2023. *CEOWORLD Magazine.* August 25, 2023. Available at: https://ceoworld.biz/2023/08/25/revealed-countries-with-the-best-health-care-systems-2023. Accessed December 25, 2023.
26. Institute for Health Metrics and Evaluation. Global Health Data Exchange. Available at: https://ghdx.healthdata.org. Accessed December 25, 2023.
27. World Bank Data Help Desk. World Bank Country and Lending Groups. Available at: https://datahelpdesk.worldbank.org/knowledgebase/articles/906519-world-bank-country-and-lending-groups. Accessed December 25, 2023.
28. Lang TA, Secic M. *How to Report Statistics in Medicine: Annotated Guidelines for Authors, Editors, and Reviewers.* 2nd ed. American College of Physicians. Available at: https://store.acponline.org/ebiz/products-services/product-details/productid/17152. Accessed December 25, 2023.
29. Gauld R. A review of public policies on Covid-19: the New Zealand experience. *Public Administration and Policy: An Asia-Pacific Journal.* 2023;26(1):10–20. https://doi.org/10.1108/PAP-04-2022-0028
30. Kung S, Hills T, Kearns N, Beasley R. New Zealand's COVID-19 elimination strategy and mortality patterns. *Lancet.* 2023;402(10407):1037–1038. https://doi.org/10.1016/S0140-6736(23)01368-5
31. Baker MG, Wilson N, Anglemyer A. Successful elimination of Covid-19 transmission in New Zealand. *N Engl J Med.* 2020;383(8):e56. https://doi.org/10.1056/NEJMc2025203
32. Huang QS, Wood T, Jelley L, NPIsImpactOnFlu Consortium, et al. Impact of the COVID-19 non-pharmaceutical interventions on influenza and other respiratory viral infections in New Zealand. *Nat Commun.* 2021;12(1):1001. https://doi.org/10.1038/s41467-021-21157-9
33. Hills T, Hatter L, Kearns N, Bruce P, Beasley R. COVID-19 border controls prevent a 2021 seasonal influenza epidemic in New Zealand. *Public Health.* 2021;200:e6–e7. https://doi.org/10.1016/j.puhe.2021.09.013
34. Kung S, Doppen M, Black M, Hills T, Kearns N. Reduced mortality in New Zealand during the COVID-19 pandemic. *Lancet.* 2021;397(10268):25. https://doi.org/10.1016/S0140-6736(20)32647-7
35. Palacio-Mejía LS, Hernández-Ávila JE, Hernández-Ávila M, et al. Leading causes of excess mortality in Mexico during the COVID-19 pandemic 2020–2021: death certificates study in a middle-income country. *Lancet Reg Health Am.* 2022;13:100303. https://doi.org/10.1016/j.lana.2022.100303
36. Loza A, Wong-Chew RM, Jiménez-Corona ME, et al. Two-year follow-up of the COVID-19 pandemic in Mexico. *Front Public Health.* 2022;10:1050673. https://doi.org/10.3389/fpubh.2022.1050673
37. Walkowiak MP, Domaradzki J, Walkowiak D. Unmasking the COVID-19 pandemic prevention gains: excess mortality reversal in 2022. *Public Health.* 2023;223:193–201. https://doi.org/10.1016/j.puhe.2023.08.004
38. Marinković I, Galjak M. Timing and toll: Europe's excess mortality in the first three years of COVID-19. *Popul Res Policy Rev.* 2024;43(3):35. https://doi.org/10.1007/s11113-024-09884-5
39. Ge Y, Zhang WB, Wu X, et al. Untangling the changing impact of non-pharmaceutical interventions and vaccination on European COVID-19 trajectories. *Nat Commun.* 2022;13(1):3106. https://doi.org/10.1038/s41467-022-30897-1
40. Shattock AJ, Le Rutte EA, Dünner RP, et al. Impact of vaccination and non-pharmaceutical interventions on SARS-CoV-2 dynamics in Switzerland. *Epidemics.* 2022;38:100535. https://doi.org/10.1016/j.epidem.2021.100535
41. Cao X, Li Y, Zi Y, Zhu Y. The shift of percent excess mortality from zero-COVID policy to living-with-COVID policy in Singapore, South Korea, Australia, New Zealand and Hong Kong SAR. *Front Public Health.* 2023;11:1085451. https://doi.org/10.3389/fpubh.2023.1085451
42. Liss DT, Uchida T, Wilkes CL, Radakrishnan A, Linder JA. General health checks in adult primary care: a review. *JAMA.* 2021;325(22):2294–2306. https://doi.org/10.1001/jama.2021.6524
43. Mularczyk-Tomczewska P, Zarnowski A, Gujski M, et al. Barriers to accessing health services during the COVID-19 pandemic in Poland: a nationwide cross-sectional survey among 109,928 adults in Poland. *Front Public Health.* 2022;10:986996. https://doi.org/10.3389/fpubh.2022.986996
44. Gasch-Illescas A, Calle-Serrano M, Vallejo-Vaz AJ, et al. Impact of the first wave of the COVID-19 pandemic on non-COVID inpatient care in southern Spain. *Sci Rep.* 2023;13(1):1634. https://doi.org/10.1038/s41598-023-28831-6
45. Forthun I, Madsen C, Emilsson L, et al. Excess mortality in Denmark, Finland, Norway and Sweden during the COVID-19 pandemic 2020–2022. *Eur J Public Health.* 2024;34(4):737–743. https://doi.org/10.1093/eurpub/ckae091
46. Moolla I, Hiilamo H. Health system characteristics and COVID-19 performance in high-income countries. *BMC Health Serv Res.* 2023;23(1):244. https://doi.org/10.1186/s12913-023-09206-z
47. Kinman G, Teoh K, Harriss A. Supporting the well-being of healthcare workers during and after COVID-19. *Occup Med (Lond).* 2020;70(5):294–296. https://doi.org/10.1093/occmed/kqaa096
48. Buonsenso D, De Rose C, Pierantoni L. Doctors' shortage in adults COVID-19 units: a call for pediatricians. *Eur J Pediatr.* 2021;180(7):2315–2318. https://doi.org/10.1007/s00431-021-03995-3
49. Strangio A, Leo I, Spaccarotella CAM, et al. Effects of the COVID-19 pandemic on the formation of fellows in training in cardiology. *J Cardiovasc Med (Hagerstown).* 2021;22(9):711–715. https://doi.org/10.2459/JCM.0000000000001185
50. Alicandro G, La Vecchia C, Islam N, Pizzato M. A comprehensive analysis of all-cause and cause-specific excess deaths in 30 countries during 2020. *Eur J Epidemiol.* 2023;38(11):1153–1164. https://doi.org/10.1007/s10654-023-01044-x
51. Yao XI, Han L, Sun Y, He D, Zhao S, Ran J. Temporal variation of excess deaths from diabetes during the COVID-19 pandemic in the United States. *J Infect Public Health.* 2023;16(4):483–489. https://doi.org/10.1016/j.jiph.2023.01.018
52. Yao L, Aleya L, Howard SC, et al. Variations of COVID-19 mortality are affected by economic disparities across countries. *Sci Total Environ.* 2022;832:154770. https://doi.org/10.1016/j.scitotenv.2022.154770
53. López-Gigosos R, Vegas-Romero M, Mariscal A, Mariscal-López E, Fang J, Gutiérrez-Bedmar M. Excess mortality in 22 European countries in 2020 and 2021: relationship with socioeconomic indicators. *Perspect Public Health.* 2023:17579139231180800. https://doi.org/10.1177/17579139231180800
54. Faust JS, Du C, Mayes KD, et al. Absence of excess mortality in a highly vaccinated population during the initial Covid-19 delta period. Preprint. Posted online September 21, 2021. MedRxiv. https://doi.org/10.1101/2021.09.16.21263477
55. Arbel R, Sergienko R, Friger M, et al. Effectiveness of a second BNT162b2 booster vaccine against hospitalization and death from COVID-19 in adults aged over 60 years. *Nat Med.* 2022;28(7):1486–1490. https://doi.org/10.1038/s41591-022-01832-0
56. Matveeva O, Shabalina SA. Comparison of vaccination and booster rates and their impact on excess mortality during the COVID-19 pandemic in European countries. *Front Immunol.* 2023;14:1151311. https://doi.org/10.3389/fimmu.2023.1151311

The Citizens Air Complaint Program: Laypeople Reporting Air Pollution Violations in New York City

Chris Hartmann, PhD

Air pollution is associated with numerous adverse health outcomes and increased mortality. Nationally, medium- and heavy-duty vehicles produce more than one half of nitrogen oxides and particle pollution, despite comprising only 6% of on-road vehicles.

Instituted in 2018, the Citizens Air Complaint Program (CACP) in New York City permits laypeople to file complaints against commercial trucks and buses that idle in excess of the legal limit. Lay complainants receive one quarter of the paid penalty. In 2024, laypeople submitted more than 124 000 complaints for alleged idling infractions.

Empowering laypeople to report environmental health code infractions and compensating them to do so is an innovative, critically important complement to public health practice that advances healthy communities. Additional steps are needed to address barriers to participating in the CACP. Lawmakers should consider layperson reporting and remuneration programs for other underenforced public health issues. (*Am J Public Health*. 2025;115(9):1529–1535. https://doi.org/10.2105/AJPH.2025.308137)

AJPH September 2025, Vol. 115, No. 9

The harmful impacts of air pollution on human health—and for climate change—are numerous and well-documented.[1] Short- and long-term exposure to air pollution is a major risk factor for chronic respiratory diseases, cardiovascular diseases, and cancers, among others, as well as increased mortality.[2,3] Annually, air pollution is estimated to cause more than 100 000 premature deaths in the United States[4] and approximately 7 million premature deaths globally.[5] Therefore, addressing air pollution remains a fundamental public health priority.

Although sources of air pollution vary across the United States, the transportation sector is a leading producer of noxious gases and fine particulate matter ($PM_{2.5}$), as well as greenhouse gas emissions.[6] Medium- and heavy-duty vehicles produce more than one half of nitrogen oxides and particle pollution, despite comprising only 6% of on-road vehicles.[7] Furthermore, exhaust from idling medium- and heavy-duty vehicle engines is a known major contributing factor to air pollution and greenhouse gases[8]; in general, diesel exhaust is associated with many short- and long-term health impacts.[9]

Since the mid-19th century, laypeople's activism and legislative changes have played an important role in improving air quality. Laypeople have monitored pollution, raised awareness of myriad health impacts from pollutants, and demanded legislative changes to limit and prevent further pollution.[10] Several significant legislative acts have contributed to reductions in air pollution, including from the transportation sector, such as the founding of the Environmental Protection Agency (in 1970), the first Clean Air Act (1970) and subsequent amendments (1977), national standards for 6 common air pollutants (1971), and phasing out leaded gasoline (1973), among others.

Still, air pollution remains a major public health problem. One novel approach to enforcing municipal air pollution regulations is the Citizens Air Complaint Program (CACP) in New York City. Recognizing air pollution as an underenforced and pervasive problem, the CACP permits laypeople to document and submit complaints against commercial trucks and buses that idle more than the legal limit and awards them a portion of the paid penalty. If a truck or bus is found in violation of illegal idling and the fine is paid, then lay complainants are entitled to 25% of the paid civil penalty. In 2024, laypeople submitted more than 124 000 complaints for alleged idling infractions; by comparison, in 2023, municipal employees submitted only 210 complaints. I provide an overview of the CACP and situate it within other citizen-led approaches to document environmental health code infractions. I also outline several ways in which the CACP may be improved to increase participation.

AIR POLLUTION IN NEW YORK CITY

In New York City, public outrage from a deadly smog event in 1966 contributed to a tightening of the municipal Air Pollution Control Codes.[11] Since then, air quality has generally improved. Between 2009 and 2022, for example, annual averages of key indicators of air pollution, including black carbon, nitric oxide, nitrogen dioxide, and $PM_{2.5}$, decreased by at least 40% across New York City.[12] Still, pollutant levels in New York City are high relative to other cities, and it remains one of the most polluted cities in the United States.[13]

Current major sources of air pollution in New York City include emissions from commercial cooking, fossil fuel combustion for residential and commercial buildings, and motor vehicle traffic.[11] Research shows that variations in air pollution across all 5 boroughs are largely attributable to motor vehicle traffic,[14] which accounts for 59% of nitrous oxide emissions, 17% of $PM_{2.5}$, and 70% of black carbon.[15] Trucks and buses account for only 6% of all vehicle miles traveled, yet they contributed the largest share of ambient $PM_{2.5}$ and nitrous oxide among all vehicles.[14]

The estimated health impacts of air pollution from all sources on New Yorkers are profound. For example, annually, $PM_{2.5}$ kills an estimated 1800 people, causes nearly 2000 emergency department visits for asthma, and leads to over 900 hospitalizations for asthma, cardiovascular, and respiratory issues.[16] Trucks and buses are responsible for most of the $PM_{2.5}$-attributable deaths each year (170 deaths).[14] Representative of long-standing environmental injustices associated with air pollution, low-income people and people of color are more likely to live in heavily polluted "microclimate" neighborhoods because of their proximity to heavily trafficked roads and industrial facilities.[17] Importantly, air pollution is particularly harmful to low-income and Black and Hispanic or Latino communities because of long-standing structural inequities like inadequate health care access, lower-quality housing, and preexisting comorbidities.[11]

THE CITIZENS AIR COMPLAINT PROGRAM

In 1971, City Council adopted anti-idling legislation, as well as other air pollution reduction policies, in an effort to improve air quality and meet new federal clean air guidelines. Since then, City Council has amended and expanded the law to prohibit many commercial trucks and buses from unnecessarily idling their engines for more than 3 minutes (Table 1); currently, the law exempts emergency vehicles and vehicles engaged in certain activities (e.g., operating a lift gate).

TABLE 1— Timeline of Notable Anti-Idling Legislation in New York City

Year	Notable Precedent or Changes
1971	No motor vehicle, including buses, is permitted to idle for more than 3 min; exemptions: emergency service vehicles and vehicles engaged in loading, unloading, or operating a processing device (sections 1403.2–11.15). Any person who is not an employee of NYC is authorized by law to serve summonses for violation of the administration code may file a complaint against a bus; the complainant is to be awarded an amount of not more than 25% of the collected proceeds from a civil penalty (sections 1403.2–15.09).
2009	No motor vehicle is permitted to idle for more than 1 min adjacent to a preschool or K-12 school. Any nonemployee of NYC is authorized to submit complaints against trucks and buses for illegal idling. In addition to NYPD and DEP, the Department of Parks and Recreation and the Department of Sanitation are given the authority to issue idling summonses.
2018	Citizen complainants will be awarded 25% of the collected proceeds from a civil penalty. DEP must make available online information about best practices for filing citizen complaints, including gathering supporting documentation for the complaint.
2023	No motor vehicle may idle adjacent to a preschool or K-12 school or inside a park under the jurisdiction of the Parks Department for more than 1 min; no motor vehicle may idle adjacent to a park under the jurisdiction of the Parks Department (delayed until 2024).

Note. DEP = Department of Environmental Protection; K-12 = kindergarten to 12th grade; NYC = New York City; NYPD = New York Police Department. For a list of complete sources, see Appendix (available as a supplement to the online version of this article at http://www.ajph.org).

In 2009, in response to 1 in every 4 New York City school-aged child having asthma, City Council reduced the legal idling time from 3 minutes to 1 minute in front of a school. (In 2024, the Department of Environmental Protection [DEP], which is tasked with overseeing the CACP, extended a stricter 1-minute idling limit to roads adjacent to municipal parks and green spaces under the jurisdiction of the Department of Parks and Recreation.) Despite these laws, DEP and the New York Police Department rarely issued summonses for idling violations, despite evidence suggesting its widespread prevalence.[18] In 2018, for example, DEP issued fewer than 5 summonses per day for complaints initiated by municipal employees. Based on the daily volume of commercial vehicles that traverse New York City—nearly 200 000 commercial vehicles enter Manhattan and Brooklyn alone[19]—and the expansive size of the 5 boroughs—there are 6300 miles of roadways across the city[20]—it is very likely that anti-idling legislation was severely underenforced.

Public concern about pervasive commercial vehicle idling pushed City Council to create the CACP in 2018. (The inclusion of the word "citizen" is a misnomer; any person, regardless of their place of residence or their immigration status, is permitted to participate in the CACP.) The legislation that created the CACP reaffirmed laypeople's right to submit complaints against commercial trucks and buses that violate the Air Code, mandated that DEP make available online information about best practices for filing lay complaints, and codified that the lay complainant was entitled to one quarter of the proceeds collected from the imposed penalty ($350–$2000), or $87.50 to $500 per paid complaint.

Laypeople may submit complaints against commercial entities for any violation of the New York City Air Code, including excessive noise, dispersal of dust particulates (e.g., construction debris), and odors; however, here I focus only on commercial vehicle idling complaints.

To submit an idling complaint against a commercial truck or bus, a lay complainant must (1) complete an online form that requires inclusion of personal information of the complainant (e.g., address), name and contact information of the company alleged to have violated the Air Code, and a brief description of the idling offense; and (2) submit a time-stamped video documenting the alleged offense plus time-stamped photos of the license plate and other identifying information of the vehicle (e.g., company address, US Department of Transportation number). Each complaint is reviewed by 2 DEP inspectors. If the complaint is accepted and pursued, then a summons is written and the Office of Administrative Trials and Hearings (OATH) schedules a hearing. The company alleged to have violated the Air Code is permitted to admit to the violation prior to the hearing or dispute the charges at the hearing. Between 2021 and 2023, the average time DEP took to review a complaint increased 56% to 113 days.[21] Currently, OATH hearings are scheduled between 3 and 15 months after DEP determines it will pursue charges; consequently, it is not uncommon for a hearing to be scheduled more than 1 year after the initial complaint is submitted. Both DEP and the alleged Air Code violator are entitled to contest the outcome of the hearing, which can prolong the process by 3 months or more.

Since 2018, the number of commercial idling vehicle complaints submitted by laypeople has increased substantially and far outpaced those submitted by New York City employees (Table 2). Few people participate in the CACP relative to the population of New York City (8.25 million people) and the metropolitan area (23.5 million people). According to data that examined the first 20 000 submissions (2018–mid-2020), 20 lay individuals submitted 85% of all complaints.[22] In 2023, more than 900 complainants submitted approximately 88 000 complaints, which resulted in 77 193 summonses for violations of the city's anti-idling law; DEP has not

TABLE 2— Number of Summonses Issued Since 2019 by Laypeople and Employees of New York City

Year	Idling Complaints Initiated by Laypeople	Idling Complaints Initiated by New York City Employees[a]
2019	9 070	1 278
2020	9 406	284
2021	11 138	383
2022	48 979	445
2023	82 615	210
2024	124 330	Not available

Source. New York City Department of Environmental Protection, New York Clean Air Collective. For a list of complete sources, see Appendix (available as a supplement to the online version of this article at http://www.ajph.org).

[a]For example, employees of the Department of Environmental Protection or the New York Police Department.

released additional information about the number of complaints submitted per complainant. Between 2019 (the first full year in which the program operated) and 2024, the number of complaints filed increased 1270%.[21] From 2019 to 2023, complaints initiated by municipal officials decreased 87%; according to the DEP commissioner, this decrease is because of officials having to spend more time processing layperson-initiated complaints.[21] It is estimated that more than 95% of complaints submitted by laypeople resulted in a summons for excessive idling.[21] To date, the summonses are largely concentrated in 2 boroughs: Manhattan (66.1%) and Brooklyn (21.9%; Figure A, available as a supplement to the online version of this article at http://www.ajph.org). For summonses issued in 2022, the most recent year for which all summonses have received at least 1 hearing, approximately 75.6% of summonses found "in violation" were paid (NYC Open Data; https://opendata.cityofnewyork.us). To date, approximately $49.2 million in air code violation fines issued through the CACP have been paid to New York City.[21] Demonstrating one of the program's vital short- and long-term impacts on air pollution and climate change, several commercial entities, including private school bus companies, have electrified a portion of their vehicle fleets to avoid further idling fines.[21]

The current compensation structure of the CACP makes it unique among environmental health enforcement. To my knowledge, the CACP is the only program in the United States that compensates complainants for reporting environmental health code violations. In New York City, laypeople can anonymously report illegal idling activity and other quality of life issues (e.g., excessive noise, illegal parking, unsafe street conditions) to the 311 Customer Service Center. However, response times to 311 complaints are often slow, only 1% of all 311 complaints responded to by DEP resulted in a violation being issued, and complainants are not compensated if a summons is issued and paid.[23] An anti-idling program in Washington, DC accepts laypeople complaints but does not compensate the complainants.[24] In 2025, the Los Angeles City Council reintroduced a motion to explore a layperson idling complaint program modeled after the CACP.[25]

Regarding the CACP, compensation is believed to be a primary driver[26] of the nearly 14-fold increase in the number of complaints submitted from 2019 to 2024 (Table 2). Compensation is a source of discord among DEP officials because published reports state that some complainants earn 2 to 5 times as much as the DEP employees who review lay-initiated complaints.[26] However, reducing compensation for lay complainants could disincentivize participation in the CACP, as happened with the city's now-decimated citizen noise complaint program.[27] Coincidentally, the success of the CACP spurred the introduction of a bill (Intro 2024–0080) to compensate laypeople for identifying violators of another major public health issue that often is underenforced: private and commercial vehicles that block bicycle lanes, bus lanes, or pedestrian infrastructure (e.g., crosswalks).

LAYPEOPLE ADDRESSING ENVIRONMENTAL HEALTH ISSUES

The CACP shares similarities with several public health approaches that center and integrate the value of contributions by laypeople to complement public health practice and advance healthy communities. Citizen science, for example, encourages laypeople to engage in research activities, including developing research questions and collecting and reporting data, typically carried out by scientists. This approach is shown to improve public understanding of science and increase participation in local environmental science decision-making.[28,29] Similarly, popular epidemiology involves laypeople in scientific research, yet is unique for emphasizing connections between lay observations and health impacts. As a social movement, popular epidemiology is notable for spurring community action, including community organizing and litigation and confrontation when deemed necessary, to address understudied or poorly understood local exposures.[30] Finally, environmental racism and justice activists elevate communities historically underrepresented in research to localize their race- and class-based inequitable exposures to toxins. Addressing their pollution burden through lay observation and community organizing has been paramount to racial and environmental justice movements.[31]

The CACP is an effective enforcement tool because it incorporates—and has the potential to further incorporate—elements of each of the aforementioned 3 approaches. Consider the role of lay observations. In documenting illegal commercial vehicle idling, laypeople play a central role in realizing the core intent of the CACP: to enforce the New York City Air Code. Lay complainants use their experiential knowledge, including knowledge of where and at what time of day violations are most likely to occur, to enforce environmental health laws. Therefore, it is not surprising that complaints initiated by laypeople far outnumber those initiated by municipal employees (Table 2) because of laypeople's knowledge of and motivation to address neighborhood problems such as air pollution as well as staffing shortages at the DEP and the incentivization model of the CACP. Further, the CACP shines light on the magnitude of illegal commercial vehicle idling and laypeople's ability and desire to address local air pollution.

Similar to participants in popular epidemiology, CACP participants have organized themselves to preserve and expand the program, frequently drawing connections between personal or neighborhood health issues and commercial vehicle idling, and engaging in litigation and confrontation against DEP. CACP participants have formed 3 groups to advance the CACP and promote environmental health equity: the Idle Warriors listserv, a private group communication platform, and the New York Clean Air Collective (NYCAC), a 501(c)(6) nonprofit organization. At the time of writing, the Idle Warriors listserv is a publicly accessible Google listserv where lay observers, especially those new to the program, seek information (e.g., best practices, rule clarification) on how to navigate the CACP. Additionally, the listserv announces and encourages participation at public hearings on legislation about the CACP and other public health, environmental, and urban planning topics. There is some evidence to suggest that the CACP is increasing public interest in promoting healthy communities through policy change. Consider that 46 laypeople provided testimony on proposed changes to the CACP in fall 2024; among 4 public hearings focused on separate issues held on the same day, fewer than 10 laypeople on average submitted testimony.[21] In their public testimony, many lay enforcers and community members discussed how commercial vehicle idling adversely affected personal, familial, or community health issues. In February 2025, the public listserv began transitioning to a private group communication platform because of concerns about privacy. Further, a subgroup of the Idle Warrior group has formed NYCAC, a dues-paying social action group that, among other activities, engages in lobbying and litigation against DEP that, from the perspective of NYCAC, aims to preserve the intent of the CACP as originally enacted by City Council and hold polluters accountable for excessive idling. For example, at the time of writing, NYCAC is lobbying against DEP-endorsed legislation that, among other outcomes, would permit buses to idle next to schools for up to 18 minutes (compared with the 1-minute limit currently in place), reduce compensation for submitting a complaint, reduce the types of commercial trucks that can be served a summons, and permit DEP to ban laypeople who do not act in a "dignified, orderly, and decorous manner" from participating in the program.[20]

In general, evidence suggests that there may be less environmental health enforcement in historically marginalized communities than in others.[32] The CACP, which is open to all laypeople, should conceivably democratize the enforcement of the New York City Air Code. WE ACT, a well-known Black-led environmental justice organization in Harlem, commented,

> [The CACP] empowers these communities to report air quality issues, advocate for healthier living conditions, and hold polluters accountable, advancing both environmental justice and public health equity.[21]

Still, Air Code enforcement through the CACP relies on gathering documentation to submit a complaint; doing so gives laypeople—not municipal employees—the responsibility to collect evidence to initiate the complaint process. Since DEP rarely advertises the CACP, raising awareness and training communities also falls to individuals and community organizations. For example, WE ACT, together with DEP representatives and a member of the Idle Warrior listserv, hosted an informational webinar in 2022.[33] Importantly, and despite the DEP commissioner stating that "an unintentional impact of this program has been to shift DEP's own enforcement out of many [environmental justice] neighborhoods,"[21] data show that more than 25% of complaints were recorded in areas designated as "disadvantaged communities," the criteria for which consider environmental burdens and climate change risks, population characteristics, and health vulnerabilities.[34] Thus, the CACP model is an important tool for vulnerable communities to hold polluters accountable.

BARRIERS TO PARTICIPATION

Although the number of summonses submitted annually continues to increase, few people participate in the CACP relative to the population of the New York City metro area. Several factors may hinder broader participation in CACP, which in turn may reproduce uneven enforcement of New York City's Air Code. First, DEP should promote the CACP more broadly, especially in communities with poor air quality as well as in communities (South Bronx and Central Queens) and boroughs (Bronx, Queens, and Staten Island) where relatively few idling complaints have been submitted (Figure A); media coverage and word-of-mouth seem to have driven participation in the CACP. Similarly, DEP should undertake frequent campaigns to remind commercial vehicle operators of the idling laws; the most recent large-scale campaign was in 2020.[35] Second, the guidelines for submitting a complaint are technical and confusing, and updated guidelines about the program are poorly communicated to lay complainants—currently, updates are posted without notice to the CACP FAQ webpage. At a minimum, DEP should provide a sample (i.e., "best practices") video of how to record an idling vehicle and inform complainants via e-mail when program requirements change.

Third, participation in the program requires digital literacy, access to a smart phone, utilization of several different computer applications ("apps"), and a stable Internet connection; developing a single app to aid lay complainants might reduce barriers to participation. Fourth, DEP should accept complaints written in languages other than English since one quarter of all New Yorkers are not English proficient. Regarding points 3 and 4, a council member attempted to submit a complaint in real time during a recent public hearing, only to find they could not because doing so was neither "simple" nor "remotely user friendly," particularly for non-English speakers; they concluded that the CACP submission process presented a "giant barrier" to enforcing the Air Code.[21]

Fifth, complainants should not be required to submit certain personal data (e.g., bank account) to collect an award on a paid summons; such requirements could be perceived as overly intrusive or impractical. Finally, the municipal government should provide additional resources to DEP to greatly reduce the timeline from complaint submission to review, which delays a timely response to the lay complainant, delays notification of the alleged idling offense to the offender and, consequently, delays potential behavior changes that would decrease air pollution and improve air quality. Addressing these barriers will broaden accessibility to the CACP, particularly for historically marginalized communities, which in turn will likely foment a more equitable and inclusive enforcement of the Air Code.

LIMITATIONS

To date, data about the CACP and its potential public health impacts are limited. There is some evidence that summonses for excessive idling are correlated with neighborhood-level truck traffic (personal communication with NYCAC, February 21, 2025); additional analyses are warranted. The rapid increase in the number of summonses issued for excessive idling suggests that excessive idling remains an underreported public health threat. However, a lack of systematic observation data hinders estimation of the frequency of unreported excessive idling across New York City. Importantly, it is not known how much truck and bus operators who have received at least 1 summons for excessive idling are deterred from future idling, although personal observation suggests that receiving at least 1 summons does decrease the likelihood of future idling. It is important to examine whether additional barriers to participating in the CACP exist. Finally, measuring the impacts of the CACP on public and environmental health should be a priority.

CONCLUSIONS

Despite improvements, air quality in New York City remains a major public health issue. The CACP provides laypeople the opportunity to report illegal commercial vehicle idling and, through financial compensation, incentivizes them to do so. The CACP is an important mechanism to include laypeople in environmental health enforcement and hold polluters accountable. Officials should address barriers to participating in the program. The CACP incentivization model should inspire efforts to address other pervasive public and environmental issues that are underenforced. AJPH

ABOUT THE AUTHOR

Chris Hartmann is with the Department of Public Health, the State University of New York (SUNY) Old Westbury, Old Westbury, NY.

CORRESPONDENCE

Correspondence should be sent to Chris Hartmann, P.O. Box 210, Old Westbury, NY 11578 (e-mail: hartmannc@oldwestbury.edu). Reprints can be ordered at https://www.ajph.org by clicking the "Reprints" link.

PUBLICATION INFORMATION

Full Citation: Hartmann C. The Citizens Air Complaint Program: laypeople reporting air pollution violations in New York City. *Am J Public Health*. 2025;115(9): 1529–1535.

Acceptance Date: March 22, 2025.

DOI: https://doi.org/10.2105/AJPH.2025.308137

ORCID iD:

Chris Hartmann https://orcid.org/0000-0002-8947-205X

ACKNOWLEDGMENTS

I am grateful to the lay complainants who participate in the Citizens Air Complaint Program (CACP) and the Department of Environmental Protection (DEP) staff who review complaints to make New York a cleaner city for all. Eric Eisenberg, Esq., provided valuable feedback on Table 1. The New York Clean Air Collective provided data gleaned from NYC Open Data. All errors are my own.

CONFLICTS OF INTEREST

I have submitted idling complaints to the Citizens Air Complaint Program and, like other lay complainants, have been awarded 25% of the paid penalties.

HUMAN PARTICIPANT PROTECTION

This article is not human participant research, so institutional review board approval was not required.

REFERENCES

1. Manisalidis I, Stavropoulou E, Stavropoulos A, Bezirtzoglou E. Environmental and health impacts of air pollution: a review. *Fron Pub Health.* 2020;8:14. https://doi.org/10.3389/fpubh.2020.00014
2. Brunekreef B, Holgate ST. Air pollution and health. *Lancet.* 2002;360(9341):1233–1242. https://doi.org/10.1016/S0140-6736(02)11274-8
3. Orellano P, Reynoso J, Quaranta N, et al. Short-term exposure to particulate matter (PM_{10} and $PM_{2.5}$), nitrogen dioxide (NO2), and ozone (O3) and all-cause and cause-specific mortality: systematic review and meta-analysis. *Environ Int.* 2020;142:105876. https://doi.org/10.1016/j.envint.2020.105876
4. Tessum CW, Apte JS, Goodkind AL, et al. Inequity in consumption of goods and services adds to racial–ethnic disparities in air pollution exposure. *Proc Natl Acad Sci U S A.* 2019;116(13):6001–6006. https://doi.org/10.1073/pnas.1818859116
5. World Health Organization. Health consequences of air pollution on populations. 2024. Available at: https://www.who.int/news/item/25-06-2024-what-are-health-consequences-of-air-pollution-on-populations. Accessed December 23, 2024.
6. US Environmental Protection Agency. Inventory of US greenhouse gas emissions and sinks: 1990–2022. 2024. EPA 430-R-24-004. Available at: https://www.epa.gov/ghgemissions/inventory-us-greenhouse-gas-emissions-andsinks-1990-2022. Accessed April 8, 2025.
7. American Lung Association. Zeroing in on healthy air. 2022. Available at: https://www.lung.org/getmedia/13248145-06f0-4e35-b79b-6dfacfd29a71/zeroing-in-on-healthy-air-report-2022.pdf. Accessed December 24, 2024.
8. Ashrafur Rahman SM, Masjuki HH, Kalam MA, et al. Impact of idling on fuel consumption and exhaust emissions and available idle-reduction technologies for diesel vehicles—a review. *Energy Cons Mgmt.* 2013;74:171–182. https://doi.org/10.1016/j.enconman.2013.05.019
9. Ris C. US EPA health assessment for diesel engine exhaust: a review. *Inhal Toxicol.* 2007;19(suppl 1):229–239. https://doi.org/10.1080/08958370701497960
10. Mohai P, Pellow D, Roberts JT. Environmental Justice. *Annu Rev Environ Resour.* 2009;34(1):405–430. https://doi.org/10.1146/annurev-environ-082508-094348
11. New York City. EJNYC: a study of environmental justice issues in New York City. 2024. Available at: https://climate.cityofnewyork.us/ejnyc-report. Accessed December 18, 2024.
12. New York City Dept of Health and Mental Hygiene. The New York City Community Air Survey Report. 2008-2022–2024. Available at: https://a816-dohbesp.nyc.gov/IndicatorPublic/data-features/nyccas. Accessed December 23, 2024.
13. American Lung Association. Most polluted cities. 2024. Available at: https://www.lung.org/research/sota/city-rankings/most-polluted-cities. Accessed September 10, 2024.
14. Kheirbek I, Haney J, Douglas S, et al. The contribution of motor vehicle emissions to ambient fine particulate matter public health impacts in New York City: a health burden assessment. *Environ Health.* 2016;15(1):89. https://doi.org/10.1186/s12940-016-0172-6
15. US Environmental Protection Agency. National Emissions Inventory (NEI) 2017 Report Dashboard. 2022. Available at: https://www.epa.gov/air-emissions-inventories/2017-national-emissions-inventory-nei-data. Accessed January 17, 2025.
16. New York City Dept of Health and Mental Hygiene. Environment & Health Data Portal. 2024. Available at: http://a816-dohbesp.nyc.gov/IndicatorPublic/Subtopic.aspx?theme_code=2,3&subtopic_id=103. Accessed December 23, 2024.
17. Carlson A. The Clean Air Act's blind spot: microclimates and hotspot pollution. *UCLA L Rev.* 2018;1036:399–457.
18. Tran K, Packenham G. *Idle Threat* [DVD]. New York, NY: Kimball Tran LLC; 2012.
19. New York City Dept of Transportation. Improving the efficiency of truck deliveries in NYC. 2019. Available at: https://www.nyc.gov/html/dot/downloads/pdf/truck-deliveries-ll189.pdf. Accessed February 24, 2025.
20. New York City Dept of Transportation. About NYC DOT. 2025. Available at: https://www.nyc.gov/html/dot/html/home/home.shtml. Accessed February 24, 2025.
21. New York City Council Meetings. Public testimony: September 18, 2024. Available at: https://citymeetings.nyc/city-council. Accessed December 23, 2024.
22. Novich J. An analysis of 20,000 idling complaints in NYC. 2021. Available at: https://jeffnovich.medium.com/an-analysis-of-20-000-idling-complaints-in-nyc-4bea2411eaeb. Accessed February 24, 2025.
23. New York City Council. Are city agencies responding to 311 calls? 2019. Available at: https://council.nyc.gov/data/311-agency. Accessed February 24, 2025.
24. Dept of Energy and Environment. Engine Anti-Idling Law. 2023. Available at: https://doee.dc.gov/service/engine-anti-idling-law. Accessed February 24, 2025.
25. Random Lengths News. CD15 briefs: policy update citizen idling complaint program motion. Available at: https://www.randomlengthsnews.com/archives/2025/02/12/citizen-idling-complaint-program/69531. Accessed February 24, 2025.
26. Kroll-Zaidi R. Among the idlers. *Curbed.* 2024. Available at: https://www.curbed.com/article/nyc-idling-law-citizen-air-complaint-program.html. Accessed March 22, 2025.
27. Fickenscher L. NYC sues Margaritaville hotel over $54k noise complaints fine, despite "vigilantes" crackdown. *New York Post.* June 14, 2024. Available at: https://nypost.com/2024/06/14/business/nyc-sues-margaritaville-hotel-over-54k-noise-complants-fine. Accessed September 10, 2024.
28. Bonney R, Phillips TB, Ballard H, et al. Can citizen science enhance public understanding of science? *Public Underst Sci.* 2016;25(1):2–16. https://doi.org/10.1177/0963662515607406
29. Mahajan S, Kumar P, Pinto JA, et al. A citizen science approach for enhancing public understanding of air pollution. *Sustain Cities Soc.* 2020;52:101800. https://doi.org/10.1016/j.scs.2019.101800
30. Brown P. Popular epidemiology revisited. *Curr Sociol.* 1997;45(3):137–156. https://doi.org/10.1177/001139297045003008
31. Sze J. *Noxious New York.* Cambridge, MA: MIT Press; 2006.
32. Konisky DM, Milyo J, Richardson Jr LE. Environmental policy attitudes: issues, geographical scale, and political trust. *Soc Sci Quart.* 2008;89(5):1066–1085. https://doi.org/10.1111/j.1540-6237.2008.00574.x
33. WE ACT. Truck idling workshop for NYC's Citizens Air Complaint Program. 2022. Available at: www.youtube.com/watch?v=XEDvm04JMqo. Accessed December 23, 2024.
34. New York State. Climate Justice Working Group. 2023. Available at: https://climate.ny.gov/Resources/Climate-Justice-Working-Group. Accessed December 24, 2024.
35. New York City Dept of Environmental Protection. Billy never idles. Available at: https://www.nyc.gov/site/dep/whats-new/billy-never-idles.page. Accessed February 24, 2025.

Promulgating Joy and Expiating Guilt: Camp and LGBTQ+ Health Education in the History of The Sisters of Perpetual Indulgence

Tyler J. Fuller, MTS, MPH

The Sisters of Perpetual Indulgence (The Sisters) have engaged in health education and promotion for more than 40 years, yet their contributions remain underexplored in public health literature. This article examines the role of camp, humor, and joy in their work by drawing on primary sources from the San Francisco, California, and Boston, Massachusetts, Sisters' archives, as well as publicly available interviews. The Sisters published one of the first safer-sex pamphlets in the United States, written by and for gay men, using camp and setting a precedent for community-led health education. Since then, they have continued to leverage public health knowledge—sourced from health professionals within their order, local health organizations, and public agencies like the Centers for Disease Control and Prevention—while using camp to make it accessible, engaging, and quintessentially queer. The Sisters exemplify how serious public health initiatives can be conducted with queer pride, humor, and joy. (*Am J Public Health*. 2025;115(9):1536–1544. https://doi.org/10.2105/AJPH.2025.308112)

AJPH September 2025, Vol. 115, No. 9

Donning nuns' habits, cocktail dresses with veils, or leather and kink gear, often painted with clown white makeup and bright colors, The Sisters of Perpetual Indulgence (The Sisters) stand out in a crowd (Figure 1). The Sisters are a contemporary order of queer,[1] clown, drag nuns who engage in community work that they call "ministry," through activism, education, entertainment, and service.[2] While The Sisters are serious about being queer nuns, they are not a religious order; across the United States, each city's "house" is its own 501(c)(3) nonprofit corporation. The Sisters are widely recognized in many queer communities across the United States because of their history of sexual health education and promotion during the HIV and AIDS crisis and their mission to "promulgate universal joy and expiate stigmatic guilt."[3] Jason B. Crawford argues, "The Sisters have been at the forefront of actions that brought awareness of HIV/AIDS and helped make health a political issue."[4] The Sisters have been engaged in health education and promotion work for more than four decades, yet there is little discussion of this among public health scholars.

There is a paucity of academic literature on The Sisters, with most of the literature published by humanities scholars. Only one article appeared in a search of PubMed for "The Sisters of Perpetual Indulgence" (search conducted on February 11, 2025). Thomas Blair discusses the legacy of The Sisters' most well-known public health pamphlet, *Play Fair!*[5] He picks up themes from earlier queer scholars who argued for grassroots sexual health education and promotion.[6] He demonstrates the importance of understanding the role of The Sisters' engagement in community-based health education and health promotion in the HIV and AIDS crisis in the 1980s. Yet, no (history of) public health articles have focused at length on how The Sisters employ camp and joy in their work during and after the crisis.

Susan Sontag describes "camp" as a sensibility and an aesthetic that is hard to define. In her seminal 1964 article, she writes, "Homosexuals have pinned their integration into society on promoting the aesthetic sense. Camp is a solvent of morality. It neutralizes moral indignation, sponsors playfulness."[7] Camp disarms and creates space for possibilities. Camp was one, of multiple,

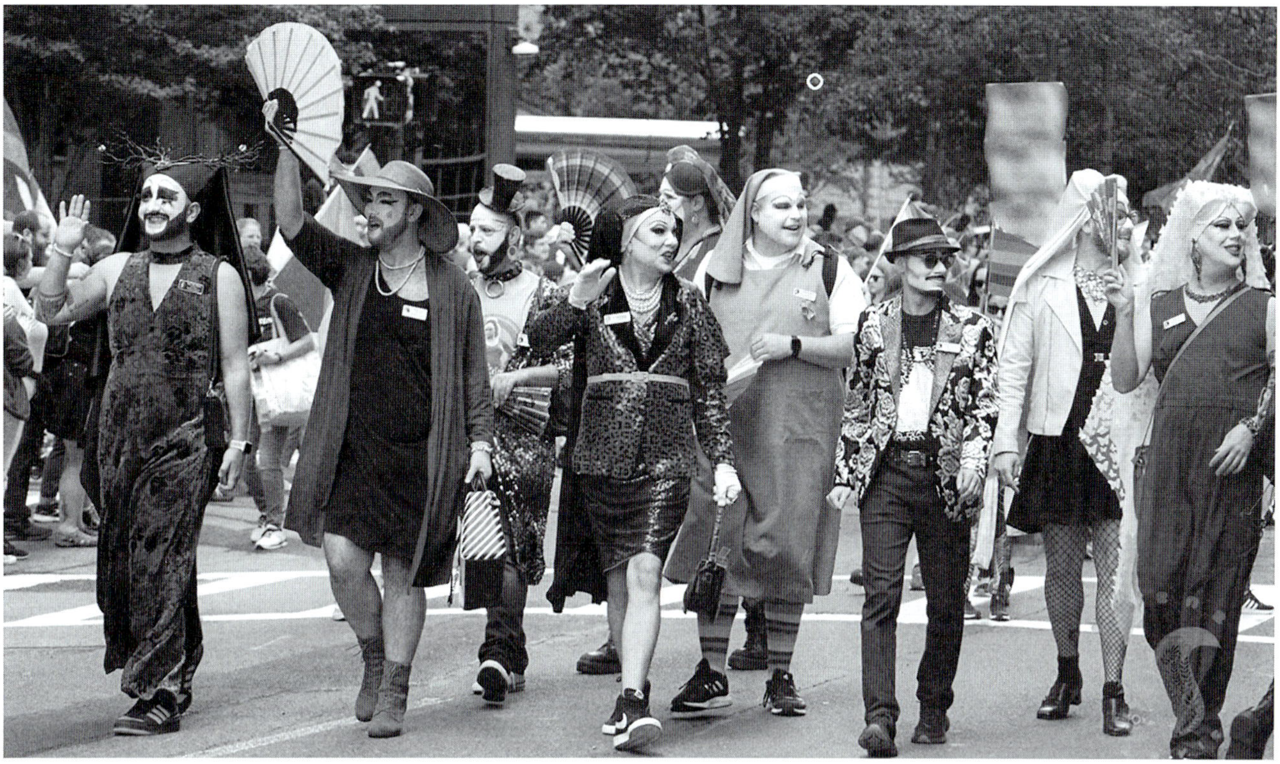

FIGURE 1— The Boston Sisters of Perpetual Indulgence Marching in the Boston Pride for the People Parade, 2023

Source. Courtesy of The Sisters of Perpetual Indulgence, Boston Convent of the Commonwealth.

aesthetics employed in the Harlem ballroom scene to embody Black queer resistance and creative empowerment that have become popular in mainstream American drag and queer culture.[8] Melissa Wilcox writes about The Sisters' employment of "camp" saying,

> Camp, in some of its forms, takes a traditional cultural object or practice that has become slightly antiquated, an object of nostalgic and even saccharine affection in some areas of mainstream culture, and reinvigorates it with an ironic, queer twist that can be respectfully subtle, cunningly subversive, or blatantly shocking.[9]

Wilcox writes about The Sisters' use of camp in their "ministry"—for even calling their community work "ministry" is an act of camp—and also theorizes "serious parody." She examines how The Sisters both parody Catholic nuns and also seriously consider themselves nuns in their community work. From the beginning, The Sisters embraced drag, camp, and joy, all of which are characteristic parts of queer history and culture.[10]

To fill the gap in the literature, I examine primary sources from the San Francisco, California, and Boston, Massachusetts, Sisters of Perpetual Indulgence archives—both physical and digital[11]—as well as sources from popular and academic media. My positionality in elucidating the history of The Sisters within public health is twofold: as a scholar and as a Sister. This work is informed by my experiences and perspectives as a fully professed member of The Boston Sisters. Through this historical research, I argue that The Sisters' joy and camp make their health education and promotion ministries more accessible, engaging, and quintessentially queer.

THE FIRST MANIFESTATIONS: 1979–1980

The Sisters' first public manifestation was Easter weekend 1979 in the San Francisco Castro. Three gay men "being extremely bored with the conformist atmosphere . . . went out into the streets to challenge the world."[12] They donned nuns' habits previously acquired for a drag troupe under the guise of a performance of *The Sound of Music,* Sister Vicious Power Hungry Bitch (now known as Grand Mother Vish-Knew) drew inspiration from the emcee in *Cabaret* and wore white pancake makeup with some rouge, and one sister even took along a toy machine gun (Figure 2).[13] They were a sight to see, these drag nuns who wandered through the Castro down to the local nude beach in the hot sun. Who, after all, would expect to see a nun walking down the nude beach with a machine gun, only to discover that this was a gay man, subverting ideas of organized religion and patriarchy. Sister Vicious Power Hungry Bitch recalled the moment saying, "We realized we had a stick of dynamite and that we should do something productive with it. We should use it as a tool for social change, for the change that we want to see."[14] The employment of camp through the drag of wearing habits in queer spaces created a rupture, one that opened up space for possibilities.

Not long after this first manifestation, The Sisters were born. The Sisters engaged in a number of ministries their first year, some which would later fall under the category of "ministry of presence," centered on spreading joy through their queer and campy presence. In October 1980, The Sisters engaged in their first fundraising event, hosting a bingo game at the lesbian, gay, bisexual, transgender, and queer (LGBTQ+)–affirming Metropolitan Community Church to raise funds to assist gay Cuban refugees coming to the United States.[15] Hosting a drag bingo was an act of camp as much as the dress and names of the sisters themselves. The Sisters took a traditional church basement game and breathed new, campy, and risqué life into it as they made sexual innuendos over the microphone. Since then, drag bingos have become a staple of The Sisters across the United States.

These bingos became a time to support nonprofit (often health) organizations as well as bring in leaders and professionals from those organizations to share information. Collaborating with other groups and raising funds for local nonprofits is a large part of The Sisters' health promotion ministry. This health promotion work does not always include health education or passing out condoms; sometimes it means supporting local organizations in their health promotion work. The Sisters are prolific fundraisers, and they partner with grassroots organizations that promote youth mental health, support unhoused populations, and care for our gay elders, just to name a few.[16] In addition, many Sister houses have spaces on their websites with information about where to find local health information or services.[17]

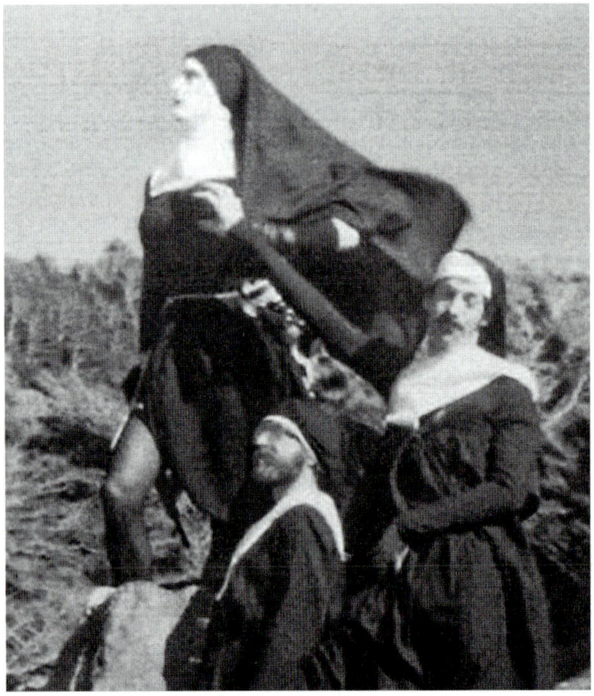

FIGURE 2— Ken Bunch (Who Would Become Sister Vicious Power Hungry Bitch), Fred Brungard (Who Would Become Sister Missionary Position), and Baruch Golden at the First Manifestation, Easter Weekend, 1979

Source. Courtesy of The Sisters of Perpetual Indulgence, San Francisco.

PLAY FAIR! AND SEXUAL HEALTH EDUCATION: 1981–1982

The Sisters maintain a stigma-free approach to sex positivity that was contextualized, in part, by the work of the National Coalition of Gay Sexually Transmitted Disease Services and the Bay Area Physicians for Human Rights.[18] Some Sisters were also connected with the Radical Faeries and blended their sex-positive views with The Sisters' goals of expiating stigma and guilt.[19] Blair provides a historical overview of how Sister Florence Nightmare and Sister Roz Erection, both registered nurses in their secular (non-Sister) lives, drew on their professional knowledge to create *Play Fair!*[20] one of the first safer-sex pamphlets in the

United States written by and for gay men (Figure 3).[21] *Play Fair!* engaged in the work of translating medical jargon into language that lay queer people could understand. Blair demonstrates this, writing

> [The National Coalition of Gay Sexually Transmitted Disease Services'] Guidelines warn that because "scented lubricants may [cause] a chemically induced proctitis (rectal inflammation), the use of hand lotions and other scented products for these purposes are discouraged." Play Fair! translated that message: "buy lubricants free of fancy perfumes . . . the chemicals can inflame your ass."[22]

The Sisters used the language of their community; gay men in the bars were not talking about "proctitis" but they were discussing how their "ass" was burning after their last hook up. In addition to using the common vernacular, the crassness of the message disarms the reader. The camp of this message comes from the reality that while this is medical information coming from registered nurses, one could hear their gay friends saying this to them over drinks.

Camp and humor can be effective tools in engaging health education and promotion. According to William Robertson, "Camp originated as a gay survival mechanism and is associated with an ironic aesthetic that queers heteronormative sensibilities."[23] Crawford writes about *Play Fair!*

> This approach to public health education used popular language, cartoon drawings and up-to-date health information delivered with campy humour. The logic inherent in *Play Fair!* and in many of the Sisters' interventions is grounded in the care of queer people's selves (mental and physical health) and is also a way of taking care of the community.[24]

Robertson corroborates Crawford's analysis and writes about camp and humor as "queer care practices."[25] He argues that the employment of camp humor in medical settings can assist in building rapport, relaxing patients, and questioning the boundaries of "bad taste" by bringing topics often not discussed publicly, including sexual encounters and sexually transmitted infections, inside the boundaries of what can be talked about.

To promote *Play Fair!*, The Sisters released a public service announcement, although it is unclear exactly where or how this was shown to audiences.[26] The video depicts several nuns wearing the full habit, frolicking up a hill to "The Hills Are Alive" from *The Sound of Music*, with a church in the background. As they lay down a pride flag as a picnic blanket and a basket of fruit, the music shifts to "Moulin Rouge," signaling the campy sex education they are about to present. They then demonstrate how

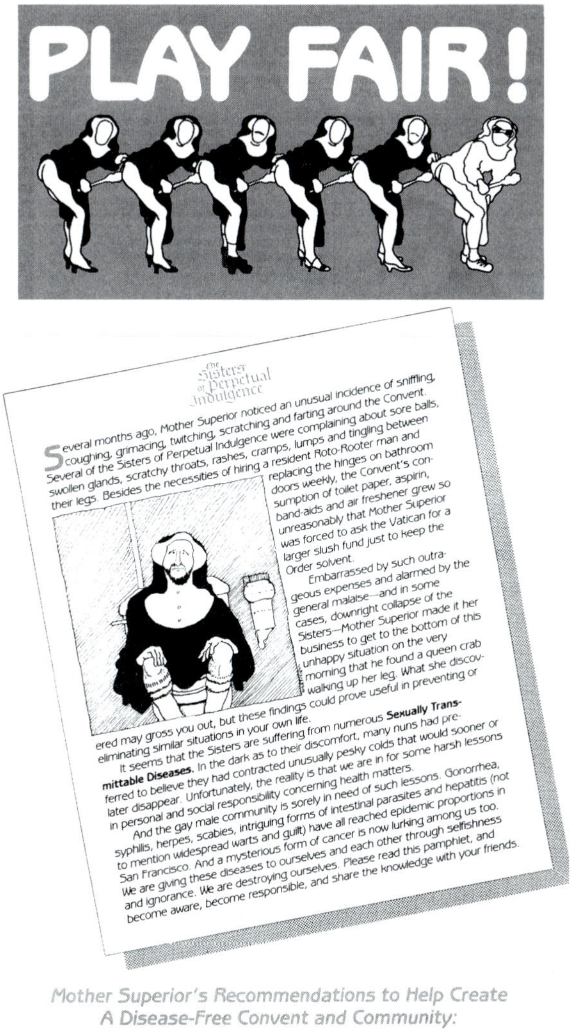

FIGURE 3— The Cover of *Play Fair!*

Source. Courtesy of The Sisters of Perpetual Indulgence, San Francisco.

AJPH September 2025, Vol. 115, No. 9

to use condoms, gloves, and dental dams as safer-sex aids on different fruits representing a penis, anus, and vagina. The video ends with a shot of the sisters jumping for joy and throwing condoms in the air as the words "Now sisters play fair!" appear. The video recalls the American trope of a high-school teacher putting a condom on a banana, but again with a humorous and campy twist that makes it not only accessible but also entertaining for gay audiences.

Several decades later, in Boston, Sister Aria Inyette, a registered nurse in her secular life, was inspired by *Play Fair!* to engage in health education through her programs "Put It in My Ask" and "Aria's Annals," which, just like her, drew their names from sexual innuendos.[27] Her goal with these programs was to "create a platform for us as a community to generate conversation and discuss those hard to talk about/taboo topics . . . and provide credible information so everyone can make decisions that work for them."[28] Put It in My Ask functioned as a virtual space to anonymously submit questions and receive direct message answers. Aria's Annals were public videos on topics Sister Aria was passionate about discussing with the community. In a personal communication, Sister Aria shared that she created these because it can be uncomfortable for queer people to ask heteronormative health care providers about sexual health, and it can be hard to find queer health care providers; in addition, she wanted to bring humor, fun, and laughter into discussion of serious topics.

THE CONDOM SAVIOR MASS: 1987–1991

After the release of *Play Fair!*, The San Francisco Sisters continued their work to promote safer sex practices, which often focused on promoting condom use among gay men. This work was especially important during the deeply conservative Reagan administration. In January 1987, The Sisters performed a public exorcism of Pope John Paul II while also canonizing Harvey Milk as a gay saint. They were angry with the Pope because of his insistence that condom use and homosexuality were intrinsic moral evils. As part of this public ritual, The Sisters invoked the status of condoms as sacred shields in the gay community and distributed communion condoms—condoms in gold wrappers to resemble Catholic Eucharist wafers. The Sisters proclaimed,

> Oh holy savior, you who can deliver us from the scourge of AIDS, you who will now [protect] the safety of our sexual play, you who will enable us to cum clean and often [crowd laughs], you who are our protector from viral infection and unplanned pregnancy, be here with us today. We now have communion wafers that will be dispensed to the crowd.[29]

This scene is preceded by three Sisters performing a cheerleader routine, highlighting that this event was not gloomy in nature; it was campy and joyful. The Sisters saw their joy as resistance to the homophobia, shame, and guilt they felt from the Pope and the Catholic Church.

In 1991, the condom communion was expanded to the first Condom Savior Mass, which was performed by the San Francisco house when they granted the status of fully professed house to the Paris, France, convent.[30] The Condom Savior Mass includes a vow to use condoms in all sexual encounters. The mass proclaims,

> We have gathered today to consecrate and receive the Holy Communion Condom. As I take it onto myself, so shall I keep its ritual sacred. The condom is part of my life—part of my responsibility now. If I desire to live, and let my sex partners live, I must sanctify my vow to hold the condom savior sacred. My seed is under siege by a horrific virus. Let me not become horrific as well with careless disregard for my life and the lives of those with whom I share the divine gift of love.[31]

For more than two decades, the Condom Savior Mass reimagined a ritual—associated with a Pope who engaged in homophobic rhetoric and discouraged evidence-based practices—into something life-giving. To reimagine the condom as a source of nourishment meant reimagining and re-embracing sex in a positive way, free of guilt or shame. The Sisters' camp, their reimagining of this ritual, spread a vital public health message.

Yet, the Condom Savior Mass must be contextualized in its own time. Wilcox writes,

> In the 2010s, with ongoing and justified concern among queer activists over the bio-political enforcement of AIDS prevention, some might cringe at terms like "responsibility" and the linkage of condom usage to one's very humanity. Yet the impact of the Mass becomes clearer when one considers the climate in gay communities in the early 1990s.[32]

Contextualized in a time before the development of highly effective combination antiretroviral treatments, prevention was the only hope for thousands of gay men whose friends and community were dying all around them. The ritual also embodies one way some Sisters interpret their mission to spread joy and relieve stigma and guilt. Some Sisters will share that "you are perfect, and as long as you are not hurting yourself or anyone else, you remain perfect." In this perspective, the Condom Savior Mass takes on new light as a ritual to prevent harm to self or others.

COCKTAILS AND CONDOMS: 2010–2019

The Sisters are no strangers to gay bars. In fact, because these bars are common social settings in the gay community, much of The Sisters' work over the past four decades has taken place in them. In their archive of reports to the community about their activities, The Boston Sisters discuss attending queer bars and parties in Boston, collaborating with health providers and educators, and starting conversations with community members. In recent years, The Boston Sisters have written about attending a monthly party for the leather, BDSM (bondage, discipline, domination, submission, sadism, and masochism), and kink communities where they collaborate with a local free health clinic that brings a mobile clinic to the parties.[33] The Sisters, who often dress in attire that is common to the context, are able to move freely within the party while they participate in the community. While the staff from the health clinic stay in the mobile clinic outside providing services, The Sisters are able to engage the community and refer people to the clinic or provide condoms.

The Boston Sisters archives describe a bar crawl ministry where The Sisters collaborated with Fenway Health clinic to raise awareness of HIV preexposure prophylaxis (PrEP).[34] While health workers from Fenway wore shirts that said, "I'm on PrEP—Ask me about it" or "Ask me about PrEP," The Sisters report a special connection they had with the community:

> Overall, the event was extremely successful. While many individuals knew about PrEP, many of them were hesitant approaching medical providers for prescriptions or felt nervous about potential side-effects. This event created a safe space for individuals to ask questions and get connected to resources in the Boston area.[35]

When it may feel difficult or embarrassing to approach a medical provider, The Sisters, in their camp, are approachable. As they expiate stigma and guilt, The Sisters strive to make others feel comfortable with themselves and accepting of their current circumstances and feelings. In this event, this connection was important because The Sisters reported that, "Fenway Health also received a small number of vouchers from Gilead covering the cost of PrEP copays which [The Sisters] distributed to individuals who indicated financial hardships."[36]

The Sisters' camp, humor, and joy are part of what makes them both effective in their work and also approachable. In an interview with Melissa Wilcox, Sister Mona Little-Moore sheds light on how bar patrons can react differently to health educators and The Sisters:

> So, like condom outreach is a really good example. As Ken, or like if I was working for [Cascade AIDS Project] and just a city guy, they're just out there in their street clothes . . . no makeup or anything on. They walk up to a [bar] table, and I used to be one of those people at the table. They'd walk up to a table and say, "Are you interested in a safe sex kit" or whatever, and we'd be like, "No, we don't need it." . . . But as Sister Mona, with the whiteface, because of that anonymity I can go up there and say, "Okay, raise of hands, who's going to go home and bone?" You know, and start these conversations. So the whiteface is just another tool of the whole thing, it's part of the habit, and allows me to do the work that I want to do.[37]

The habit and makeup that The Sisters wear and the personas they perform do work at the interpersonal level when they engage in health education and promotion. The Sisters perform multiple roles depending on the need and the context. Sometimes a sister is a jester, a clown who uses humor to point out something that others are not able to openly discuss. Sister Vicious Power Hungry Bitch explained this when she said,

> We're not making fun of nuns or the church. We're trying to make them confront certain issues, such as sexism and the fear of homosexuality. Humor is a good way to communicate ideas.[38]

Sister Mona took on this role when she bluntly asked who was having sex that evening. A health educator might be presuming that some people will be having sex and, thus, might benefit from a safer-sex kit. But, as the jester, Sister Mona can point out what she sees as obvious, that someone at that table is going to be having sex later. Where a simple "No, thank you" might have shut down a health educator, Sister Mona does not even offer the chance. She calls out what she sees and starts a conversation about it. With a name like Sister Mona Little-Moore, she creates an interaction that is sex-positive from the moment she introduces herself.

The Sisters also bring camp and high energy to events hosted by other organizations. For several years, Northeastern University in Boston hosted Condom Couture, a fashion show of "outrageously gorgeous condom outfits" that also featured games and prizes.[39] Through these events, students learned about sexual health and safer sex practices, and got comfortable seeing and talking about condoms. The Sisters' role in making the space comfortable and accessible is highlighted in the university's promotional materials, which encourage students to "laugh yourself into oblivion with the glitteringly fabulous MCs (Boston's chapter of the Sisters of Perpetual Indulgence)."[40] In their archives, The Sisters describe one of their roles at the event as providing "witty banter"[41] and "colorful commentary."[42] Their second role in the 2015 Condom Couture was to host sexual health trivia and a game where students learned "the proper use of external condoms, internal condoms, and dental damns [sic] through a 3-person relay race."[43]

HIV/AIDS LESSONS IN CURRENT WORK: 2020–2024

The Sisters began their public ministry on the eve of the HIV and AIDS crisis, and their work in educating the public about HIV and promoting safer sex practices has shaped how they engage in their work to this day. In an interview, Sister Purrr Do shared with Lauren Pond how The Sisters' experiences with HIV and sexual health education and promotion during the HIV and AIDS epidemic prepared them to respond to the COVID-19 pandemic:

> [The Sisters have] operated in the midst of a pandemic for the past 40 years . . . This is our space. We understand what to do in regards to service . . . when we show up, when we are visible, [we], through being present, are a reflection of beauty and joy.[44]

The lessons learned about how camp lowers the barriers of stigma and guilt and opens space for joy, education, and action continue to inform The Sisters' practice, even for health concerns that are not related to sexual health.

Sisters around the country have engaged with issues including COVID-19, mpox, *Shigella*, and naloxone use for overdoses. The San Francisco Sisters shared a media campaign to promote six feet of distance between people in physical spaces while COVID-19 was spreading, with photos of Sisters in masks with the hashtag #PracticeSafeSix, a play on "practice safe sex."[45] Even in the midst of an international

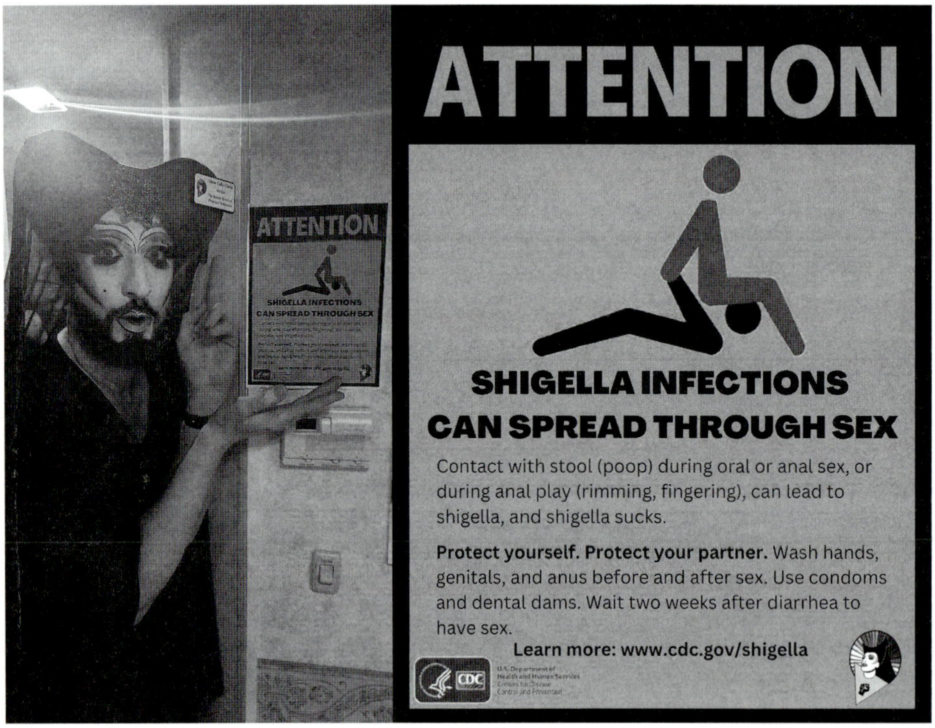

FIGURE 4— **Sister Lida Christ Modeling Next to a Poster The Boston Sisters Created to Share Information About *Shigella***

Source. Courtesy of The Sisters of Perpetual Indulgence, Boston Convent of the Commonwealth.

pandemic, The Sisters kept their wit and camp in service of the community. Sisters from around the United States engaged in virtual events meant to keep up spirits and help people feel less isolated during the pandemic, a serious concern for mental health.[46]

During mpox and the *Shigella* outbreaks, The Boston Sisters drew on their former condom and sexually transmitted infection and HIV testing promotion techniques to advocate for mpox vaccinations and safer sex practices that could prevent virus transmission. One report from The Boston Sisters describing their presence at a queer party states, "As always there was medical on site for things like HIV testing and COVID boosters. We got to spread awareness of shigella to friends old and new."[47] They created public service announcement flyers, modeled after those from the Centers for Disease Control and Prevention (CDC) and with the information from the CDC website, but with The Sisters' special campy twist to them that made them fun to read, while maintaining the accurate information (Figure 4).[48] These were posted around gay bars and parties in Boston that The Sisters attended.[49]

As members of the community, The Sisters are aware of how substance use and the presence of fentanyl has impacted the gay community. The Sisters and drag friends are encouraging people, especially club goers, to carry naloxone because it is hard to predict when it will be urgently needed.[50] In Provincetown, Massachusetts, Sister Lida Christ has worked with AIDS Support Group of Cape Cod to inform the community about access to free naloxone and fentanyl testing strips.[51]

LOOKING TOWARD THE FUTURE

The Sisters have been part of the health education and promotion community for more than four decades. They draw on public health knowledge from the health professionals within their order, from local health organizations and providers, and from public sources like the CDC. Then they use camp to make it accessible, engaging, and quintessentially queer. This is powerful in the context of health education and promotion, where stigma and guilt are barriers to gaining knowledge or lasting behavior change.[52] The Sisters demonstrate that serious public health initiatives can be conducted with LGBTQ+ pride, humor, and joy. AJPH

ABOUT THE AUTHOR

Tyler J. Fuller is with the Graduate Program in Religion, Boston University, Boston, MA.

CORRESPONDENCE

Correspondence should be sent to Tyler J. Fuller, MTS, MPH, CHES, 145 Bay State Rd, Boston, MA 02215 (e-mail: tjfuller@bu.edu). Reprints can be ordered at https://www.ajph.org by clicking the "Reprints" link.

PUBLICATION INFORMATION

Full Citation: Fuller TJ. Promulgating joy and expiating guilt: camp and LGBTQ+ health education in the history of The Sisters of Perpetual Indulgence. *Am J Public Health*. 2025;115(9): 1536–1544.

Acceptance Date: March 9, 2025.

DOI: https://doi.org/10.2105/AJPH.2025.308112

ORCID iD:

Tyler J. Fuller https://orcid.org/0000-0002-6766-2231

ACKNOWLEDGMENTS

I am indebted to several Sisters for their assistance in helping me navigate the archives and giving feedback on this article. Thank you to Sister Betty Esém, Sister Mary Media, Sister Brother Freddie Anne Willing, Brother Gary Cruter, Sister Aria Inyette, Sister Luvinya Always, and Sister Lida Christ.

CONFLICTS OF INTEREST

T.J. Fuller is a volunteer member of The Sisters of Perpetual Indulgence, Boston Convent of the Commonwealth.

ENDNOTES

1. The term "queer" has taken on different definitions across scholarly history. I use the term "queer" in the colloquial sense I experience most frequently in Boston, Massachusetts. Queer is an inclusive adjective that describes individuals and communities who do not fit a cisgender, heterosexual mold. I sometimes use it interchangeably with the acronym "LGBTQ+."
2. The Sisters of Perpetual Indulgence, Boston, "Our Mission – The Boston Sisters of Perpetual Indulgence," https://www.thebostonsisters.org/about (accessed October 24, 2024); for a robust description of The Sisters' founding, procedures, and organizational structures see Melissa M. Wilcox, *Queer Nuns: Religion, Activism, and Serious Parody*, *Sexual Cultures* (New York: University Press, 2018).
3. Yet, I recognize that queer communities within San Francisco, Boston, and the United States at large are not monolithic. Each city may have multiple queer communities, some of whom are knowledgeable about The Sisters' history and work, others who are not aware of it yet. Mission statement quote from The Sisters of Perpetual Indulgence, San Francisco, "Sistory," https://www.thesisters.org/sistory (accessed October 21, 2024).
4. Jason B. Crawford, "Feeling of/Feeling for Queer Community: The Social Activism of the San Francisco Sisters of Perpetual Indulgence," *Conexión Queer: Revista Latinoamericana y Caribeña de Teologías Queer* 1, no. 1 (2018): 54, https://repository.usfca.edu/conexionqueer/vol1/iss1/3
5. Thomas R. Blair, "Safe Sex in the 1970s: Community Practitioners on the Eve of AIDS," *American Journal of Public Health* 107, no. 6 (2017): 872–879, https://doi.org/10.2105/AJPH.2017.303704.
6. Douglas Crimp, "How to Have Promiscuity in an Epidemic," *AIDS: Cultural Analysis/Cultural Activism* 43 (1987): 237–271, https://doi.org/10.2307/3397576
7. Susan Sontag, "Notes on 'Camp,'" in *Camp: Queer Aesthetics and the Performing Subject: A Reader* (Edinburgh: Edinburgh University Press, 1999), 64, https://www.jstor.org/stable/10.3366/j.ctvxcrp56
8. The Harlem Ballroom scene has influenced much of contemporary American drag culture and, by extension, queer culture. *Paris Is Burning*, Documentary (Off White Productions, 1990); Constantine Chatzipapatheodoridis, "Strike a Pose, Forever: The Legacy of Vogue and Its Recontextualization in Contemporary Camp Performances," *European Journal of American Studies* 11, no. 3 (2017), https://doi.org/10.4000/ejas.11771; Brian C. Stephens, "Never Too Much: Notes on Black Camp and the Politics of Black Excess" (PhD Dissertation, Riverside, CA, University of California, Riverside, 2023).
9. Wilcox, *Queer Nuns*, 96.
10. Jason B. Crawford, "'Go Forth and Sin Some More!' A Performance Geography of the San Francisco Sisters of Perpetual Indulgence" (PhD Dissertation, Montreal, Quebec, Canada, Concordia University, 2011).
11. See: Itza A. Carbajal and Michelle Caswell, "Critical Digital Archives: A Review from Archival Studies," *The American Historical Review* 126, no. 3 (September 1, 2021): 1102–1120, https://doi.org/10.1093/ahr/rhab359; Adam Nix et al., "Archival Research in the Digital Era," in *Handbook of Historical Methods for Management* (Edward Elgar

Publishing, 2023), 156–172, https://www.elgaronline.com/edcollchap/book/9781800883741/book-part-9781800883741-19.xml
12. The "conformist atmosphere" that The Sisters reference in their "sistory"—a play on "sister history"—is the stereotype of the "Castro clone," a style characterized by tight jeans, a tight t-shirt or plaid button-down shirt, and often a mustache. The Sisters of Perpetual Indulgence, San Francisco, "Sistory."
13. Wilcox, *Queer Nuns*, 31–33.
14. As quoted in Wilcox, 33.
15. The Sisters of Perpetual Indulgence, San Francisco, "Sistory"; Wilcox, *Queer Nuns*, 43–44.
16. There are only a few examples of programs where The Sisters have supported local nonprofits and health organizations. The Sisters of Perpetual Indulgence, Boston, "Fenway Health Men's Event – The Boston Sisters of Perpetual Indulgence," March 11, 2017, https://www.thebostonsisters.org/fenway-health-mens-event-2 (accessed October 22, 2024); The Sisters of Perpetual Indulgence, Portland, "Hand Up Project Has Received Another Grant from The Sisters of Perpetual Indulgences of Portland," https://www.handupproject.org/sisters-of-pdx (accessed October 22, 2024); The Sisters of Perpetual Indulgence, Boston, "Point Nun Report: Prime Timers Anniversary Party 9/17/2 – The Boston Sisters of Perpetual Indulgence," August 28, 2024, https://www.thebostonsisters.org/point-nun-report-prime-timers-anniversary-party-9-17-2 (accessed October 22, 2024); The Sisters of Perpetual Indulgence, Boston, "Point Nun Report: Salem Survivor Program 7/20/2024 – The Boston Sisters of Perpetual Indulgence," July 25, 2024, https://www.thebostonsisters.org/point-nun-report-salem-survivor-program-7-20-2024 (accessed October 22, 2024).
17. The Sisters of Perpetual Indulgence, Los Angeles, "RESOURCES," Mysite, https://www.lasisters.org/resources-1 (accessed October 22, 2024); The Sisters of Perpetual Indulgence, San Francisco, "Joy," https://www.thesisters.org/joy (accessed October 22, 2024).
18. Blair, "Safe Sex in the 1970s."
19. The Sisters of Perpetual Indulgence, San Francisco, "Sistory"; Wilcox, *Queer Nuns*, 35.
20. Blair, "Safe Sex in the 1970s."
21. Sister X, Sisters of Perpetual Indulgence "Condom Savior Mass," interview by Phil Tarley, Video, n.d., AIDS Activist Videotape Collection, Manuscripts and Archives Division, The New York Public Library, Astor, Lenox and Tilden Foundations.
22. Blair, "Safe Sex in the 1970s," 875.
23. William J. Robertson, "The Butt of the Joke: Humour and Queer Care at an Anal Dysplasia Clinic," *Medicine Anthropology Theory* 11, no. 2 (2024): 9, http://www.medanthrotheory.org/article/view/7278.
24. Crawford, "Feeling of/Feeling for Queer Community," 63.
25. Robertson, "The Butt of the Joke": 1.
26. Play Fair PSA, https://vimeo.com/178198717 (accessed October 22, 2024).
27. The Sisters of Perpetual Indulgence, Boston, "Aria Inyette – The Boston Sisters of Perpetual Indulgence," August 11, 2016, https://www.thebostonsisters.org/?post_type=member_page&p=5896 (accessed November 1, 2024); The Sisters of Perpetual Indulgence, Boston, "Aria's Annals – The Boston Sisters of Perpetual Indulgence," https://www.thebostonsisters.org/arias-annals (accessed November 1, 2024).
28. The Sisters of Perpetual Indulgence, Boston, "Aria's Annals – The Boston Sisters of Perpetual Indulgence."
29. Scene begins around minute 33:14. *Exorcism of Pope John Paul 2 and Sainting of Harvey Milk - 1987*, 1987, https://vimeo.com/294854310 (accessed October 22, 2024).
30. Wilcox, *Queer Nuns*, 75.
31. *Condom Savior Mass*, 2009, https://www.youtube.com/watch?v=8x5fa6L2O70 (accessed October 22, 2024); Wilcox, *Queer Nuns*, 75–77.
32. Wilcox, *Queer Nuns*, 77.
33. The Sisters of Perpetual Indulgence, Boston, "Point Nun Report: Fascination 3/6 – The Boston Sisters of Perpetual Indulgence," March 13, 2023, https://www.thebostonsisters.org/point-nun-report-fascination-3-6 (accessed October 22, 2024); The Sisters of Perpetual Indulgence, Boston, "Point Nun Report – Fascination at Legacy 6/5 – The Boston Sisters of Perpetual Indulgence," June 20, 2023, https://www.thebostonsisters.org/point-nun-report-fascination-at-legacy-6-5 (accessed October 22, 2024).
34. The Sisters of Perpetual Indulgence, Boston, "PrEP Awareness Bar Ministry – The Boston Sisters of Perpetual Indulgence," April 18, 2015, https://www.thebostonsisters.org/prep-awareness-bar-ministry (accessed October 22, 2024).
35. The Sisters of Perpetual Indulgence, Boston, "PrEP Awareness Bar Ministry – The Boston Sisters of Perpetual Indulgence."
36. It does not appear that the vouchers were unique to this specific event, but that Fenway Health already had these available to distribute. The Sisters of Perpetual Indulgence, Boston, "PrEP Awareness Bar Ministry – The Boston Sisters of Perpetual Indulgence."
37. Wilcox, *Queer Nuns*, 98.
38. As reported by Theresa Keeley, "Clothes Make the Nun? Feminism, Fashion, and Representations of Catholic Sisters in the 1980s," *Gender & History* 31, no. 2 (2019): 493. Keeley attributes this to a 1987 *Philadelphia Daily News* article by Scott Flander, but I was unable to locate the original source.
39. Northeastern University, "Condom Couture 2015," Northeastern University, https://calendar.northeastern.edu/event/condom_couture_2015 (accessed October 22, 2024); Northeastern University, "Condom Couture," Northeastern University, https://calendar.northeastern.edu/event/condom_couture_9675 (accessed October 22, 2024).
40. Northeastern University, "Condom Couture."
41. The Sisters of Perpetual Indulgence, Boston, "Condom Couture – Northeastern University – The Boston Sisters of Perpetual Indulgence," March 29, 2015, https://www.thebostonsisters.org/condom-couture-northeastern-university (accessed October 22, 2024).
42. The Sisters of Perpetual Indulgence, Boston, "Condom Couture – The Boston Sisters of Perpetual Indulgence," February 23, 2014, https://www.thebostonsisters.org/condom-couture (accessed October 22, 2024).
43. The Sisters of Perpetual Indulgence, Boston, "Condom Couture – Northeastern University – The Boston Sisters of Perpetual Indulgence."
44. Lauren Pond, "Queer Nuns and Digital Dragtivism in the Age of COVID-19," *The Revealer* (blog), September 3, 2020, https://therevealer.org/queer-nuns-and-digital-dragtivism-in-the-age-of-covid-19 (accessed October 22, 2024).
45. The Sisters of Perpetual Indulgence, San Francisco, "Joy."
46. The Sisters of Perpetual Indulgence, Boston, "A Meditation on a Year with Covid-19 – The Boston Sisters of Perpetual Indulgence," March 9, 2021, https://www.thebostonsisters.org/a-meditation-on-a-year-with-covid-19 (accessed October 23, 2024).
47. The Sisters of Perpetual Indulgence, Boston, "Point Nun Report," March 13, 2023.
48. The Sisters of Perpetual Indulgence, Boston, "Shigella – The Boston Sisters of Perpetual Indulgence," https://www.thebostonsisters.org/shigella (accessed October 23, 2024).
49. The Sisters of Perpetual Indulgence, Boston, "Point Nun Report," March 13, 2023.
50. Lauren Harvey, "Fentanyl Is Contaminating S.F. Club Drugs. Here's How the City's Nightlife Is Responding," *San Francisco Chronicle*, August 27, 2024, sec. Arts & Entertainment, https://www.sfchronicle.com/entertainment/article/narcan-fentanyl-sf-overdose-19594990.php (accessed October 23, 2024); The Sisters of Perpetual Indulgence, Boston, "Point Nun Report: Provincetown 7/04/24 – The Boston Sisters of Perpetual Indulgence," July 18, 2024, https://www.thebostonsisters.org/point-nun-report-provincetown-7-04-24 (accessed October 23, 2024).
51. The Sisters of Perpetual Indulgence, Boston, "Point Nun Report," July 18, 2024.
52. Lorraine T. Benuto et al., "The Behavioral Model of Health: Education, Behavioral Health Factors, and Stigma as Predictors of Help-Seeking Attitudes," *Community Mental Health Journal* 56, no. 7 (October 1, 2020): 1275–1283, https://doi.org/10.1007/s10597-020-00601-y; Meghan Romanelli and Kimberly D. Hudson, "Individual and Systemic Barriers to Health Care: Perspectives of Lesbian, Gay, Bisexual, and Transgender Adults," *American Journal of Orthopsychiatry* 87, no. 6 (2017): 714–728, https://psycnet.apa.org/buy/2017-51519-002; J. Whitehead, John Shaver, and Rob Stephenson, "Outness, Stigma, and Primary Health Care Utilization Among Rural LGBT Populations," *PLoS One* 11, no. 1 (January 5, 2016): e0146139, https://doi.org/10.1371/journal.pone.0146139; Mark L. Hatzenbuehler et al., "Structural Stigma and LGBTQ+ Health: A Narrative Review of Quantitative Studies," *The Lancet Public Health* 9, no. 2 (2024): e109–e127, https://doi.org/10.1016/S2468-2667(23)00312-2; Monique Tarver, "No Shame, All Gain: A Feminist Study of the Influence of Sex Positive Learning on the Sexual Health of Black Women" (PsyD dissertation, San Francisco, CA, Alliant International University, 2024), https://www.proquest.com/docview/3049557712/abstract/4776719137704B12PQ/1

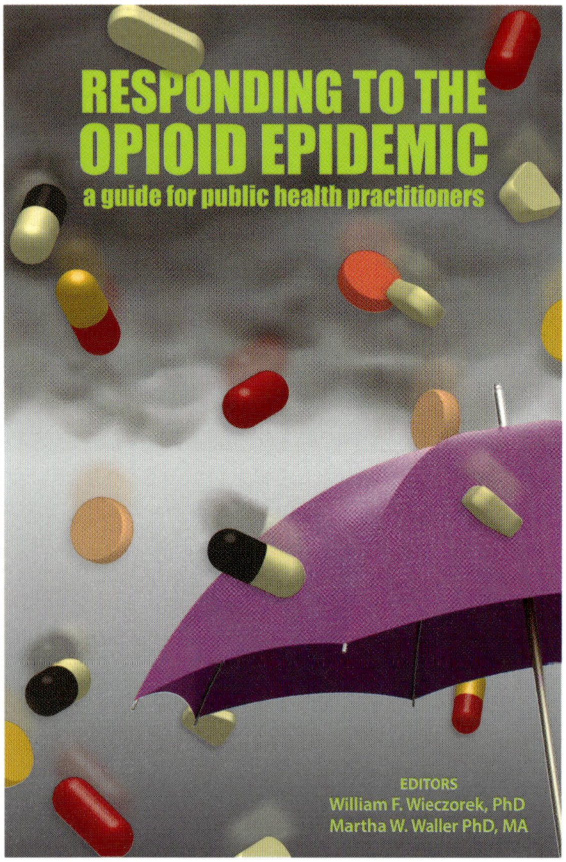

Responding to the Opioid Epidemic: A Guide for Public Health Practitioners

Edited by: William F. Wieczorek, PhD and Martha W. Waller PhD, MA

ISBN 978-0-87553-344-5, 400 PP., 2024,
SOFTBOUND/PRINT-ON-DEMAND

It's impossible to completely prevent the substance misuse defining the opioid epidemic, and it's impossible to treat the problem away. This reality requires a continuum of care (COC) approach, which includes promotion, prevention, case-finding, treatment, and recovery. This book presents research-informed interventions aligned with the COC approach to guide how communities, first responders, lay persons, medical providers, policymakers, treatment providers, and others can respond to the opioid epidemic at an individual, community, state, and national level.

APHABOOKSTORE.ORG

APHA PRESS

AN IMPRINT OF AMERICAN PUBLIC HEALTH ASSOCIATION